Achievement-Based Curriculum Development in Physical Education

Achievement-Based Curriculum Development in Physical Education

Janet A. Wessel, Ph.D.
Michigan State University

Luke Kelly, Ph.D.
University of Virginia

 Lea & Febiger   Philadelphia   1986

Lea & Febiger
600 Washington Square
Philadelphia, PA 19106-4198
U.S.A.
(215) 922-1330

Library of Congress Cataloging in Publication Data

Wessel, Janet A.
  Achievement-based curriculum development in physical education.

  Bibliography: p.
  Includes index.
  1. Physical education and training—United States—
Curricula. 2. Curriculum planning—United States.
I. Kelly, Luke.   II. Title.
GV365.W47 1985   375.6137′0973   85-12854
ISBN 0-8121-0958-9

Permission is granted to the users of this book to reproduce the activity sheets, worksheets, and evaluation forms for academic use without charge.

PRINTED IN THE UNITED STATES OF AMERICA

Print No.   4   3   2   1

PREFACE

This text is an outgrowth of curriculum projects funded by federal, state, and local educational agencies. Based on research and school experiences, an instructional model was developed. Instructional processes that consistently improved the learning experience for students in a school or class were identified to plan, implement, and evaluate the model. Our purpose is to share these findings with those who are, or will be, responsible for teaching in regular or special education: students (future teachers), teachers, curriculum planners, supervisors, administrators, policy-makers, or educational researchers.

Our goal is to help improve the quality of instructional programs in physical education. High quality programming is the precursor to superior results—student achievement. The five-step Achievement-Based Curriculum (ABC) Model presented will help teachers develop their own personal techniques of teaching. The steps are: (1) to define program goals and objectives; (2) to assess students' performance on objectives taught; (3) to prescribe instruction based on students' preassessment strengths and needs; (4) to teach and manage time effectively; and (5) to evaluate student and program effectiveness.

Strong research evidence from effective schools and instruction led to the recognition of the powerful effects this model has for improving the quality of physical education for all students. Each step in the process makes a unique contribution to the quality of instruction and to the desired outcomes of learning. These steps also share five characteristics. *First,* they relate to three important student behaviors that impact on student achievement: student involvement (time on task), success in learning, and teaching and testing objectives (content) to be achieved. *Second,* they help orchestrate and integrate teacher behaviors in planning, managing, and in instruction focused on the strengths and needs of students. *Third,* they are alterable and their effects can be observed within a relatively short time. *Fourth,* they can be used effectively to carefully plan and sequence essential learnings at any program or lesson level or with individual students. *Fifth,* the model does not require sophisticated equipment; it is cost-effective in terms of time and energy, and easily identifies, incorporates, or supplements ongoing effective instructional practices.

Mastering the ABC model presented in this book will help students and teachers develop professional competencies and improve their effectiveness. Reading this text will help develop an understanding of the appropriateness of this model and how to adapt it to different types of students. It will explain how the model works, how it can be integrated into the instructional working place, and how it can be adapted to provide individualized instruction for all students. No matter how skillfully these concepts and procedures are presented, however, they are still only inert ideas on paper. Their full potential is realized when students or teachers acquire a high degree of skills and practice these concepts and procedures in the workplace immediately following skill development. Only by applying these new skills can improved instructional programs and student achievement be transferred to the workplace.

Individualizing instruction and adaptation, as used in this book, does not require major changes in class. Teachers are directed to know the strengths and needs of all their students. Emphasis is placed on student behaviors that impact on student success and motivation to "learn how to learn," and is highly correlated with the effectiveness of instruction. Students' characteristics are not examined according to specific handicapping conditions, but are viewed on a continuum across personal-social, physical and motor, and learning needs. Teachers can adapt instruction to students' strengths and needs within the framework of group instruction. The Achievement-Based Curriculum Model provides a technology of teaching to help students and teacher meet these challenges.

This book may appear to be a radical departure from existing texts in physical education in general, and particularly from texts in adapted or special physical education. We believe, however, that it is one of the first books to step toward the twenty-first century and reflect changing attitudes and focus on excellence in physical education. We also believe that all students have a basic right to quality and individualized physical education. Instructional models in physical education must accommodate a wide range of diverse student backgrounds, interests, and abilities. Such models must be based on the best we know today and be designed to grow with future findings and developments from research and promising practices.

East Lansing, Michigan   Janet A. Wessel
Charlottesville, Virginia   Luke Kelly

SCOPE AND SEQUENCE

To provide the reader with an overview of the scope and sequence of this text, we have divided the book into three distinct parts: Part I, Individualization; Part II, Implementation; and Part III, Evaluation.

Within these parts we further divided the text into chapters that answered the key questions asked by physical education teachers, teachers of special education students, curriculum coordinators, and administrators in the workshops and leadership training institutes we have attended.

These questions and the relevant chapters are outlined to provide a ready reference as to the scope and sequence of the text.

Part I	Nine Key Questions	Chapter Response	Chapter
INDIVIDUALIZATION	1. What are the characteristics and mandates for quality programs for all children?	The Professional Imperative	1
	2. How can we individualize instruction to improve the quality of physical education?	Achievement-Based Curriculum Model: ABC	2
	3. What are the significant student characteristics influencing the instructional learning process?	Know the Learner	3
Part II IMPLEMENTATION	4. What content should be taught? Why? When? Where?	Program Planning	4
	5. How does the teacher know the entry performance of students on the content to be learned and the sequence of instruction required by students to progress toward achieving desired learning outcomes?	Assessment	5
	6. What are the effective teaching and time management strategies to improve student achievement?	Instructional Planning	6
	7. What techniques can teachers foster to motivate and develop appropriate student behaviors in learning?	Motivation and Class Management	7
Part III EVALUATION	8. How does the teacher know what each student has learned? How can these results be communicated to parents, students, and administrators? Is the program effective or should it be modified?	Student and Program Evaluation	8
	9. What are the challenges and how do we meet them with today's focus on excellence and concern for quality?	The Quest for Quality: Shaping Up	9

Utility is the chief criterion for the text and activities that accompany each chapter. To increase the readability of the text and save space, specific references are not cited. General and specific reference material is listed in the Resources for Teachers section in each chapter. A Glossary, Case Study report, and Subject Index are provided at the end of the text.

A chapter outline appears on the opening page of each chapter with the definition of the chapter title followed by descriptive statements. Text development in a question format correlated with decision aids follow. Activities related to each chapter appear following the text. Each activity provides "hands-on" experience that implements the key concepts and skills in the text.

The activities are numbered by chapter for easy reference. In Chapter 1 the activities are numbered 1–1, 1–2, and in Chapter 2 they are 2–1, 2–2, and so forth. Each activity is introduced with a statement of the activity objective, a listing of materials needed, specific directions, and in some instances variations of the activity and supplemental resource material. Worksheets are included for each activity and numbered accordingly.

The activities allow for flexibility and can be modified to meet particular needs. For example, they can serve as a model for the class group to design different activities to achieve the same objective. Teachers can use their daily classes to implement the activities or use Staff Development Days to accomplish some of the activities with their colleagues. Although the activities are organized sequentially by chapters, activities can be selected from different chapters for designing workshops, leadership institutes, or be correlated to other courses such as student teaching, measurement and evaluation, curriculum, and teaching methods.

The activities are designed to be assigned individually and/or to a small group. They provide an opportunity for students to work together, cooperatively making instructional decisions to solve day-by-day teaching and programming problems. Immediate feedback and self-correction features are incorporated into the activities through peer review and interaction to achieve the objective of the activity. Peers provide continuous feedback and reinforcement. The team approach, with a consensus-forming technique to resolve differences, generates a "learning how to learn together" effect for all members of the group. In this way, the activities provide a learning situation that provides a high degree of motivation for all concerned: students, teachers, and class group.

ACKNOWLEDGMENTS

Many people and organizations make a book such as this possible. Research and demonstration projects, supported in part by the United States Department of Education, Special Education Programs, and the Department of Education, State of Michigan Instructional Program Specialist and Special Education Division, to a large extent provided the time and money that helped us formulate our ideas and test them in practice. Special acknowledgment must go to M. Appell, W. Hillman, M. Kaufman, and M. Mueller, Special Education Programs; and Ted Beck, Wanda Jubb, and Muriel Van Patten of the Special Education and Instructional Program Specialist Division. We also thank the many teachers and students who worked with us in field-testing many of the procedures and concepts underlying the Achievement-Based Curriculum Model known as ABC.

Specifically, we want to thank the following colleagues whose enthusiasm and encouragement aided our endeavors.

Dr. Patricia L. Austin, a former Canadian colleague and friend, a pioneer in the preparation of teachers of physical education, who helped us find better ways to teach students with handicapping conditions; a forerunner in the advocacy of the Achievement-Based Curriculum Model whose writing and courses influenced the focus of this book.

Dr. Claudia J. Knowles who provided assistance in editing sections of the manuscript, exchanged points of view on teaching and learning, contributed to many chapters of the book, and shared in many other ways.

Dr. Julian Stein who provided valuable reviews on sections of the manuscript and helped to clarify ideas and concepts related to legislative mandates.

Betty Lessard, Sharon Bacon, Karen Knowlton, and Larry Carmichael who helped field-test and disseminate Project I CAN, the forerunner of the ABC model. Our special thanks to Paul Vogel who helped develop, implement, and evaluate Project I CAN and assisted us in clarifying ideas and procedures described in program planning and evaluation.

Carol Brody for her editorial assistance, secretarial skills, and patience in the preparation of the many drafts of the text. Special thanks to Jackie Peek for her help with numerous activities associated with the final manuscript.

Eileen McElroy Kelly for her inspiration and assistance throughout the development of the final manuscript.

For the many colleagues and friends who helped by reviewing the manuscript and who exalted in its successful completion.

J.A.W.
L.K.

CONTENTS

PART I

Individualization

The professional imperative, quality education, has set us in pursuit of instructional programs that can be provided and delivered to all students. This section consists of three chapters that provide the basis for our program. Chapter 1 introduces quality programming and the professional imperative. Quality program issues—individualization, accountability, effective practices, and a definition are discussed. Meeting this challenge is the professional imperative, which is quality programs for all students. An achievement-based curriculum model is presented to meet design criteria for quality program models; it accommodates the needs, performances, and interests of a diverse group of students.

Chapter 2 presents the achievement-based curriculum model for quality programming. Five steps to plan, implement, and evaluate the model are identified. The usefulness of the model for delabeling students, for detecting learning difficulties early, for adapting to meet the unique needs of all students, and the benefits of the model for all participants in the educational process are presented.

Chapter 3, Know the Learner, gives an overview of the characteristics of students, not labels. Key student characteristics that interact with instruction are identified in three categories: learning, personal-social, and physical and motor needs. These characteristics provide essential criteria to help in instructional decision-making—successes in learning for all students.

CHAPTER 1

The Professional Imperative

QUALITY PROGRAMMING: THE PROFESSIONAL IMPERATIVE
THE LEGISLATIVE MANDATES
  Appropriate Education
  Individualized Education Program (IEP)
  Least Restrictive Environment (LRE)
MEETING THE CHALLENGE
  I. A Definition of Quality Programs
  II. Effective School Practices
  III. Criteria for Designing a Model for Quality Programming
SYNOPSIS
ACTIVITIES
    1–1. Examine PL 94-142 and Section 504 of the Vocational Rehabilitation
          Act of 1973: Rules and Regulations published in the Federal Register.
    1–2. Examine local school or school district's plan to implement your state's
          Annual Plan in Special Education for regular class settings.
    1–3. Review effective practices and definition of quality programs and rate
          perceived importance to improving physical education instruction for
          all students.
    1–4. Review the design criteria identified to select, select/adapt, or develop
          quality program models in physical education for all students.

What is the Professional Imperative?	
The professional imperative is threefold. First, it defines quality programs. Second, it provides quality programs—individualized and accountable—for all children. Third, it documents student achievement, demonstrating effective programs.	

What is Quality Programming for All Children?	Decision Aids
1. What is a quality program? What can it do? Why for all children?	Definitions Equity/Quality Issues
2. Why and how is individualized instruction discernible in the accountability movement? Criterion-referenced measurements? Quality programs?	Definitions Purposes Student achievement
3. What are the legal and policy mandates underlying appropriate education for all handicapped children?	Legal and policy mandates —Free appropriate public education for all —Individualized education programs —Least restrictive environment —Physical education —Related services —Accountability/Evaluation
4. How will quality physical education be provided for all children in our programs?	
5. Professional commitment Equality/Quality	Legal and policy mandates—instructional program model

Our professional drive to instructional excellence in physical education for all children is already under way. To help every child—the handicapped, the gifted, the disadvantaged, and the average—develop to the fullest of his or her interests and abilities in physical education is our professional commitment. Our greatest challenge is to provide quality education for all children. Equality of opportunity in physical education is meaningless unless instruction is relevant and of the highest quality appropriate for each child's learning needs.

The demand for quality programs for all children is increasing, not decreasing. Strong pressures are making schools responsible for thinking through what kind of instruction is appropriate for each child. A well-informed and demanding public is determined to see more effective instruction—what did the child learn and what did it cost? Support for programs is increasingly based upon clearly demonstrated student achievement on what is taught in the program. Physical educators must respond with valid, educationally defensible instructional programs. These programs must demonstrate their effectiveness in meeting the diverse needs of all children as they progress toward achieving the desired learning outcomes.

This chapter begins with an overview of two concepts—individualized instruction and accountability. Both of these concepts characterize quality programming in physical education for all. Significant features of the provisions of Public Law 94-142, Education for All Handicapped Children, underline free, appropriate public education and have implications for quality programs and physical education. These provisions as well as ways to meet the challenge for quality programming in physical education are presented.

QUALITY PROGRAMMING: THE PROFESSIONAL IMPERATIVE

A basic principle of quality education has always been to focus on the individual. Quality education is appropriate education for every child. Instruction, not students, must be adaptable to individual differences. Only in this way can we provide appropriate physical education for all students. The first step is a major one. It starts us on the course of increasing personalized instructional approaches to programming in physical education. Individualized instruction has long been singled out as a viable means of providing quality education for all children in that they are unique individuals who differ only in the nature of their learning needs. Individual differences are described in terms that are directly relevant to instruction, not labels. Individualization requires us to stop typecasting the learner with labels such as special education, disadvantaged, poor gifted, or typically average. This approach has set us in pursuit of how to provide and deliver individualized instruction to meet every child's needs.

Real individualization in physical education must begin with the acceptance of the learner as the central focus of concern. In the past, the major focus of our concerns had been fitting the student to the program, not the program to the student. Teaching in physical education school programs today does not often provide the opportunity for individualization such as:

- assessing students' needs and abilities;
- setting students' learning tasks based on prior assessment data;
- prescribing and teaching based on assessment data;
- modifying instruction and learning tasks assigned based on students' achievement on objectives taught and covered in the lessons; and
- involving students in planning, monitoring, and reporting results of instruction and parents in decision-making activities.

Emphasis on every student's right to quality education will become more pronounced in this decade. Strong pressures emerging at both national and state levels are calling for thorough and efficient education and equating these terms to quality education. Accountability has become one of the most easily identified features of quality education. In this sense, accountability is a key concept of this decade.

It is relatively easy to focus on getting all children into some kind of physical education program designed to meet their needs. It is more difficult to ask whether or not this program works or how we measured its effectiveness—student's achievement of definitive goals of instruction.

Individualization is observable in much of the accountability movement. Accountability refers to the current trend in education to hold schools responsible for producing demonstrable learning in students on stated goals. Accountability, when correctly implemented, can be an effective means for improving student learning, which is to provide impetus to discard what does not work and adopt new input approaches.

Accountability is a tool, a systems-analysis approach to planning and evaluating instruction. It is focused on the desired student behaviors or "outputs" of the program. These "outputs" are cast in terms of observable and measurable results of instruction. Evaluation of the effectiveness of the instructional program is based on these outputs—what did the student learn in the class? Measurements of "outputs," criterion-referenced levels of mastering objectives taught in the class, are being viewed as an effective strategy to improve schools. These measurements provide teachers with valuable feedback information that is critically needed in the process of individualizing instruction to meet the needs of the students in the class.

Evaluating the effectiveness of the program in terms of student achievement will influence many decisions in state and local physical educational programs. By demanding that we focus attention on the results of our programs, careful analyzing and documenting is assured. We must know:

- what our program goals are;
- what objectives should be achieved to reach these goals;
- what strategies we will use to plan and manage instruction for each learner to achieve desired outcomes;
- what our needs are to support quality programs.

In the final analysis, the philosophical basis for equity and quality education for all is the value placed on each individual in our society. In developing this rationale, we have increasingly emphasized the right of every child to quality programs—instructions appropriate to each child's learning needs. Physical education for a child who has special needs is not a charity. It is not a desired extra in school programs. It is a fundamental right to which a child and the child's family are entitled. Although the following section deals specifically with legal and policy mandates that require greater individualization and accountability for handicapped children, our professional imperative is to develop quality programs, individualized and accountable, for all children as we step toward the twenty-first century.

THE LEGISLATIVE MANDATE

For more than a century American society has prided itself in its free public education as a basic human right for all children. This philosophy was based on the belief that the foundation of any nation lay in the education of all its children. The single most significant feature of The Education for All Handicapped Act, Public Law 94-142, is that it reaffirms this basic human right for all handicapped children, regardless of the nature or severity of a child's handicap.

The Act is the most important piece of educational legislation in this century. With Public Law 94-142, Congress made it a basic *legal* right to provide free *appropriate* education to all handicapped children. Educators, parents, legislators, and others are meeting this challenge and finding ways to implement both the intent and mandates of the Act. With its far-reaching implications for free appropriate education—individualized and accountable—as a basic legal right, the Act highlights the quest for equity and quality education for all children. The Act states that no matter what race, background, sex, or ability, all children have the right to equal access to quality education.

The roots of the Act can be found in the Civil Rights Movement of the 1960s. The same rationale of the detrimental effects of segregation of the Civil Rights Movement influenced the thinking of advocates for the handicapped. A strong coalition of parents, legislators, lawyers, and public servants fought the denial of education to handicapped children, and then they fought the emerging practice of segregated classes. Their work culminated in the powerful mandate of Public Law 94-142.

Congress had already enacted antidiscrimination protections for handicapped people of all ages in the Rehabilitation Act of 1973. Section 504 of that Act guarantees the right of handicapped individuals to jobs and services in schools and colleges, health care facilities, social service agencies, physical accessibility to buildings, and other activities receiving federal funds. The Act is popularly known as the Civil Rights Act for the Handicapped.

NONDISCRIMINATION UNDER FEDERAL GRANTS

"Sec. 504. No otherwise qualified handicapped individual in the United States, as defined in Section 7(6), shall, solely by reason of his handicap, be excluded from the participation in, be denied the benefits of, or be subjected to discrimination under any program or activity receiving Federal financial assistance."

In Public Law 94-142 Congress spelled out Section 504's education guarantees for school age children including incentives for early childhood programs. The

Statement of Purpose section of the Act clearly spells out the intent of the mandate. The Act is designed to accomplish four far-reaching goals for all handicapped children:

1. Assure that all students can have available free appropriate public education to meet their needs and abilities.
2. Assure that the rights of students and their parents or guardians are protected.
3. Assist states and localities to find and educate all handicapped children within their jurisdiction, regardless of the nature or severity of the child's handicap.
4. Assist and assure the effectiveness, accountability, of efforts to educate all students.

Federal and state definitions of the term "handicapped" are categorical and traditional. *To qualify for special education services, a student must have characteristics that interfere with the student's learning.* The laws defining eligibility for special education and related services are designed to ensure that students who require such services receive them, and to prevent the inappropriate or discriminatory labeling of students who do not require special education. Each state has formulated evaluation processes and definitions of the term "handicapped" which serve as eligibility criteria for receiving special education services.

The mandate for free appropriate public education for all students with handicapping conditions has markedly increased the categories used to define or describe the range of handicapping conditions and made the criteria more specific for eligibility. The term "handicapped children" defined by the federal mandate includes: deaf, deaf-blind, hard of hearing, mentally retarded, multihandicapped, orthopedically impaired, other health impaired, seriously emotionally disturbed, specific learning disability, speech impaired, and visually handicapped, *who, because of those impairments, need special education and related services.* These labels describe the major categories or classification systems into which handicapped students have been traditionally placed.

Although handicapping labels are useful for eligibility, funding, and teacher certification decisions, they are neither constructive nor valid for making student placement or instructional decisions. For example, if a child is labeled deaf or so-called normal, the label tells you nothing about the child's needs or physical and motor abilities. The deaf student could have exceptional motor skills, and the so-called average child could have great needs in this area. Individualizing instruction to meet student needs becomes the paramount directive of free appropriate education for all children.

How many students require special education? Some authorities have estimated that between 7 and 8 million children from ages 3 to 21 years are handicapped. In general, the figure is somewhere between 5.7% and 9.4% of the total elementary- and secondary-school enrollment. These percentages are distributed according to the traditional categorical labels in special education. For those interested in the number and percentages of children by categorical groups, federal and/or state special education divisions can be contacted. These sources have national figures, state figures, and local school district figures. What is of interest in instructional planning is knowing the placement of the children in the feeder schools for a particular school's program. Knowing the number of children and having a record of their prior achievements and needs helps in making instructional decisions.

Reference to instruction in physical education as part of the definition of special education spells out the intent of Congress to ensure that physical ed-

TABLE 1–1. *Highlights of the Rules and Regulations for PL 94-142 Regarding Definitions of Physical Education*

Special Education: The term "special education" means specially designed instruction, at no cost to parents or guardians, to meet the unique needs of a handicapped child, including classroom instruction, **INSTRUCTION IN PHYSICAL EDUCATION** (emphasis added), home instruction, and instruction in hospitals and institutions.

Physical Education: The term means the development of:

—Physical and motor fitness

—Fundamental motor skills and patterns

—Skills in aquatics, dance, and individual group games and sports (including intramural and lifetime sports)

The term includes:

—Special physical education

—Adapted physical education

—Movement education

—Motor development

(From Sections 121.a14 and 121a.13, Federal Register, August 23, 1977, pp. 42479-42480.)

ucation is a direct service for all handicapped children. Table 1–1 highlights the definitions of direct and related services of the Act.

Emphases of these definitions of physical education are important for two reasons. *First,* many students were being excluded from physical education. In some cases, therapeutic modalities and/or a free play period were considered to be physical education. Physical education as defined in the law is clearly a part of specifically defined instruction in the mandate. It must be provided to all handicapped students.

Second, some orthopedically impaired children who do not need specially designed instruction in the academic program were excluded from physical education most often because they were not considered to be in special education, or because it was thought they would not be able to benefit from physical education. Under PL 94-142 these students could be considered in special education solely based on their specific physical and motor needs as defined in terms of *physical education.* Physical education, specially designed instruction if necessary, must be made available to every handicapped child receiving a free appropriate public education. Table 1–2 provides a summary of the Rules and Regulations for PL 94-142 regarding instruction in physical education.

Significant features of the Act having direct implications for quality education and physical education are discussed under the following topics: appropriateness, individualization, and placement. These topics were selected for one reason. As we reach the midpoint of the 1980s, physical education's most profound inequality is unequal student access to quality education.

APPROPRIATE EDUCATION

One requirement is the immediate concern of the regular physical education teacher, for much of this requirement will be carried out in regular physical education classes for most students. This requirement is the *appropriate physical education program.* Appropriateness of the instructional physical education program for each student is determined by the degree to which it addresses objectives specified in the *Individualized Education Program* and is carried out in the *Least Restrictive Environment.*

The goal of PL 94-142 is to provide all children with an appropriate education

TABLE 1–2. *Highlights of the Rules and Regulations for PL 94-142 Regarding Instruction in Physical Education*

(a) General. Physical education services, specially designed if necessary, must be made available to every handicapped child receiving a free appropriate public education.

(b) Regular physical education. Each handicapped child must be afforded the opportunity to participate in the regular physical education program available to nonhandicapped children unless:

(1) The child is enrolled full time in a separate facility; or

(2) The child needs specially designed physical education, as prescribed in the child's individualized education program.

(c) Special physical education. If specially designed physical education is prescribed in a child's individualized education program, the public agency responsible for the education of that child shall provide the services directly, or make arrangements for it to be provided through other public or private programs.

(d) Education in separate facilities. The public agency responsible for the education of a handicapped child who is enrolled in a separate facility shall insure that the child receives appropriate physical education services in compliance with paragraphs (a) and (c) of this section.

(From Section 121a.307, Federal Register, 42(163), August 23, 1977, p. 42497.)

within the least restrictive environment. The many specific regulations spelled out in the Rules and Regulations are, for the most part, responsibilities of administrators who must certify that these Rules and Regulations are being followed. Teachers are referred to the Federal Register documents as the primary source for Rules and Regulations of PL 94-142 and for any changes that might occur in the educational processes. All school districts should have copies of these federal regulations. All teachers should read and review them carefully.

Each state is required to have an Annual Plan for Special Education. The plan must detail how the state and school districts intend to implement the mandates. These plans—local, intermediate, or state—must be available to the public for review and comment before they are adopted by state boards of education. Hearings are posted for geographic sites. Written comments are accepted. The state plans include a description of priority educational areas for allocation of monies. Know your State Plan. Know your District Plan. Know how the plan is implemented in your school.

Appropriate educational decisions require a complete and nondiscriminatory evaluation of the student's educational needs. This evaluation must be made before the child is placed. The evaluation requires an examination into everything related to the suspected disability, including where appropriate, health, vision, hearing, social and emotional status, general intelligence, academic performance, communicative status, and physical and motor abilities. The evaluation must not involve tests that discriminate against children on the basis of race, culture, language, or sensory disability. The evaluation must provide the basis for determining eligibility, development of the Individualized Education Program (IEP), and objective evaluation procedures to determine the effectiveness of the program, including placement decision.

INDIVIDUALIZED EDUCATION PROGRAM (IEP)

The individualized education program represents the primary vehicle in PL 94-142 for assuring that the individual needs of each student are the paramount concern for instructional programming and placement. This provision is intended to provide quality education for every student. That right is most clearly reflected in the specified content in the individualized education program. The program is a written management tool. It must include the following:

1. Statement of child's present levels of educational performance.
2. Statement of annual goals including short-term instructional objectives.
3. Statement of specific special education and related services to be provided to the child and the extent to which the child will be able to participate in the regular education program.
4. Projected dates for initiation of services and anticipated duration of the services.
5. Appropriate objective criteria and evaluation procedures and schedules for determining, on at least an annual basis, whether the short-term instructional objectives are being achieved.

Physical education must be addressed when developing an Individualized Education Program. Key questions and answers regarding instruction in physical education and the implementation of PL 94-142 related to the Individualized Education Program are presented in Table 1–3.

Other requirements of the law relating to the Individualized Education Program are those designed to ensure *parent* participation, due process, nondiscriminatory evaluations, and reporting. Each teacher who receives the student placed in a regular class setting should be part of the proceedings. If there are questions or concerns about instruction, progress or placement of the student, the teacher should request conferences with designated special education support personnel.

The Individualized Education Program is a tool for planning, managing, and evaluating the student's instructional program. The intent is to ensure that each student is provided an appropriate program—quality education regardless of the placement. As such, it serves five major purposes. It provides:

- A permanent source of information on each student's instructional plan that can be shared with parents, teachers, and other personnel responsible for implementing the student's program. The program therefore promotes continuity and consistency.
- An objective reference regarding instructional decisions made for a student's program; replaces blanket instructional activities calculated to achieve program goals and objectives in accordance with individual student needs, status, rate of learning, and learning style.
- A cumulative record of student performance based on annual goals and short-term instructional objectives tailored to the needs of individual students; short-term instructional objectives are outcomes or milestones for indicating progress in meeting annual goals and are not intended to address specific activities in daily or weekly instruction plans.
- A base for determining program effectiveness in individual student terms, i.e., the appropriateness of regular and/or special class placement.
- A communication tool to ensure that IEP participants know what a child's learning needs are, what will be provided, when and where, and what the anticipated outcomes may be.

To meet this challenge, school programs in physical education must change to provide for a greater diversity of students' abilities and needs in the regular classes. Individualizing instruction, accountability, and communicating results to all participants in the educational process on a regular schedule underlie the requirements for individualized education programs.

TABLE 1–3. *Highlights of a Position Paper on the Individualized Education Program and Instruction in Physical Education*

> *If modifications are necessary for a handicapped child to participate in a regular education program, must they be included in the IEP?*
>
> Yes. If modifications (supplementary aids and services) to the regular education program are necessary to ensure the child's participation in that program, those modifications must be described in the child's IEP (e.g., for a hearing impaired child, special seating arrangements or the provision of assignments in writing). This applies to any regular education program in which the student may participate, including physical education, art, music, and vocational education.
>
> *When must physical education (PE) be described or referred to in the IEP?*
>
> Section 300.307(a) provides that "physical education services, specially designed if necessary, must be made available to every handicapped child receiving a free appropriate public education." The following paragraphs (1) set out some of the different PE program arrangements for handicapped students, and (2) indicate whether, and to what extent, PE must be described or referred to in an IEP:
>
> a. *Regular PE with nonhandicapped students.* If a handicapped student can participate fully in the regular PE program without any special modifications to compensate for the student's handicap, it would not be necessary to describe or refer to PE in the IEP. On the other hand, if some modifications to the regular PE program are necessary for the student to be able to participate in that program, those modifications must be described in the IEP.
>
> b. *Specially designed PE.* If a handicapped student needs a specially designed PE program, that program must be addressed in all applicable areas of the IEP (e.g., present levels of educational performance, goals and objectives, and services to be provided). However, these statements would not have to be presented in any more detail than the other special education services included in the student's IEP.
>
> c. *PE in separate facilities.* If a handicapped student is educated in a separate facility, the PE program for that student must be described or referred to in the IEP. However, the kind and amount of information to be included in the IEP would depend on the physical-motor needs of the student and the type of PE program that is to be provided.
>
> Thus, if a student is in a separate facility that has a standard PE program (e.g., a residential school for the deaf), and if it is determined—on the basis of the student's most recent evaluation—that the student is able to participate in that program without any modifications, then the IEP need only note such participation. On the other hand, if special modifications to the PE program are needed for the student to participate, those modifications must be described in the IEP. Moreover, if the student needs an individually designed PE program, that program must be addressed under all applicable parts of the IEP. (See paragraph "b" above.)

(From Federal Register 46(12), January 19, 1981.)

LEAST RESTRICTIVE ENVIRONMENT (LRE)

A primary thrust of PL 94-142 is the right of each student to be educated in the least restrictive environment (LRE). The law makes it clear that students should be removed from the mainstream of school only if the student is not able to function in the regular classroom. When a student is in a separate program, every effort should be made to provide as many contacts with peers as possible.

The key word in the provision for an "appropriate public education in the least restrictive environment" is "appropriate." This provision does not automatically mean that all students will be placed in a regular physical education class, full- or part-time. It does mean that the school districts should offer a variety of alternative settings. Student placements must be made on the basis of individual needs. Many students are able to participate in the regular class settings without any special aids or accommodations. For some students, placement in regular classes may require some accommodations. For example, modifications might include:

• Using adaptive equipment such as flotation devices in swimming.

- Using paraprofessional, peer tutors, buddy systems, volunteers, and others to provide support as needed.
- Following health and safety precautions in moving from place to place; more time for dressing and undressing or getting to and from classes.
- Selecting and/or adapting instructional activities for all students to participate according to their abilities.
- Adapting or modifying instructional objectives to meet unique needs such as throwing a ball from a wheelchair.

For other students, it may mean spending most of the time in separate classes with as much opportunity as possible to participate with peers. For a few it may mean living and learning in special centers, close to home.

The term mainstreaming, placement in regular class setting, is often used in place of least restrictive environment. This use is inappropriate unless the following interpretation is applied to both terms:

1. An assumption that the child can best be served through placement with peers in regular class settings when appropriate.
2. Assigning primary instructional responsibility to regular class teachers who received students.
3. Providing support services to the regular class teachers as a means of helping students when special assistance is required.
4. Providing direct support services on a part-time basis to the student only if the regular class teacher is unable to provide an appropriate program through assistance from support personnel.
5. Making assignment to special classes or separate programs as a last alternative.
6. Considering placement a dynamic, not static, event for each student, it is not engraved in stone but changes as students change at different stages in their schooling.

The important point to stress about the least restrictive environment provision is that it *does not imply the wholesale placement of all students in regular physical education classes;* nor does it mean doing away with regular physical education classes. It does stress the importance of appropriate placement decisions to meet the needs and abilities of the student. It does opt for integrated classes, combined with concrete assistance and support services for the regular physical education teacher or the student when necessary. It does identify the need for shared decision-making with school personnel in planning, implementing, monitoring, and evaluating the student's progress to and/or from the placement setting. It does mean that *a continuum of alternative placements in physical education should be provided* by the school district.

Each school district should have physical education placement alternatives. Each placement decision must be tailored to meet the individuual needs of students at any given time during the students' school careers. A placement continuum is shown in Figure 1–1.

The continuum ranges from regular class placement to very intensive special physical education services. In the first four placement options, the student remains in a regular physical education class for all or a portion of the yearly instructional program. In these placement selections, the regular physical education teacher has primary responsibility for the student's instructional program. Needed back-up support and services provided by special education personnel and/or related support personnel may take place in the regular classroom or in a designated work area, such as a resource or adapted physical education room.

In option four, the student attends a regular classroom part-time and an

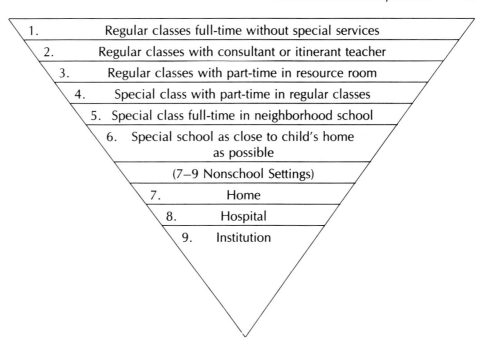

1. Regular classes full-time without special services
2. Regular classes with consultant or itinerant teacher
3. Regular classes with part-time in resource room
4. Special class with part-time in regular classes
5. Special class full-time in neighborhood school
6. Special school as close to child's home as possible

(7–9 Nonschool Settings)

7. Home
8. Hospital
9. Institution

Figure 1–1. *A continuum of alternative physical education placement options.*

adapted special class part-time. The amount of time spent in the regular class is dependent on the student's ability to *profit* from regular class instruction. The student may spend a near-equal amount of time in each setting or the student may spend the majority of the time in the adapted class and is selectively included in the regular physical education class activities for a specific instructional unit. In options five, six, seven, eight, and nine, comprehensive services needed by the more seriously involved or multihandicapped are provided in special settings.

Placement of the student is a local determination. The decision is part of the Individualized Education Program planning process. The Act does place the *burden of proof* on the schools to justify and document placement decisions in which the student is served outside of regular physical education class. There are conditions that facilitate appropriate placement decisions. Each teacher should be knowledgeable about these conditions in their school setting. Three major conditions are:

1. The thrust of all decision-making is to meet the learner's instructional needs, not the legislative or special education categorical labels—placement in a learning-disabled class because the student has been so labeled.
2. Alternative program placement and supplemental service personnel exist who will help teachers with students who have learning or adjustment problems in the regular setting (such as consulting teachers, itinerant teachers, resource room teachers, special education personnel, methods and materials specialists, and related support personnel).
3. Assessment and evaluation are continuous processes. Testing must be oriented to individual benefits and to assist school personnel in making instructional decisions. From this point of view, the purpose of the test is to analyze what each child has to offer, so that placement can be individualized. The benefit of this type of testing is to ensure that each student is offered quality physical education at all stages of schooling.

We must now redirect our professional energies away from where we educate the child to more substantive concerns of how we plan and implement quality

TABLE 1–4. *A Summary of the Ten Basic Principles Related to the Delivery of "Appropriate" Physical Education Services*

1. The Individualized Education Program is a management tool designed to facilitate instructional planning and student achievement.
2. The Individualized Education Program is a plan, not a contract. It does not constitute a guarantee that the student will progress at a specified rate or achieve specific performance levels in the skills making up the physical education program. It merely projects realistic student performance expectations.
3. Instructional physical education must be included to meet the needs of handicapped students regardless of placement.
4. The individual student's physical education instructional needs and the capability of the class placement to meet these needs must be considered in determining the appropriateness of the placement.
5. The placement of students in regular physical education must be aided where necessary with concrete assistance for the regular physical education teacher. Resource materials, special aids, and modified equipment, support services for the teacher and/or student, all or in part, may be appropriate.
6. Inservice training programs must be developed for teachers with focus on appropriate programming and placement, on testing and evaluation, and open communication across all school personnel.
7. Students (preschool and secondary) should be enrolled in the regular physical education class for as much of the time as appropriate, given their unique needs. For some students, this may mean that they are in regular class all the time, in a special adapted physical education class all the time, or somewhere between these extremes.
8. The regular class teacher is responsible for the instruction, grading, and reporting for all students placed in the regular class. The teacher regularly screens and evaluates all students' achievement and makes referrals when needed for any student who has special needs.
9. The regular physical education teacher should participate in, or contribute to, the assessment of the student's progress and jointly plan appropriate instruction with support personnel for a student placed in a regular class setting.
10. The least restrictive environment concept should, when properly implemented, effectively unite the skills of the regular physical education teacher and the special educator, thus providing maximum assistance to the student and for the teacher in regular physical education programs.

programs for all students. We must individualize instruction to meet each student's needs in the class setting.

The ultimate question is: "Can students achieve desired learning outcomes in this class setting? A summary of the basic facts and principles underlying the intent of PL 94-142, The Education for All Handicapped Children Act, is presented in Table 1–4.

Understanding the underlying concepts of the legal and policy mandates as they apply to handicapped children is a major step forward in the delivery of quality physical education programs for all students. Although these mandates do not apply to nonhandicapped children, the concepts of free, *appropriate* public education, parent involvement, individualized educational programs, and evaluation of the effectiveness of the program in terms of student achievements on clearly stated program goals and objectives of instruction underlie our continuing quest for equity and quality education for all children in physical education.

MEETING THE CHALLENGE

Quality in physical education is a widely accepted goal of this decade. Individualization is no longer a catch word. It is a viable approach to providing quality programs for all students. Many school districts are attempting to assess individual capabilities and match instruction as nearly as possible to these assessments. State educational agencies, if they have not already done so, are in the process of setting student performance standards on essential skills for promotion and graduation competencies. Furthermore, state and other educational agencies have, or are considering, teaching competency qualifications for certification and promotion. These efforts indicate the sustained and growing urgency that exists to improve the quality of education. Our challenge is to make quality education an answer to equality, opportunity, and excellence for all.

A sustained and growing urgency to improve physical education now exists. This challenge comes during a time when we have witnessed tremendous growth in educational technology and pedology. At the same time, this is a period of *doing better with less.* Vast increases in the quality, quantity, and availability of research on improving schools and effectiveness of instruction have resulted in an increasingly rich educational resource. Combined with instructional technology, the systematized use of effective practices, these resources can provide a key to improving the quality of our programs. Because of these considerations and the demand for programs with demonstrated effectiveness, the time is ripe to identify and translate into action what research on effective schooling tells us.

How can we begin to do this? There are three steps we can take. *First,* to define a quality school program in physical education for all students. *Second,* to identify key practices of effective schooling most likely to have direct effect on outcomes as reflected in assessed pupil performance. *Third,* to determine criteria to select, select/adapt, or design a general model of instruction for quality programs.

I. A DEFINITION OF QUALITY PROGRAMS

The definition of a quality school program in physical education must be determined. This definition must be clear, reliable, and stated in operational terms. It must address the effectiveness issue—that it be accountable for all students to learn the essential skills identified for the program. The definition must permit schools with different purposes, and instructional focus in physical education, to be able to qualify as having quality programs to meet their purposes. The definition must be relevant to research on effective schools and teaching; all such research studies look at measured student achievement as the outcome on which to judge effectiveness.

With these considerations in mind, a definition of a quality school program in physical education follows . . .

> The aims of the physical education program—the goals and objectives of the intended program must be clearly stated by grade or multi-program levels.
> A high (90% plus) proportion of all students should be able to demonstrate mastery of the program objectives at stated levels.

To use this definition, schools need achievement scores for students in the physical education program. These achievement scores must be based on a locally specified standard of mastery of the objectives of the program—meaningful and realistic.

Student achievement scores are used to assess the effects of the program. These scores are used to evaluate the effectiveness of instruction, and help determine what needs to be changed, why, and when. The scores also help school personnel and members of the school community to allocate resources—human and/or material—to sustain or improve the school program. Three proposals have been put forth to improve the quality of physical education school programs. These proposals highlight the definition of quality programs and the need for documented evidence of its effectiveness:

    A. No instructional program should be undertaken or continued in the absence of evidence of its effectiveness in producing learning.

    B. Each school physical education system should publish annually the results of the systematic assessment of pupil achievements in learning.

    C. Each teacher should submit evidence of the learning achievements of pupils in the class periodically.

II. EFFECTIVE SCHOOL PRACTICES

The *second* step is to identify key practices from effective school and teaching research studies. School improvement studies measure student achievement as the outcome on which to evaluate effectiveness. There are different lists of effective practices. Compelling evidence exists that teachers do make the difference. In all lists, teachers and students are the primary resources that are consistently related to student achievement in the learning setting.

The following section briefly describes key practices compiled from effective schools and teaching reports. Each practice represents a cluster of practices. It should not be presumed that other effective practices that do not appear are rejected. Administrative structure is an important characteristic of effectiveness that does not appear in this list. Other sets of effective practices that depend on school boards and the central administration are listed. The practices selected are controlled primarily by local school personnel, in particular, teachers. These practices are aligned with the definition of quality programs. If you, your school, school district, or professional organization extend or change this list, that is a professional judgment.

Each practice is presented and followed by a brief description. These practices are not listed in any order or priority, and although they have come from effective schools and teaching studies, their application here is to physical education.

A. Instructional Focus and Direction: Goals and Objectives

There is a clearly articulated focus and direction to the program. Documented program goals and relevant objectives by grade or program level to achieve these goals are provided by a long-term program plan. The staff share an understanding of and a commitment to the instructional goals, priorities, assessment procedures and accountability, and contribution of the program to the school's mission.

A quality program has a clearly developed mission. The mission is focused and clear for teachers, students, parents, and other school community members. The goals and objectives are clearly defined to identify the contributions of the instructional program to the school's mission. The physical education staff use their program plan to make decisions in allocation of scarce resources, such as instructional time itself, which will remain fixed or become even scarcer.

The program objectives organized over youngsters' school years operationally define the long-term program goals on a continuum of essential skills for all students to achieve. These objectives, stated in behavioral terms, clearly define performance standards, mastery expectations for all students.

B. High Expectancies: All Students Expected to Achieve

There is a climate of expectation for all students. Teachers believe and demonstrate that all students can attain mastery of essential skills. Teachers believe they have the capability to help all students. Teachers believe that students can take responsibility for their work behaviors and their achievements. Peer models and tutors who have mastered the standards of conduct and skills help others to succeed. No student remains isolated in his endeavors to achieve.

Teachers do make the difference. Teachers who believe that their role is to teach all students, who fully expect to conduct such instruction within the class, who proceed on this premise, fulfill this prediction. On the other hand, if teachers believe that, for whatever reason, some students cannot learn and proceed on this premise, the prediction is not realized.

C. Teaching-Learning: Task-Oriented, Orderly, Motivating, Safe

There is an orderly, purposeful learning climate. Teaching-learning climate is task-oriented, free of threat of failure on assigned learning tasks. Class is organized to maximize available instructional time with students engaged in learning assigned tasks.

All teaching and learning activities reflect a sense of purposefulness. Students and teachers know the objectives of instruction. The lesson is organized to maximize instructional time for learning assigned tasks. High-interest activities are provided to engage students in learning assigned tasks. The learning tasks assigned are challenging—not too difficult nor too easy—providing a high degree of success for all students. The setting is relatively clean, safe from physical threat or harm, and accessible to all students. Students know what is expected of them and the imposition of discipline is uniform for all. Help is provided to students with learning difficulties. Teachers supply feedback-reinforcement as soon as possible. Student progress is monitored continuously and instructional activities are adapted accordingly. Students are presented directives by teachers. Drill, practice, and organized game-time activities are provided to the whole class group and assigned as independent learning contracts according to students' abilities. Students are actively involved in planning, coaching skills, reporting results, and helping each other for at least 60% of the instructional time.

D. Monitoring Student Progress and Using Measures of Student Achievement as the Basis for Program Evaluation

Student progress is measured and reported frequently. The results of assessments are used to improve individual student performance and to improve the instructional program.

The feedback from assessment of student performance is a valuable source of information for teachers when teachers believe that student achievement is derived largely from instruction.

The teachers use student achievement data as the basis of program effectiveness: whether or not to continue the program or teaching-learning activity. Teachers are willing to accept the fact that the best way to evaluate student progress is to collect measures of pupil performance frequently. The measures of performance do not rely on teacher judgment alone or on teacher judgment in combination with grades assigned for a unit of activity. Although useful, such measures do not provide adequate curriculum-based assessments of skill mastery. Multiple measures need to be used, which should reinforce one another.

Criterion-referenced measurements are preferred to norm-referenced measurements. A norm-referenced measurement is a standardized achievement test. This measurement communicates little about the student's actual skills and performance levels on what is taught in the class. It answers the questions: "How much has Tom improved since last year" and "Is his achievement at, above, or below that of a representative sampling of students his age, grade, sex, state, or region?". The criterion measures permit teachers to individually analyze each student's progress. Students are not evaluated in comparison with each other.

They are evaluated in comparison to the uniform standard of mastery to which all students are expected to rise.

Criterion-referenced evaluation procedures can be used by teachers in four different types of testing programs. *First,* criterion-referenced tests are used for preassessment of students on objectives taught in instruction. *Second,* criterion-referenced tests are used concurrently with instruction for the purposes of checking the progress of students so teachers can help students who are having difficulties when necessary. *Third,* they are used to modify components of instruction for student objectives and instructional procedures. *Fourth,* criterion-referenced tests are used at the end of the instructional unit, grade, or program level to determine whether students have achieved the criterion levels of objectives taught.

It is recommended that criterion-referenced measures be locally validated, curriculum-based standardized measures. These measures ensure that students are tested on what they are taught. The measure is validated to be certain that the description of mastery is an acceptable level of mastery for all students in the school program. The measure is standardized so as to eliminate teacher subjectivity as a possible source of error or unfairness in assessing student progress.

E. Parent Involvement and Other Citizens in the Educational System

Positive experiences with active parent involvement in education resulted in communities establishing broader education coalitions. These coalitions become more deeply involved in broader educational processes and develop positive feelings and support for school program goals and objectives.

To improve quality education, effective schools deem it essential to strive to foster mutual school-community relations. Every effort is made to actively involve parents and other citizens in the educational processes: planning the program, implementing the program, evaluating the effectiveness of the program, and communicating results of the program to the community-at-large. Parents and other citizens can be involved as:

1. Decision Advisors.   Many federal and state guidelines recommend or require parental involvement in programs receiving federal or state funds. Because of this requirement, more parents have become involved in assisting with decision-making. Encouraging parents in this role brings about shared responsibility for decisions and the change to quality decisions is increased.

2. Educational Monitors.   Parents are informed through regular communication procedures of happenings in the school district or of a particular program. They are encouraged to attend board of education meetings, advisory meetings, and to participate as members of planning committees.

3. Community Organizers.   Many parents and other citizens excel in organizational skills for a common purpose. These individuals can reach people in many organizations and other agencies, inform them of issues related to quality education, or recruit others to help to improve the school program. They can link the school programs with resource people in the community who can assist teachers in enriching the curriculum through presentations or availability of community resources.

F. Instructional Leadership and Support Services

The instructional leader can effectively communicate the mission of the school and the individual programs within the school to the staff, parents, students, and community-at-large. The leader understands and applies the characteristics of instructional effectiveness in the management of the instructional program.

The leader ensures open communication and organized support services for all involved in schooling.

Accepting the premise that the instructional program is directed toward accomplishing specific goals and objectives, then it follows that teachers and the school-community-at-large expect certain leadership qualities and behaviors from the principal: goal-setting, assessment and accountability, support, information, supervision, and building a working consensus of quality programs for all students.

Communication focuses on the "what" and "why" of instructional programs, effective practices, assessing school and teaching effectiveness, and determining inservice education needs to improve competence and productivity. The principal of the school or facility provides organized support services and effective delivery of these services to both teachers and students. Effective school programs depend on the acceptance and cooperation among teachers, administrators, parents, and students as well as the availability and allocation of physical resources and equipment.

The design of strategies for delivering these needed supports to teachers is a major leadership task in implementing effective programs. Teachers may require training in effective use of available support services to maximize their effectiveness in meeting the needs of all students. Teachers are challenged to become broadly resourceful in maintaining more flexible and diverse learning environments, seeking and collaborating with others who have expertise in meeting special needs. If the instructional program is to be effective, leadership must be provided and consideration must be given to specifying the kind and extent of supportive services that are needed to best serve the teachers and *all* the students in the regular class.

III. CRITERIA FOR DESIGNING A MODEL FOR QUALITY PROGRAMMING

Criteria for designing quality programs are derived from three major sources: definition of quality programs, effective practices, and benefits for all participants involved in the educational process. The participants include students, teachers, parents, administrators, boards of education, legislators, and other members of the school community. Six major criteria were derived for designing quality programs. These criteria are analogous to categories. Within each category there are specific statements of specifications. Some of these specifications have been identified for each criterion. These criteria are listed below.

A. Flexibility

1. Clearly defined program goals, common to all students, with a wide range of content exemplified by objectives to meet unique needs of individual students, districts, schools and/or classrooms.
2. Objectives pursued within a given class group are readily adaptable to meet unique needs of learners at all levels.
3. Instructional activity options to meet the unique needs of learners within a given class are readily available to all students at all levels.

B. Accountability

1. The program provides for systematic monitoring of student progress and frequent reporting of student achievement results to all members of the school community.
2. The program provides systematic procedures for using the results of instruction (student achievement on stated learning outcomes), to improve individual student performance as well as the program.
3. The program provides for criterion levels of objectives to help teachers

individually analyze each student's progress on a uniform standard of mastery to which all students are expected to rise.

C. Communication

1. The program's mission, instructional focus and direction, is clearly articulated and readily communicated to students, parents, administrators, colleagues, and other relevant members of the school community.
2. A program plan, documented program goals and relevant essential objectives by grade or multilevels to achieve these goals, serves as a communication tool for establishing common agreement and understanding between teachers, students, parents, and administrators.
3. The program plan serves as a communicating tool for students to understand specific instructional requirements, diminish their anxiety, and improve self-confidence. All students are expected to learn essential skills.
4. The program plan provides a structure for parent involvement, namely, by understanding the specific instructional requirements and student expectancies, resources needed to support the program, and reinforcing goals of the program.
5. The program structure clearly defines the teaching competency requirements to effectively implement instruction for all students alike.

D. Compliance

1. The program must provide for full compliance with state and federal legal mandates and policies, and professional guideline standards.
2. The program affords a structure to facilitate continuous updating of instructional processes with new educational and technologic research and development practices.

E. Efficiency

1. The program goals and objectives serve to organize and provide sequential, progressive nonredundant program content maximizing the available instructional time and resources—equipment, materials, and support services for teachers and students.
2. The program provides a student data base on clearly defined objectives to help teachers plan, implement, and evaluate the effectiveness of their instruction—student achievement.
3. The program provides a consistent framework to yield data—units of improvement—to properly document programmatic needs—improve quality and/or defend the program.

F. Effectiveness

1. The teachers must demonstrate the stated level of mastery of the teaching behaviors required to implement the program as intended.
2. The program must result in a significant number of students (high proportion) demonstrating mastery on the essential skills specified for instruction.

Using these criteria to select, select/adapt, or design a quality program, a curriculum model that invariably emerges is based on objectives for instruction and evaluation. The focus of the model is student achievement. An achievement-based curriculum model represents, in essence, the rationale for this book. Chapter 2 examines the components of the model and their relationship to quality programs—individualization and accountability for all students.

SYNOPSIS

The professional imperative challenge is quality programs for all students in physical education. Two quality issues are individualization and accountability. Three concrete approaches to meet the challenge are (1) defining quality programs in objective terms, (2) identifying key practices of effective schools and teaching, and (3) specifying criteria to design a model for quality programs in physical education. The six criteria are flexibility, accountability, communication, compliance, efficiency, and effectiveness. Using these criteria, a curriculum model ultimately emerges that is based on objectives for instruction and evaluation. The focus of the model is student achievement. An achievement-based curriculum model to develop and/or improve program and teacher effectiveness is the purpose of this book.

RESOURCES FOR TEACHERS

American Alliance for Health, Physical Education, Recreation and Dance: Shaping the Body Politic. Legislative Training for Physical Educators, 1900 Association Drive, Reston, VA 22091, 1983.

Ballard, J., Ramierez, B., and Weintraub, F.: Special Education in America: Its Legal and Governmental Foundation, 1980. The Council for Exceptional Children, Department 5509, 1900 Association Drive, Reston, VA 22091.

Berman, P.: Educational change: An implementation paradigm. *In* Improving Schools: Using What We Know. Edited by R. Lehming and M. Kane. Beverly Hills, CA. Sage Publications, 1981.

Duckett, L., et al.: Why do Some Schools Succeed? The Phi Delta Kappa Study of Exceptional Elementary Schools. Bloomington, IN, Phi Delta Kappa, 1980.

Duckworth, K.: Specifying Determinants of Teacher and Principal Work. Center for Educational Policy and Management, University of Oregon, Eugene, OR, 1983.

Fraley, A.E.: Schooling and Innovation: The Rhetoric and the Reality. New York, Tyler Gibson Publishers, 1981.

Legislation and Regulations

Superintendent of Documents, U.S. Government Printing Office, Washington, D.C. 20040
—Public Law 94-142, 94th Congress, S.6
November 29, 1975
An Act
—Vocational Rehabilitation Act of 1973
Public Law 93-112 as amended by the Rehabilitation Act
Amendments of 1974, Public Law 94-516, 29 U.S.C.794 Section 504 of the Act

Federal Register, 1100 L Street, N.W., Washington, DC 20002
These are located in the public documents sections of libraries. The rules and regulations for PL 94-112, Section 504, are published in the Federal Register, May 4, 1977, Part IV, Vol. 42, No. 86. The rules and regulations for PL 94-142 are found in the Federal Register, August 27, 1977, Vol. 42, No. 163.

State Guidelines

Contact your school district office, State Department of Education, or school principal.

National Advisory Committee on Handicapped: The Individualized Program: Key to Appropriate Education for Handicapped Children. 1977 Annual Report. 400 Maryland Ave., S.W., Washington, DC 20202.

National Commission on Excellence in Education: A Nation at Risk: The Imperative for Educational Reform. Washington, DC, Government Printing Office, 1983, Stock #065-000-00177-2.

Reynolds, M., and Birch, J. (Eds.): Teaching Exceptional Children in All America's Schools. Rev. Ed. The Council for Exceptional Children, Department 5509, 1900 Association Drive, Reston, VA, 1983.

Squires, D.C., Huitt, W.G., and Segars, J.K.: Effective Schools and Classrooms: A Research-Based Perspective. Association for Supervision and Curriculum Development, 225 N. Washington St., Alexandria, VA 22314, 1983.

United States Commission on Civil Rights: Accommodating the Spectrum of Individual Abilities. Clearing House Publication 81, Washington, DC, September 1983.

Wessel, J.A. (Ed.): Planning Individualized Education Programs with Examples from I CAN Physical Education. Northbrook, IL, Hubbard, 1977.

ACTIVITY 1–1. Examine PL 94-142 and Section 504 of the Vocational Rehabilitation Act of 1973: Rules and Regulations published in the Federal Register.

Objective: To introduce and gain an understanding of the rules and regulations directly related to physical education and recreation for the handicapped student.

Materials: Federal Registers are located in the public documents section of libraries.

The rules and regulations for PL 94-112, Section 504, are published in The Federal Register dated May 4, 1977, Part IV, Vol. 42, No. 86. The following sections are of particular interest:

   84.34—Educational Setting
   84.47—Nonacademic Services

The rules and regulations for PL 94-142 are found in The Federal Register dated August 23, 1977, Vol. 42, No. 163.

The following sections are of particular interest:

   121a.14—Special Education
   121a.306—Nonacademic Services
   121a.307—Physical Education
   121a.346—Content of IEP
   121a.532—Evaluation Procedures
   121a.533—Placement Procedures
   121a.550—Least Restrictive Environment

WORKSHEET 1–1

Directions: **1.** Using the preceding references, answer the following questions. Cite from these references the sections that support your answer.
2. Be concise, and write your answers on Worksheet 1–1.

Variations: **1.** Make up questions other than the ones provided, or add questions. Answer them concisely, using a worksheet similar to the one provided.
2. Use the questions provided, interview professionals in the field—teachers of physical education in regular and/or special class settings; state department personnel; local or school district administrative personnel; and special education personnel. Record answers on Worksheet provided or design another one.
3. If there are new rules and regulations published, compare the sections with any new policies published. Draw conclusions with regard to impact on implementation. Interview professionals in the field and compare findings. A worksheet similar to the sample worksheet 1–1 can be designed for this purpose.

SAMPLE WORKSHEET 1–1.   Comparison of Changes

PUBLIC LAW 94-142 REGULATION REVISION CATEGORY	CURRENT LANGUAGE	LANGUAGE CHANGES	RESPONSES IMPLEMENTATION CHANGES RESULTING
Evaluation Procedures			
Individualized Education Program: IEP			
Least Restrictive Environment			
Parent Involvement Due Process			
Physical Education			
Related Services			
Special Education			

WORKSHEET 1–1. *Legal and Policy Mandates*

QUESTIONS	ANSWERS
1. What is the probability of a wheelchair paraplegic being hired for a public school physical education position?	
2. May an entire special education class consisting of students homogeneously grouped according to a specific handicapping condition be sent as a group to physical education?	
3. Will the regular classroom teacher be responsible for the handicapped child's physical education if there is no physical education program in the school district?	
4. A severely physically involved child in our school could benefit from swimming. There are no pools in any of the schools; therefore, swimming is not currently available to any students in our system. How can swimming be made available to meet the specific and special needs of this student?	
5. Since aquatic activities are included within the definition of physical education, does this mean we have to provide such a program for handicapped students?	
6. What are the implications for applications of PL 94-142 and Section 504 in states where physical education is not required at all, or not at certain grade levels?	
7. Must physical education be in every handicapped child's IEP?	
8. If the regular or special education classroom teacher uses motor, physical, or recreational activities as methods to teach certain students, has the physical education requirement been satisfied?	
9. What, then, is the role and how are therapies such as physical and occupational therapy considered?	
10. Does this mean that the local education agency must actually provide the specially designed physical education program when it does not have facilities or staff?	
11. Do the provisions of the law apply to children who are obese, malnourished, possess low levels of physical fitness, or have a poor level of motor development?	
12. If a child is receiving homebound instruction through an IEP, must physical education be made available?	
13. Define the following terms included in Public Law 94-142, using a separate sheet of paper.	

Free Appropriate Public Education
Least Restrictive Environment
Nondiscriminatory Evaluation Procedures
Parent Involvement: Due Process Procedures
Physical Education
  Definition
  Accommodation
  Specially Designed Instruction
  Placement Options
Types of Handicapped Children Identified in the Act

ACTIVITY 1–2.	Examine local school or school district's plan to implement your state's Annual Plan in Special Education for regular class settings.
Objective:	To understand the process for delivering physical education services to special education students.
Materials:	Contact local school district or administrative personnel, or the State Department of Education–Special Education Personnel, or State Director of Physical Education.
	Obtain a copy of the Individual Education Program Process including IEP forms and schedule of phases during implementation and evaluation.

WORKSHEET 1–2.

Directions:	1. Using the materials listed, answer the following questions.
	2. Be concise. Write answers on Worksheet 1–2.
Variations:	1. Make up questions other than the ones provided. Answer them concisely, using a worksheet similar to the one provided.
	2. Use the questions provided, interview professionals in the field who are involved in the IEP process, and complete forms. Collect sample IEP forms from different local or intermediate school districts. How do they view and report physical education services?

WORKSHEET 1–2. *Individual Education Program Process and Forms*

Questions	Answers
1. How are students with handicapping conditions defined for potential special education services?	
2. How are referrals made for special education? For physical and motor needs in physical education skills?	
3. What evaluation procedures are used to determine placement and progress?	
4. What IEP form or record was used?	
5. How often is the IEP reviewed? By whom?	
6. What is the role of the regular physical education teacher in the referral process? the evaluation process? the planning process? the implementation process?	
7. How are parents involved in the IEP?	
8. What is the schedule—flow chart—depicting each phase of the IEP process? Who are the key personnel (positions) involved at each phase?	
9. What is the involvement of the regular physical education teacher in each phase of the IEP process?	
10. How are physical and motor needs evaluated?	
11. How is physical education defined?	
12. Who can provide physical education to students with handicapping conditions in regular and special education settings?	
13. What child-find procedures are used in your school district to locate a handicapped child?	
14. How many children will be served in your district according to the federal and/or state categorical definitions?	

15. How many children will be served in your physical education program according to the categorical definitions:
    Regular Class in Physical Education?
    Adapted Physical Education
    Other Physical Education Options?	

ACTIVITY 1–3. Review effective practices and definition of quality programs and rate perceived importance to improving physical education instruction for all students.

Objective: To identify perceptions of the importance for improving quality programs of the proposed definitions of quality programs and effective practices.

Materials: Material presented in the chapter.
Recommended resources listed for the chapter.

WORKSHEET 1–3

Directions: **1.** Review the material in the chapter.
2. Use Worksheet 1–3 and rate perceived importance for improving the quality of physical education programs.

Variations: **1.** Use Worksheet 1–3 and interview professional personnel in the field. Do one for teachers of physical education, one for principal, and one for a parent. Compile findings. Make comparisons with each item in terms of respondents to the interview.

WORKSHEET 1–3. *Quality Programs: Factors*

Rate each of the following factors as to perceived importance to improve the quality of physical education programs for all students K–12.

Rating Scale: 1 = none; 2 = little; 3 = moderate; 4 = considerable; 5 = high.

FACTORS	PERCEIVED IMPORTANCE	COMMENT
A. *Definition of Quality Programs*		
1. Program goals and objectives stated by grade or multi-grade levels.	1 2 3 4 5	
2. A high (90%) proportion of all students should be able to evidence mastery of these objectives at stated grade levels.	1 2 3 4 5	
B. *Three Proposals to Improve Programs*		
3. No instructional program should be undertaken or continued in the absence of its effectiveness in producing stated learning outcomes.	1 2 3 4 5	
4. Each school should annually publish the results of a systematic assessment of pupil achievements in stated learning outcomes.	1 2 3 4 5	
5. Teachers should periodically submit evidence of the learning achievements of the pupils in their classes.	1 2 3 4 5	
C. *Effective Practices—School-Improvement Studies and Research on Teaching*		
1. Instructional focus and direction: goals and objectives defined, staff committed to priorities, assessment procedures, and accountability.	1 2 3 4 5	
2. High expectancies: all students to achieve stated learning outcomes.	1 2 3 4 5	
3. Teaching/learning task oriented, safe, orderly, motivating. Teachers and students know objectives for instruction and evaluation of achievement.	1 2 3 4 5	
4. Monitor student progress and frequently report results of instruction in terms of student achievement to evaluate program effectiveness.	1 2 3 4 5	
5. Instructional leadership, communication, and organized support system to help teachers and students achieve stated learning outcomes.	1 2 3 4 5	

Grand Total Points =

ACTIVITY 1–4. Review the design criteria identified to select, select/adapt, or develop quality program models in physical education for all students.

Objective:	To identify perceptions of the importance of these criteria to designing quality programs in physical education for all students.
Materials:	Materials presented in the chapter.
	Recommended resources listed for the chapter.

WORKSHEET 1–4

Directions:
1. Review the materials in the chapter.
2. Define each criterion in one sentence or less on Worksheet 1–4.
3. On Worksheet 1–4, rate perceived importance for designing quality programming models for instruction in physical education.
4. Draw conclusions and make recommendations: Are the design criteria all-inclusive? Clearly stated? Are the criteria listed under each criteria category clear? Should more be added? Deleted? Overlap with other criteria categories?

Variations:
1. Use Worksheet 1–4 or design a new worksheet in questionnaire form. May use definition as listed or subcriteria listed in the book to describe each criteria. Interview professional personnel in the field and other members of the school community: physical education teacher, parent, and principal. Compile findings. Make comparison with each criteria in terms of respondents to the interview.
2. Identify different criteria essential to design and/or evaluate the quality of program models in instruction for physical education.

WORKSHEET 1–4. *Quality Programs: Design Criteria*

Describe in one sentence or less each of the following criteria.

Rate each of the following criteria as to perceived importance to designing and/or evaluating the quality of programs in physical education for all students.

Rating Scale: 1 = none; 2 = little; 3 = moderate; 4 = considerable; 5 = high.

CRITERIA	DESCRIPTION/DEFINITION	PERCEIVED IMPORTANCE				
1. Flexible		1	2	3	4	5
2. Accountable		1	2	3	4	5
3. Communicable		1	2	3	4	5
4. Compliant		1	2	3	4	5
5. Efficient		1	2	3	4	5
6. Effective		1	2	3	4	5

Conclusions and Recommendations:

_____

_____

_____

_____

_____

_____

_____

_____

_____

_____

_____

_____

_____

_____

CHAPTER 2

Achievement-Based Curriculum Model (ABC)

ACHIEVEMENT-BASED CURRICULUM MODEL (ABC)
  Overview
  Characteristics of the Model
    Individualized Instruction and Accountability
    Other Positive Features
      Delabeling of Students
      Early Detection of Potential Learning Difficulties
      Meeting Special Needs of Individual Students
  Implementation of the Model
    Components of the Model
      Plan
      Assess
      Prescribe
      Teach
      Evaluate
THE RELATIONSHIP OF THE MODEL TO PARTICIPANTS
  Students
  Parents
  Teachers
  Administrators
  School Boards
OFTEN ASKED QUESTIONS AND RECOMMENDATIONS
SYNOPSIS
ACTIVITIES
  2–1. Rate perceived importance of the ABC model for quality program.
  2–2. Examine ABC model components and subcomponents for quality programming in physical education for all students in the class.
  2–3. Survey current status of the achievement-based curriculum model for quality programming in physical education.

What is an Achievement-Based Curriculum Model?
An Achievement-Based Curriculum Model is a systematic process to sequentially plan, implement, adapt, and evaluate an instructional program based on essential educational goals and objectives. This process can be used for any length of instructional time (one lesson, one unit, one year, or multiyears) and for an entire class, a school, or an individual student.

What is the Rationale for the Model in Physical Education for all Children?	**Decision Aids**
1. What is it? What can it do? What does it not do?	Goal Functions Quality Issues
2. What is the relationship between the model and quality programming for all children? Individualizing instruction? Accountability? Effective practices? Adaptability?	Characteristics Seven key questions Meeting special needs Delabeling of children Early detection of learning problems
3. What are the components of the model? How do these components relate to the five-step procedural guide to implement the model?	Model components Five-step implementation guide
4. What are the possible benefits for persons involved in the physical educational process: students, parents, teachers, administrators, and boards of education?	Relationship of the model to persons involved in the educational process
5. Is the model worth the effort?	Some questions and recommendations

Individualized instruction, which adapts instruction to accommodate individual differences, has received considerable attention in both special and regular education. Individualization is the personalization of instruction. Although not necessarily different for each student, it must be appropriate for each. In this context, appropriateness refers to the degree of correspondence between the capabilities of the student and the objectives of instruction. The best approach is to think of individualizing instruction as a way of accommodating the needs of individuals in a class, preferably a group.

The extent to which the needs of all students in a class are met is viewed as an important determinate of quality programs. Teachers are now required to plan and teach students with instructional needs outside of the narrow confines of "average" performance. Faced with increasingly heterogeneous student populations, teachers must find ways to effectively instruct all students to achieve the stated objectives and goals of the program.

In this chapter, we present a general rationale for using an achievement-based curriculum model. Reasons for using the model are examined from five perspectives: relationship of the model's characteristics to the quality issues, delabeling of students, early detection of students with learning difficulties, meeting special needs of individual children, and benefits of the model to all persons involved in the process. The components of the model, steps to implement the model, are described briefly. Some conclusions are drawn relative to effort required to implement the model.

How can individualization best be accomplished? To search for a perfect individualized program, fitted to the needs of each student in a particular class, is a fantasy. To realistically respond to this problem, teachers need to be familiar with curriculum models. A model is a procedural guide for the design, implementation, evaluation, and improvement of instruction. It does not propose to tell teachers what they should teach, or what specific instructional activities they should apply in the teaching-learning process to ensure acquisition of skills taught in the program. It is not a curriculum. It does provide a framework for planning instruction and activities to help students achieve stated learning outcomes of instruction. It does provide an invaluable tool in helping teachers to individualize instruction and more effectively teach all students.

A model consistent with the concepts of quality programs, individualized instruction and accountability, is the achievement-based curriculum model. The ABC model focuses on student achievement. The model has been validated experimentally over the past several years from research and development done by us and others.

ACHIEVEMENT-BASED CURRICULUM MODEL (ABC)

OVERVIEW

The ABC model is based on two key ingredients that are receiving increased interest as an approach for systematic curriculum improvement focused on student achievement. They are: (1) objectives for instruction and evaluation; and (2) a systems approach to implement the model.

With objectives for instruction and evaluation, the model provides a systematic curriculum improvement process. We need a process of curriculum improvement especially designed to articulate content (goals and objectives) from grade to grade and school to school. The process has a way of focusing teachers' efforts to improve the program. In this context, the term *curriculum* refers to that portion of the program that meets two criteria: essentiality and structure. Essential objectives are core learnings for all students. Structured learning requires careful planning, sequencing, and articulation if the essential skills are to be mastered by the students.

Since Chapter 4 is devoted to the detailed examination of objectives, we will not take time here to describe the continuum of educational objectives in the model. An example of a program goal, program objective, and instructional objectives is given in Table 2–1 to establish understanding of these terms.

The ABC model is a procedural guide, a process model. It is based on a technology of instruction. The term technology comes from the Greek word meaning systematic treatment. In the implementation of the ABC model, this means the systematic application of scientifically based and empirically derived instructional procedures to plan, assess, prescribe, teach, and evaluate the student and program. These procedures are completely distinct and separate from curricular content or methods of teaching. Such procedures come with the unwritten guarantee that, when systematically applied, learning will occur. Students do achieve stated objectives of instruction. If not, the systems approach allows for review and study of the program and instruction, including the effectiveness of the model itself.

More specific assumptions of the model are that most effective individualization of instruction occurs when:

1. Program goals and objectives for instruction and evaluation for all students are precisely identified and stated before instruction begins: long term over school years, multiyears, yearly, unit, or lesson.
2. A sequential hierarchy of program objectives organized over the school years operationally defines the program goals and objectives of instruction on a continuum of essential skills for all students.
3. Maximum communication exists between teachers and students regarding the objectives of the lesson and goals of the program.
4. Instructional objectives clearly specify evaluative measures to assess student's entry performance and progress toward achieving the stated learning tasks of the objective and sequencing of the learning tasks.
5. Instructional objectives tailored to the needs and capabilities of the students are provided for planning instruction.

TABLE 2–1.   *An Example Goal, Program Objective, and Instructional Objective Statements*

Instructional Purpose	Goal and Objective Statement
Intent	Program Goal: To demonstrate competence on selected fundamental motor skills.
Content	Program Objective: To demonstrate a functional overhand throw.
Specification Skill Level	Instructional Objectives: A. Given a demonstration and a verbal request, the student can throw a tennis ball at least 40 feet three consecutive times in the following manner:
Learning Tasks	(1) side orientation with weight on the rear leg to initiate the throw; (2) near complete extension of throwing arm to initiate the throw; (3) weight transfer to the foot opposite the throwing arm with marked hip and spine rotation during the throwing motion; (4) a follow-through well beyond ball release; (5) smooth (not mechanical or jerky) integration of the above.
Skill Level	B. Given a demonstration, a verbal request, and a practice trial, the student will throw a ball, using skill level standards above and
Learning Tasks	(1) hit a 6' target located 1' off the ground and number of hits recorded out of 10; (2) hit the target 10 out of 10 times.

6. Instructional activities are prescribed and lessons implemented to help students achieve learning tasks based on each student's assessed needs.
7. Continuous monitoring of student's progress, feedback, and reinforcement are carried out during the lessons and activities modified based on student's needs until an acceptable level of mastery of the objective is achieved.

Obviously, there are many deterrents to the implementation of individualization. Some of these include: the diversity of students within a class, the class size, the limited resources and support assistance available to teachers and students, or lack of teacher knowledge of effective instructional models. Even though it is not possible for instruction to reflect all of the above assumptions, the model can be used effectively to guide teachers through the major steps to improve the quality of instruction by using the systems approach to planning, carrying out, and evaluating instruction. The model does provide an overall structure for teachers and others to view, evaluate, and continually update the instructional processes.

CHARACTERISTICS OF THE MODEL

The major premise underlying the model is quality programming focused on effective instruction—students do achieve what teachers teach. The model is applicable to all program levels in physical education—preschool, elementary, middle school, and secondary. The model is applicable to any length of instruc-

TABLE 2–2. *Characteristics of an Achievement-Based Curriculum Model: Objectives for Instruction and Evaluation*

Question	Development of Achievement-Based Curriculum Model Characteristics
1. What content should be taught and why?	1. Documented goals and program objectives that specify the content to be learned.
2. When is the student to learn the content?	2. The objectives that operationally define each goal are sequentially arranged into appropriate levels of the program.
3. What is the student's present level of skill and what are the student's needs?	3. Program objectives divided into subskill levels (instructional objectives) that range in skill level from near-zero to functional competence provide the criteria for (1) the assessment of student performance, (2) the sequential learning tasks for instruction, and (3) class and student expectations on acceptable standards of mastery.
4. What are the most appropriate instructional experiences to influence student learning?	4. Instruction is prescribed in accordance with the assessed needs of students on the instructional objectives.
5. How does the teacher know what each student has learned?	5. Student achievement can be documented through reassessment during and at the end of instruction.
6. Is instruction effective or should it be modified?	6. Continuous monitoring and on-going evaluation documenting the student's progress on target objectives is facilitated with the use of an ABC model because of the specification of objectives and program organization and implementation.
7. How can the results of the instruction be communicated to parents, students, and administrators?	7. Student performance data documenting both entry and progress on target objectives provide the basis for comprehensive reporting and/or communication.

tional time—one hour, one week, one semester, one year, multiyear, or total program plan over a student's school years.

Individualized Instruction and Accountability

Seven key questions must be answered to select, select/adapt, or design a model for quality programming. These questions incorporate the concepts consistent with quality programs, individualized instruction and accountability. With the ABC model, the teacher and others involved in curriculum development have a systematic approach, a procedural guide, to answer these questions. The characteristics of the achievement-based curriculum model and their relationship to these questions are portrayed in Table 2–2. To the right of each question are the characteristics of the model that provide answers to the stated question.

Other Positive Features

Three other positive features of the model need to be highlighted: delabeling of students, early detection of potential learning difficulties, and adaptability in meeting special needs of individual students. Each is briefly described below.

1. Delabeling of Students. The model helps to eliminate most of the adverse effects of labeling students by special education or any other label. The program goals of physical education tied to the common goals of education apply equally to all students. All students need to master essential skill objectives encompassed by these goals. The assessment of each student's entry level performance and continuous monitoring of progress toward stated objectives are criterion-referenced. Mastery of the objectives, acceptable level of performance, is known to all students and teachers. Each student's performance is measured directly on instructional objectives taught in the program. The student's learning needs to achieve objectives do not depend on diagnosed labels. With student assessment data, teachers plan appropriate instructional activities and evaluate their effectiveness. The emphasis, therefore, is on assessment of the student's strengths. What can the student do? What does the student bring to instruction? Emphasis is on the student's needs rather than on categorizing and labeling.

2. Early Detection of Potential Learning Difficulties. The model provides early identification of potential student learning problems on what is taught. By relating instruction to assessment, teachers have a constant flow of information to use in evaluating student progress and the effects of instruction. Objectives for instruction and evaluation allow teachers to concentrate on those areas where difficulties exist. Teachers can identify students having achievement problems. Referrals can be made or assistance requested. Immediate feedback and corrective procedures can be initiated to correct or ameliorate the problem. Early intervention of appropriate instructional activities is likely to be more effective than activities based on remedial approaches. A greater amount of success in learning, as well as development of positive feelings toward learning and self, can be expected. In particular, it is at the early elementary program level that early detection of potential learning problems and appropriate instruction best prepare students for success in learning and in achieving the more complex and demanding skills of the later grades.

3. Meeting Special Needs of Individual Students. The model provides teachers with a systematic approach to adaptation of the instruction to meet the special needs of individual students at all program levels. The adaptability of the model is based on the use of objectives for instruction and evaluation for all students:

- Program goals of physical education tied to the common goals of education apply to all students in the school program.
- Essential objectives can be selected from a wide range of objectives so that all students can learn to function effectively in socio-leisure activities and to maintain health and fitness.
- A body of literature exists which indicates that individuals learn physical and motor, personal and social behaviors in approximately the same order.
- Objectives (representative of physical education content) can be sequenced according to the "normal" developmental order and on the basis of empirically verified instructional sequence.
- Objectives defined in terms of measurable student behaviors become criterion-referenced assessment instruments to evaluate student's entry performance, progress, achievement, and the effectiveness of instruction.

In later chapters, specific task-analysis procedures that adapt objectives to meet student needs in instruction are presented. For purposes of this section, Table 2–3 lists examples of adaptation to establish understanding of the task-analysis process.

IMPLEMENTATION OF THE MODEL

Implementation of an achievement-based curriculum model is a series of five steps. A flow diagram showing the five step implementation of the model's components is presented in Figure 2–1. Each component of the model contains instructional procedures required to implement the model as intended. Each component can be considered independently from all others; however, the components are closely related and are mutually dependent in terms of sequence. No single activity will produce the results desired. Instead, the instructional procedures should be planned for the total long-term program and used systematically on a daily basis.

TABLE 2–3. *Examples of ABC Model Adaptations: Program and Instructional Objectives*

Objective	Type of Adaptation	Example of Adapting Downward	Example of Adapting Upward
1. Program objective	Number selected	Decrease number of program objectives to operationalize a goal area	Increase number of objectives to operationalize a goal area
2. Instructional objective	Level of achievement	Lower level of achievement for realistic student expectations	Raise level of achievement for realistic student expectations
3. Instructional objective	Skill level	Decrease step size: identify more elementary ones or split steps into smaller ones	Increase step size or complexity of task
4. Instructional objective	Performance standard	Alter or reduce criteria to assure success	Alter or add criteria to increase requirement for success
5. Instructional objective	Conditions	Increase number of cues, prompts, or assisting devices	Decrease number of cues, prompts, or assistance

On the following pages, each component of the model is explained briefly. Several of the major factors to consider at each step are presented. The materials provide an overview of the instructional procedures. In subsequent chapters, each component of the model is discussed more completely, particularly as it relates to the "how-to" information to implement the model.

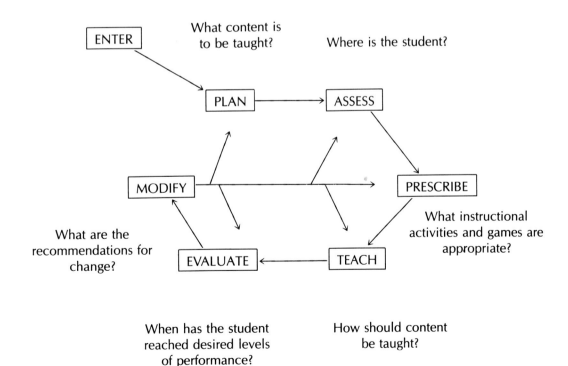

Figure 2–1. *Five-step procedural guide to implement the ABC model components.*

Components of the Model

Plan

Step One—Knowing What to Teach and When. The first step is to identify and sequence appropriate content for the instructional program. This step requires the establishment of program goals and objectives. Goals set the purpose of the program. Objectives operationalize goals and when organized sequentially by program level, provide the instructional intent. In establishing goals and objectives, priority is given to those knowledges, skills, and attitudes that contribute to the mission of the school, are unique to physical education, and are valued by students, teachers, parents, administrators, and other members of the school community as program goals and objectives.

The program objectives are sequentially arranged by program level, preschool through secondary. Instructional time, personnel, equipment, facilities, and other scheduling variables are all considered in determining what objectives and how many objectives can be included in the program. The program goals and objectives compose a written program plan. In turn, objectives for the year or multiyear are selected and sequenced. From these objectives, instructional units are developed.

Assess

Step Two—Knowing Where the Students Are Before Deciding Where They Should Go and What to Teach. Initially, the program plan is designed to meet the needs of the majority of students. The plan must, however, meet the needs of all students. To accomplish this task, preassessment prior to beginning a unit of instruction is conducted. Assessment is based on the specific instructional objectives of the unit. Using criterion-referenced measures, teachers assess students on objectives to be taught to determine:

- how much they already know;
- the capabilities of achieving the objectives;
- instructional activities and games that should be prescribed;
- how students should be grouped for instruction.

The results of assessment indicate whether any students need objectives to be modified, deleted, or added, and what specific instructional activities need to be prescribed for a particular student. Class and student expectations are set prior to instruction for each instructional objective.

Prescribe

Step Three—Knowing Where Students Are on Objectives To Be Taught and Where They Are Going and Planning the Instruction To Get Them There. After students are assessed and adjustments made in the objectives as necessary, planning instruction is next. Planning instruction involves the following procedures: (1) identifying specific instructional objectives that students are to learn, and grouping students for the lesson; (2) selecting instructional activities, games, and equipment to be included in the lesson; and (3) developing sequential lesson plans for the unit that appear to be most efficient for achieving stated objectives. The lesson prescribed according to initial assessment data may be taught over a period of one day, one week, or even one month or more. Modification of the lesson planned is based on continuous monitoring and reassessment of students prior to, during, and at the end of the unit of instructional time.

Teach

Step Four—Knowing the Prescription, Managing a Class to Maximize On-Task Time so that Learning Takes Place. Teaching the prescribed activities and games as planned for the lesson involves implementing effective practices of instruction, such as:

- physically engaging students in instruction, drill, practice, and game situations to maximize on-task time on objectives to be learned;
- feedback and reinforcement;
- motivating, high-interest activities provided for learning;
- managing disruptive behaviors;
- continuous monitoring progress and helping students who have problems learning;
- using aides, peer tutors, and other assistance when available.

Evaluate

Step Five—Knowing Where Students Are at the End of Instruction; Making Needed Modifications to Improve Instruction. Students completing a unit of instruction are evaluated to determine whether the instruction was effective in achieving the unit's objectives. The evaluation procedures involve gathering data to make decisions related to these questions:

1. Did the class and individual student achieve expectations established before instruction began on the objective?
2. If the class and/or student did not achieve target objectives, why not?
3. What changes need to be made to allow for achievement for the class? for individual students in the class groups?

Changes in objectives, instructional activities, and expectations are made on the basis of the evaluational activities, and expectations are made on the basis of the evaluational results. Changes are made to enable students to achieve mastery or as near-mastery as possible. As indicated by the feedback loop in the flow diagram, changes can be made in any component of the model: plan, assess, prescribe, teach, and evaluate. Class and student expectancies and achievement results are reported on a specified unit of instructional time: unit, semester, year, multiyear. The student report is based on objectives prescribed and achieved for class and/or individual students.

The feedback loop serves another purpose. In addition to making changes based on observed results, modifications in the model components or model evaluation can be made on the basis of new research and development findings in instructional technology, equipment, or promising practices and changing values of the members of the school community. The effects of these changes can be systematically implemented, evaluated, and reported.

THE RELATIONSHIP OF THE MODEL TO PARTICIPANTS

Implementing the model benefits everyone involved in instruction, particularly students, teachers, parents, administrators, and school boards. The purpose of this section is to illustrate how an objective-based instructional model applies to those individuals involved with the school's physical educational process.

STUDENTS

- Objectives help students understand specific requirements of a unit or course, reducing the amount of generalized anxiety about requirements.
- Objectives accommodate all students, including special needs of students, and ensure continuous progress toward program goals and objectives so that all students succeed to an acceptable level of mastery.
- Objectives given directly to students: the exact behaviors desired and conditions under which the behaviors are to be demonstrated are specified; students do not have to guess what is expected of them in instruction.
- Objectives given directly to students: students can help each other learn,

provide feedback and reinforcement for each other as they progress toward achieving stated levels of mastery on objectives.

- Objectives given directly to students: indicate practical situations for teaching the objective.

PARENTS

- Parents are increasingly concerned with quality of physical education in the schools, and are therefore more involved with their children's achievement, growth, and class problems. Parents may elect to help their children achieve objectives, knowing what behaviors are expected.
- Periodic reporting of objectives of the program and actual objectives achieved by a student is a marked improvement over the grade report card procedure commonly used. Parents can help guide the progress of the student and become involved in maintaining the proper levels of achievement.
- Conferences with teachers, as well as with their children, about achievement can take place in concrete terms and, in some instances, indicate areas where the students need special help outside of the class.
- Specification of essential objectives can help parents emphasize and reinforce the program goals sought by the teacher in physical education, as well as provide support for allocation of school resources and additional resources needed to improve the quality of the program.

TEACHERS

- Value to the teacher will be dependent on the countless variables of the school system related to the instructional environment. There are, however, five values that remain constant:
  1. Objectives help teachers determine the essential skills for all students to learn.
  2. Objectives help provide teachers with confidence that the objectives being taught are of major importance to the mission of the school and the contributions of physical education to this mission.
  3. Objectives provide teachers with objective measures of pupil progress, reporting, evaluation of the effectiveness of instruction, and sound decision-making for improving instruction.
  4. Objectives help teachers to systematically evaluate their teaching competencies and determine their inservice and staff development needs to improve instruction.
  5. Objectives help teachers meet the legal and policy mandates for individualizing instruction over a wide range of functional skill levels for all students in regular classes.

ADMINISTRATORS

- Objectives help administrators responsible for planning and coordinating the curriculum (with instructional staff) to ensure that content is covered adequately and that there is minimal overlap between courses or grade levels.
- Objectives help administrators design more effective allocation of resources and create better staff and time arrangement schedules to ensure a favorable instructional environment for students to progress toward achieving program goals.
- Objectives help administrators to respond effectively to legal and policy mandates for providing appropriate instruction to meet needs of all students in regular classes.

- Objectives help administrators responsible for supervising and evaluating teachers by ensuring support for teachers, identifying teacher needs, and planning staff development activities.
- Objectives help administrators effectively coordinate with staff to set realistic grade or multiyear student expectancies using criterion-referenced measures, and reporting results to members of the community.

SCHOOL BOARDS

Objectives have a *communicative* and persuasive value to the school board by concretely demonstrating the content of the program at any program or unit level, precisely documenting what learning achievements occur in a given class or program level, and providing a framework for cost-effectiveness analyses and sound decision-making.

OFTEN ASKED QUESTIONS AND RECOMMENDATIONS

The rationale reviewed the why and what questions: Why use an achievement-based curriculum model to develop and/or improve program and teacher's effectiveness? What is it designed to do? The implementation of the model in actual school settings over the last decade provides information to help answer questions most frequently asked.

1. *Does the model change class instructional and teaching behaviors?* A universal finding is that when the model is implemented as intended, instruction is different. The environment becomes more sensitive to the individual differences of students. There is a better match between instruction and the students' capabilities to learn objectives taught. When the model is implemented as intended, both students and staff are generally more satisfied. Simply adopting a new schedule, a label, or some different way to group or assess students will not necessarily change anything. Table 2–4 lists the key elements descriptive of objective-based instruction identified by teachers implementing the model.

2. *Is the model a great deal of effort?* It can be. It often is more effort than some teachers are willing to put forth. The problem is greater when a whole school or school district decides to implement the model all at once. Even a simpler approach, a single class, calls for additional teacher effort to implement effectively.

3. *Does the model increase the amount of record-keeping needed?* Yes. The model requires knowing more about students in the class. Lack of individualization on the part of teachers is never all due to disinterest. Teachers simply do not have the time to follow students and the procedures to collect information. Implementation of the model does provide teachers with a potential for gathering more information which requires more recording and interpreting. No completely satisfactory solution has yet been devised for addressing this problem. In the future, the computer will be able to assist in the process. Currently there are only partial solutions, which are discussed later in the book.

4. *Do students achieve more under this model?* This is a difficult question to answer. The answer must be related to what actually occurs in the class instruction and how student achievement is measured. There have been many examples of student-achievement gain when what is tested reflects what has been taught: criterion-referenced assessment. Using more generalized achievement measures, the results may be less than positive. There have been very few instances reported in which students have not done as well as those receiving traditional instruction. There is evidence to suggest that

TABLE 2–4. *Key Elements of Teacher Behaviors: ABC Model Class*

Subjective Teacher Behavior	Objective Teacher Behavior
1. Preassessing students on instructional objectives of the lesson, assigning stated objectives —Teacher and student know objectives and mastery criteria for achievement —Activities and games reinforce learning tasks on objectives —Students on task working individually, small groups or partner —Feedback and reinforcement on assigned learning tasks	1. Class Performance Score Sheets Lesson Plans
2. Selecting instructional objectives for the lesson related to program goals and objectives of instruction	2. Objective based program plan —Lesson Plan —Instructional Unit Plan —Yearly Plan —Long-Term Plan
3. Setting class and student achievement expectancies prior to instruction, evaluating effectiveness of instruction	3. Class Performance Score Sheets
4. Ongoing assessing and recording student performance and adapting instruction based on student performance	4. Class Performance Score Sheets Lesson Plans
5. Periodically evaluating and reporting student achievement on specified essential objectives by unit of instructional time	5. Individual and Class Records documenting instruction in terms of student achievement and reporting to: parents; administrators; community

other student benefits, such as the development of a positive self-concept toward physical educational experiences and helping one another achieve, can be obtained without sacrificing achievement.

5. *Is the model really worth the effort?* This is the bottom line. The question can only be answered by the individual teachers, school, or school district. Many teachers say it is worth it. Many who have not tried it, and some who have, say it is not. This question is critical now since there is an increasing demand for quality programs and they are considered a basic legal right for all children. More importantly, it is our continuing professional commitment to instructional excellence for all. Although the benefits to all participants involved in the educational process have been discussed, the following list gives some suggestions about what should be considered:

- Recognize that the model, although focusing on the achievement of desired outcomes, is a decision-making model to improve the quality of the program.

- The model is intended to provide a structure to facilitate a difficult and time-consuming but ultimately rewarding system for planning, implementing, and evaluating the effectiveness of instruction for all children in the program. It is a guide to help teachers individualize and structure teaching of essential skills that make up the school learnings necessary for success in the school for all students, and to reach all students they teach more effectively. It is not to be viewed as an alternative curriculum nor as a special physical education curriculum to be used exclusively with children requiring specially designed instruction or accommodations in regular classes.

- Using the model as a base, teachers have developed computer competencies as well as improved instructional competence to implement the model. Self-paced, teacher-training programs can be developed for both preservice education teachers and for inservice education of teachers using micro-computer technology.

- The model provides a structure to develop school or district-wide teacher support and management systems. In particular, the model can be used for constructing student profiles of progress and reports documenting student and class expectancies and achievement gains, and coding effective instructional practices to student characteristics to assist in instructional planning.

- When the decision to implement the model for a school or a district is made, do not try to do it all at once. Careful preparation and phased implementation is a more effective strategy than a single crash adoption across all classes in a school or all schools in a district.

- The evaluation plan must be designed as an integral part of implementing the model in a single school or school district. Implementation cannot take place without evaluation. Program goals and objectives of essential skill learnings for all students by grade and over a period of time, the school years, need to be defined. Criterion-referenced test items for each objective need to be constructed so that all teachers agree on the content to be taught as well as the mastery criteria of acceptable levels of performance on each objective. Data need to be gathered on students and expectancies set by grade for continuous progress toward achieving goals of the program. Teachers need to be trained to criterion level of mastery on identifiable competencies required to implement the model for unit and lessons comprising the unit for a school year. Evaluation of effectiveness of instruction in terms of student achievement is instituted when teachers have achieved stated mastery.

- Individual teachers can decide to implement the model for a class on a daily basis. The materials presented have been used by teachers for self-training at the class level. Teachers monitor their own implementation skills. With mastery of each implementation skill, they have implemented the instruction and evaluated effects in terms of student achievement. Figure 2–2 illustrates the components and steps needed to implement the model at the instructional unit level.

- The model contributes to the systematic development of a continuing inservice education program for teachers implementing the program. It has built-in features to monitor the teacher's mastery level on each identifiable teaching competency and relate these competencies to student achievement. The model incorporates the educational concepts of master teachers and student achievement criteria as promotional gates from level to level and for graduation.

- The model and its implementation are no substitute for effective teaching. No model can substitute for the teacher's knowledge of the student in planning instruction. Nor can it provide a substitute for lack of instructional leadership, poorly organized support assistance for teachers and students, and little or no communication between and among all participants in the educational process. The model's primary goal is to help teachers teach what and how they want to teach as effectively as possible for all students in the class.

SYNOPSIS

A model consistent with the concepts of quality programs, individualized instruction and accountability, is the achievement-based curriculum model. The focus of the ABC model is student achievement. The model is based on two key

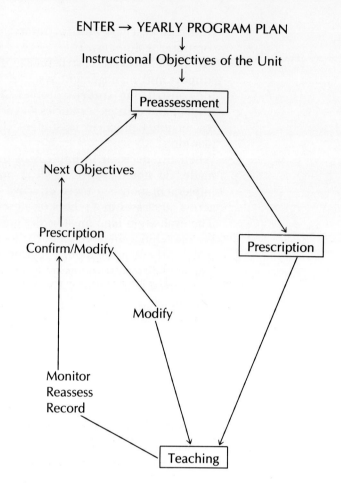

ENTER → YEARLY PROGRAM PLAN
↓
Instructional Objectives of the Unit
↓
Preassessment

Next Objectives

Prescription
Confirm/Modify

Prescription

Modify

Monitor
Reassess
Record

Teaching

Figure 2–2.   *Implementation of the ABC model at the class level.*

ingredients: (1) objectives for instruction and evaluation, and (2) a systems approach for effective implementation of the model. Positive features of the ABC model are: individualizing instruction, accountability, delabeling students, early detection of learning difficulties, and adaptability in meeting special needs of students. The components of the model are to plan, assess, prescribe, teach, and evaluate. These components are systematically applied in a series of sequential steps to implement the model. They identify teaching competencies required to implement the model effectively. The implementation of the ABC model benefits all participants involved in physical education. Following is a synthesis of the key concepts of the ABC model:

The Goal of the Model: Effective instruction in regular physical education classes for all students to achieve desired learning outcomes.

Functions of the Model: Structure to specify those skills, knowledge, and attitudes that make up the essential physical education learnings necessary for success in school for all students.

Guide to facilitate a difficult, time-consuming but ultimately rewarding system for planning, implementing, and evaluating the effectiveness of instruction.

Guide to help teachers individualize and modify the instructional plan to meet the assessed needs of the students in the class.

Structure to study, evaluate, and continuously improve instruction.

Consistent with Quality Issues —Individualization
—Performance accountability
—Effective practices
—Student achievement
—Benefits to all participants in the educational process

RESOURCES FOR TEACHERS

Gagne, R.M.: Educational objectives and human performances. *In* Learning and the Educational Process. Edited by J.D. Drumbolts. Chicago, Rand McNally, 1965.

Kibler, R.J., et al.: Objectives for Instruction and Evaluation. 2nd Ed. Boston, Allyn and Bacon, 1981.

Mager, R.F.: Preparing Instructional Objectives. 2nd Ed. Belmont, CA, Fearon Publishers, 1975.

Popham, W.J.: Criterion-Referenced Instruction. Belmont, CA, Fearon Publishers, 1973.

Popham, W.J., and Baker, E.L.: Planning an Instructional Sequence. Englewood Cliffs, NJ, Prentice-Hall, 1971.

Singer, R., and Dick, W.: Teaching Physical Education: A Systems Approach. Boston, Houghton-Mifflin, 1974.

Tyler, R.W.: Basic Principles of Curriculum and Instruction. Chicago, The University of Chicago Press, 1950.

Wessel, J.A. (Ed): I CAN Instructional Resource Materials, Achievement-Based
> I CAN Preprimary Motor and Play Skills. East Lansing, MI, Instructional Media Center Marketing Division, Michigan State University, 1980.
> I CAN Primary Skills. Northbrook, IL, Hubbard, 1976.
> I CAN Sport, Leisure and Recreation Skills. Northbrook, IL, Hubbard, 1979.
> Adaptation Manual for Teaching Physical Education to Severely Handicapped Individuals Preprimary Through Adulthood. East Lansing, MI, Instructional Media Center Marketing Division, Michigan State University, 1980.

Wessel, J.A.: Quality programming in physical education and recreation for all handicapped persons. Annu. Rev. Adapted Phys. Act., *1*, 1982.

Wessel, J.A. (Ed.): Planning Individualized Education Programs in Special Education with Examples from I CAN Physical Education. Northbrook, IL, Hubbard, 1977.

ACTIVITY 2–1. Rate perceived importance of the ABC model for quality program.

Objective:	To gain awareness of the components of the ABC model and perceived importance of the model for quality programming in physical education
Materials:	Worksheet 2–1 provided
	Design criteria discussed in Chapter 1

WORKSHEET 2–1

Directions:
1. Using Worksheet 2–1, rate perceived importance of each component of the model for quality programming: planning, assessing, prescribing, teaching, and evaluating.
2. For any item rated less than 4 or 5, state your rationale: indicate why this is of no importance to implementing a quality program model in physical education.

WORKSHEET 2–1. *Quality Program Design Criteria Related to the ABC Model Components*

Six Design Criteria and Definition of Quality Programs	Relationship to Model—Characteristics, Features, Instructional Procedures to Implement the Model
1. Flexible	
2. Communicable	
3. Accountable	
4. Efficient	
5. Effective	
6. Compliant	
7. Quality Program Definition	

ACTIVITY 2–2. Examine ABC model components and subcomponents for quality programming in physical education for all students in the class.

Objective:	To gain awareness of the ABC model components and perceptions of the importance of the model for quality programs
Materials:	Worksheet 2–2 provided. Materials discussed in this chapter

WORKSHEET 2–2

Directions:
1. Using the Worksheet provided, rate perceived importance of each model component and subcomponent: planning, assessing, prescribing, teaching, and evaluating.
2. After completing the ratings, add scores for each component and divide by the total points possible to calculate an average for component.
3. Record average score for each component in appropriate place. If any component received an average score of less than 4 or 5, make a statement of why. Provide alternative activities for this component or suggestion.

Variations:
1. Use the Worksheet to interview teachers who are mainstreaming students with special needs in regular classes. Then ask the same questions of teachers who do not have students with special needs. Compare your answers.

WORKSHEET 2–2. *ABC Model for Quality Programming—Self Perceptions*

Rate perceptions of importance of the model for quality programming.

Rating Scale: 1 = 0; 2 = little; 3 = moderate; 4 = considerable; 5 = high

IMPLEMENTATION SKILLS/KNOWLEDGES	PERCEIVED IMPORTANCE FOR QUALITY PROGRAMS				

Step 1 Plan the Program: Goals and Objectives

1. Identify relevant physical education program goals and state them in appropriate terms.   1   2   3   4   5

2. Select program objectives that operationalize the selected physical education goal statements.   1   2   3   4   5

3. Organize the objectives into sequential program levels: unit, yearly, multilevel.   1   2   3   4   5

4. Arrange the objectives into a teaching order by instructional unit for yearly program.   1   2   3   4   5

Step 2 Assessment

1. Select criterion-referenced test items to assess students' performances on objectives of the instructional unit or yearly program plan.   1   2   3   4   5

2. Be able to organize assessing activities for the class or for individual students in the class.   1   2   3   4   5

3. Know how to adapt or modify objectives to assess individual students using task analysis procedures.   1   2   3   4   5

4. Be able to reliably assess student performance on selected instructional objectives of the unit or yearly program plan.   1   2   3   4   5

5. Be able to monitor and reassess student's progress on stated learning tasks of the instructional objectives during instruction.   1   2   3   4   5

6. Be able to select and implement record-keeping procedures for class and individual students—not time-consuming.   1   2   3   4   5

Step 3 Prescription: Instructional Planning

1. Select appropriate learning tasks stated in the instructional objectives for students and class based on preassessment data.   1   2   3   4   5

2. Identify instructional activities and games appropriate for teaching assigned learning tasks for class and individual students as needed.   1   2   3   4   5

3. Arrange the identified activities and games into a written daily lesson plan.   1   2   3   4   5

4. Be able to set student and class expectancies—achievement gains on instructional objectives of the unit.   1   2   3   4   5

Step 4 Teaching: Implementing the Prescription					
1. Demonstrate working knowledge of a variety of strategies for teaching within a selected instructional activity.	1	2	3	4	5
2. Describe and/or demonstrate procedures for maximizing on-task time.	1	2	3	4	5
3. Demonstrate the appropriate use of selected motivational strategies.	1	2	3	4	5
4. Demonstrate the appropriate use of effective practices in managing behaviors, feedback, and corrective procedures.	1	2	3	4	5
5. Demonstrate procedures for monitoring reassessing, and recording students' progress during instruction.	1	2	3	4	5
6. Demonstrate the ability to teach and manage an objective based instructional model class: preassess, assign learning tasks, prescribe instruction based on need, teach, monitor, and modify instruction as needed during the lessons.	1	2	3	4	5
Step 5 Evaluation of Student and Program					
1. Determine the degree to which significant student achievement gains have been made for class and individual students based on established expectancies set prior to the teaching of the instructional unit.	1	2	3	4	5
2. Be able to establish a rationale between observed student achievement gains and "why" they occurred or did not occur, and make appropriate instructional adjustments: objectives, assessment, prescription, teaching, and evaluating.	1	2	3	4	5

3. Demonstrate an appropriate procedure for reporting and maintaining records of class and student achievement for:
     parents
     administrators
     teachers receiving the student
     significant others as identified
	1	2	3	4	5

4. Demonstrate working knowledge of kind and degree of instructional leadership, communication, and support assistance required to effectively implement the program and support teachers' and students' efforts in achieving stated learning outcomes.	1	2	3	4	5
5. Demonstrate working knowledge of kind and degree of training needs for the teacher to continue implementing the model.	1	2	3	4	5

RATIONALE STATEMENTS

Average Score	ABC Model Components	Rationale Statements with Alternative Suggestions
_____	Plan the Program	
_____	Assessment	
_____	Prescription	
_____	Teaching	
_____	Evaluating	

ACTIVITY 2–3.	Survey current status of the achievement-based curriculum model for quality programming in physical education.
Objective:	To gain understanding of the current status of the achievement-based curriculum model in a school program.
Materials:	Materials discussed in this chapter
	Contact professional personnel—teachers of physical education in a local school or a director at local, intermediate, or state level.

WORKSHEET 2–3

Directions:	1. Using the Worksheet provided as an interview form, have the person rate each question as to the current status of his or her program in relation to each question.
	2. After completing this rating, have them rate other physical education programs in similar settings in the district or school.
	3. On a separate piece of paper, tell each person to list two barriers to implementing this kind of program and two benefits significant to the profession for doing so.

WORKSHEET 2–3. *Current Status: Implementation of Achievement-Based Curriculum Model for All Students*

Directions: Rate each of the following questions as it relates to the current status of physical education in relation to: A—you and your program; and B—other staff as a whole and their programs.

Teachers of regular physical education should compare themselves and their programs to other physical educators in similar settings in the district or school. Classroom teachers should compare themselves and their physical education programs to other classroom teachers with similar settings and their programs.

0 = unable to rate; 1 = low; 5 = high

QUESTIONS—CURRENT STATUS OF PE IN RELATION TO:	(A) YOUR PROGRAM	(B) SIMILAR STAFF AND THEIR PROGRAM(S)
1. The degree to which the PE program is based upon an established curriculum of goals and objectives: yearly, multiyearly, or units.	0 1 2 3 4 5	0 1 2 3 4 5
2. The degree to which PE instruction is provided in accordance with the PE curriculum: goals and objectives.	0 1 2 3 4 5	0 1 2 3 4 5
3. The degree to which students are assessed prior to instruction on objectives to be taught in the unit.	0 1 2 3 4 5	0 1 2 3 4 5
4. The degree to which student assessment data are used in prescribing instruction for the class.	0 1 2 3 4 5	0 1 2 3 4 5
5. The degree to which student performance data are used to evaluate student progress.	0 1 2 3 4 5	0 1 2 3 4 5
6. The degree to which student performance data are used to set class and student expected achievement gains in the instructional unit.	0 1 2 3 4 5	0 1 2 3 4 5
7. The degree to which student performance data are used to evaluate effectiveness of instruction.	0 1 2 3 4 5	0 1 2 3 4 5
8. The degree to which student achievement data are used to define the quality of the program: percent of students achieving stated learning outcomes.	0 1 2 3 4 5	0 1 2 3 4 5
9. The degree to which student achievement data on goals and objectives of the physical education curriculum are documented and reported periodically to the community.	0 1 2 3 4 5	0 1 2 3 4 5
10. The degree to which students know the objectives of instruction and mastery levels to achieve these objectives.	0 1 2 3 4 5	0 1 2 3 4 5

Know the Learner

3–1. Developing a student needs profiling instrument.

3–2. Identifying and categorizing common characteristics of handicapping conditions.

3–3. Administration and interpretation of data collected with a student needs profiling instrument.

3–4. Identifying key personnel who provide support services for teachers in regular education in the school program and what placement options are available for students with special needs in physical education programs.

3–5. Identifying and evaluating the program and building accessibility for students with special needs.

3–6. Identifying and evaluating medical forms and procedures for collecting and managing student medical data.

Who Are Your Students and What Are Their Needs and Abilities?
Students' characteristics are on a continuum within and across learning, personal-social, and physical and motor needs. Teachers must understand these characteristics and deal with them on an individual need basis to make and implement appropriate instructional decisions so that all students can achieve desired learning outcomes.

How is it Done?	*Decision Aids*
1. Determine what student needs must be addressed to ensure quality instruction for all students.	Student characteristics Individual differences in instruction
2. Assess individual student needs to make appropriate instructional and placement decisions.	Needs profile
3. Communicate student needs to significant others (teachers, parents, administrators, and related support personnel).	Profiling and the individualized education program and placement
4. Identify student medical needs and the limitations imposed on performance in physical education.	Preparing medical release forms Managing student medical information

---

To plan and implement quality programs for all students, teachers must know their students. The student's race, sex, socioeconomic status, or handicapping condition does not determine success in learning. It is the individual student's needs, performance, and background, as well as the teacher's skill in adapting instruction to meet these individual needs that result in quality programs—student achievement of desired learning outcomes.

This chapter addresses the teacher's need to know individual student characteristics and how these characteristics interact with instruction and student achievement. Procedures are presented to assist in identifying significant student characteristics by using a needs profiling technique. The final section of the chapter addresses medical concerns that should be considered in physical education. Procedures are provided to assist in obtaining and managing pertinent medical information on the students in the teacher's classes.

INDIVIDUAL DIFFERENCES

Teachers have long recognized that considerable differences exist between students both within and across grade levels. Individual students differ in their ability to learn, and in their physical and motor needs, interests, motivation, self-confidence, self-concept, and anxiety level. Even within grades, widely different levels of student ability and achievement on specified objectives of instruction exist. In the regular elementary physical education class there can be a span as great as four to five years in the range of student achievement. Greater variability in achievement can exist at the higher grade levels.

Individual differences are the primary concern of teachers and others making planning and instructional decisions. How teachers manage to assess individual differences among students in their class and use these differences to guide their instructional plans and decisions is what the procedural concerns of individualizing instruction—quality programming—are all about. A more meaningful way to view students in planning programs and in instructional decisions is in determining their strengths and needs in the following areas: learning, personal and social, and physical and motor. These need areas describe the type of information teachers need to plan, manage, and deliver quality instruction to meet their students' needs.

Areas	*Descriptive Elements*
1. Learning	ability to understand instruction, follow directions, and communicate
2. Personal and Social	attitudes, feelings, interests, motivations, reactions, self-control, cooperativeness
3. Physical and Motor	performance, mobility/equipment, health/safety

Traditional handicapping categories and other types of labeling of student characteristics have been omitted to highlight the need to focus on individual student needs, not labels, that interact with instruction. Table 3–1 compares some general characteristics that may be associated to some degree with students labeled *emotionally impaired* and *learning disabled* in each of the major need areas. It is immediately apparent that there is a tremendous overlap between the characteristics attributed to the two groups. It should be noted also that no two students labeled emotionally impaired or learning disabled would have the same combination of needs or the same degree of need within a given characteristic.

Analysis and comparison of handicapped and other students' characteristics in the areas of learning, personal and social, and physical and motor strengths and needs will produce similar findings. Students who have similar learning, personal and social, or physical and motor needs may not have the same type of handicapping label or even be "handicapped."

Definitions and descriptions of various handicapping conditions can be found in a variety of general adapted physical education books. Table 3–2 contains a summary of the handicapping conditions addressed in several of these books. Although these definitions and descriptions typically provide teachers with basic facts about the various conditions (age of onset, cause, incidence, general characteristics), which are important prerequisites for understanding a student's needs, they do not provide sufficient information to allow teachers to make sound instructional decisions. Unfortunately, these general descriptions frequently produce stereotypical expectations on the part of teachers (e.g., all hearing-impaired students have balance problems, all learning-disabled students have midline problems), which could result in inappropriate instructional decisions.

INDIVIDUAL DIFFERENCES IN INSTRUCTION

To serve all students effectively in the regular physical education setting using the ABC model, teachers need to "know the learner" in terms of important learning, personal and social, and physical and motor characteristics. How these characteristics influence student learning is critical to effective teaching. The effective teacher must adapt instruction to student needs in both content and approach.

Individualizing instruction in an entire class setting is extremely challenging and depends on the teacher's ability, range of student needs, resources, and staffing. It is essential, however, that teachers realize that knowing the student is not only feasible but has direct implications for effective instruction for *all* students. Individualizing instruction does not necessarily require major changes in the class or school. Teachers can adjust existing instructional approaches to student's learning, personal and social, and physical and motor abilities within their own classrooms and within existing constraints. A variety of planned and spontaneous instruction cues to guide the student can be used (e.g., verbal and nonverbal prompts, drills and practice, games). Different groupings can be organized such as small groups, peer-partner, peer-tutor, and one-to-one, as needed during the instruction. Games and sports can be modified so all students, of varying abilities, can participate (e.g., changing boundaries, modifying rules, using different types of equipment). Motivation, positive reinforcement, and

TABLE 3–1.   *Comparison of Emotionally Impaired and Learning Disabled—
General Characteristics*

EMOTIONALLY IMPAIRED	LEARNING DISABLED
Need Area: Learning	
Distractible Hyperactive or hypoactive Inability to follow directions May use alternative modes of communication—speech Lacks perseverance to complete tasks Short attention span Poor work habits Inability to learn at a rate commensurate with his or her intellectual development May exhibit low motivation to learn May fail to talk even when skill to talk is present	Distractible Hyperactive or hypoactive Inability or remember and follow directions May have difficulties in communication—speech and language Perseverations, difficulty in shifting attention Short attention span Impulsive Problems in recall and memory skills
Need Area: Personal-Social	
Difficulty in interacting with peers; plays alone May be disruptive Impulsive Inappropriate emotional responses Lacks self-confidence; has poor self-concept May lack self-control May exhibit erratic behavior May appear disorganized, confused May exhibit lag in social and emotional development Overly aggressive, hostile Timid, afraid to try new ideas Withdrawn, disinterested Follows rather than leads May demand constant attention	Problems with interpersonal relationships May be disruptive Impulsive May overact to ordinary events Lacks self-confidence; has poor self-concept Exhibits erratic behavior May appear disorganized, confused Poor social adjustment Irritable
Need Area: Physical and Motor	
General awkwardness or clumsiness Inconsistency in motor skill performances Poor eye-hand, eye-foot coordination Difficulty with spatial, directional, and time relationships	General awkwardness or clumsiness Inconsistency in motor skill performances Poor eye-hand, eye-foot coordination Difficulty judging space, distance, direction, and time relationships Difficulties in fine and gross motor coordination Poor balance May not recognize right and left (laterality) May exhibit delayed rate of motor skill development

TABLE 3–2. *Major Handicapping Conditions Covered in Eleven Books Commonly Used in Adapted Physical Education*

MAJOR HANDICAPPING CONDITIONS	ADAMS/DANIELS MCCUBBIN/RULLMAN	BLECK/NAGEL	CRATTY	CROWE/AUXTER PYFER	FAIT/DUNN	FRENCH/JANSMA	KALAKIAN EICHSTAEDT	SEAMAN/DEPAUW	SHERRILL	WINNICK	WISEMAN
Amputations in Children	DI	D	D	D	DI	DI		D	DI	DI	D
Arthrogryposis		D			DI			D	D		
Asthma	DI	DI	DI	DI	DI	DI	DI	D	DI	DI	D
Autism			DI	D	D		DI	D	DI	D	D
Cancer	DI	DI									
Cerebral Palsy	DI	DI	DI	DI	DI	DI	DI	D	DI	DI	
Spasticity	D	D	D	D	DI	D	DI	D	DI	DI	
Athetosis	D	D	D	D	DI	D	DI	D	DI	DI	
Rigidity	D	D	D	D	DI	D		D	D	DI	
Ataxia	D	D	D	D	DI	D	DI	D	D	DI	
Tremor	D	D	D	D	DI	D		D	D	DI	
Mixed	D	D	D	D	DI	D		D	D	DI	
Convulsive Disorders	DI	DI	D	DI	DI	DI	DI		DI	DI	DI
Cystic Fibrosis	DI	DI	DI		DI		D	DI	DI		
Deaf–Blind					DI	D		D	D		
Diabetes Mellitus	DI	DI	DI	DI	DI	DI	DI	D	DI	DI	D
Emotionally Disturbed		DI	DI	DI	DI	DI	DI	D	DI	DI	DI
Hearing Disorders	DI	D	DI	DI	DI	DI	DI	DI	DI	D	DI
Heart Disease in Children		DI	D	DI	DI	DI	DI	D	DI	DI	
Hemophilia	DI	DI	DI		DI		DI	D	DI		
Language Disorders		D	DI		D			D		D	
Learning Disabilities			DI		DI	D	D	D	DI	D	
Mental Retardation		DI	DI	DI	DI	DI	D	D	DI	DI	DI
Down Syndrome		D	D		DI	D	D	D	DI	DI	D
Mild			D		DI	D	D	D	DI	D	D
Moderate			D		DI	D	D	D	DI	D	D
Severe			D		DI	D	D	D	DI	D	D
Profound			D		DI	D	D	D	DI	D	D
Multiple Sclerosis			D		DI			D	DI	DI	D
Multiply Handicapped		DI		D		D		D			
Muscular Dystrophy	DI	DI	D	DI	DI	DI	DI	D	DI	DI	D
Obesity in Children	DI		DI		DI	DI		D	DI		
Orthopedic Conditions	DI	DI	DI	D	DI	DI	DI	D	DI	DI	DI
Foot	DI	DI	D		D	D			DI		D
Lower extremities	DI	DI	DI	D	DI	DI	DI	D	DI	DI	
Head-Trunk	DI	DI	DI	D	DI	D	DI	D	DI	DI	DI
Poliomyelitis		D	D		DI			D	D	DI	DI
Rheumatoid Arthritis	DI	DI	DI	D	DI		DI	D	DI		
Scoliosis		DI	DI	D	DI	D	DI	D	DI	DI	DI
Speech Disorders		D	DI			D		D			
Spina Bifida	DI	DI	D	DI	DI	DI	D	D	DI	DI	D
Spina Muscular Atrophy	DI	DI	D							D	D
Respiratory Disorders	D				DI				D		
Visual Disorders	DI	D	DI	DI	DI	DI	DI	D	DI	DI	DI

D = Condition described   I = Instructional implications provided

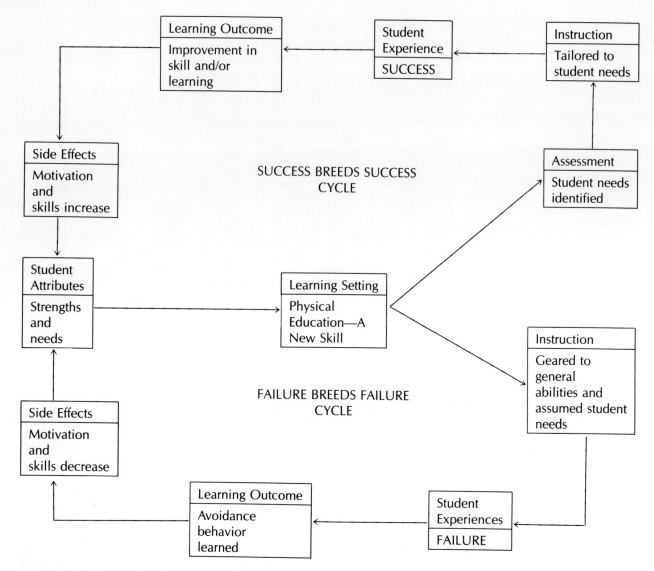

Figure 3–1. *Success breeds success—failure breeds failure cycles.*

feedback meaningful to students can be selected. Students can be given opportunities to become mutual planners by helping to assess, monitor, and record results with the teacher to achieve specified objectives.

Teachers know that there are many student characteristics (strengths and needs) and instructional procedures that affect student success in achieving instructional objectives. To plan, manage, and deliver quality instruction effectively, the teacher *first* must know the student characteristics that have the greatest effect on student achievement in the instructional setting. *Second,* the unique needs of students must be identified. *Third,* instructional procedures believed to have the greatest effect on learning for all students must be planned and incorporated into teaching. *Fourth,* the effectiveness of these instructional procedures must be evaluated in terms of student achievement to determine whether to continue or modify these procedures.

If instruction is tailored to meet the students' needs, they will eventually enter the "success breeds success" cycle depicted in Figure 3–1. Failure to consider students' needs and abilities prior to making instructional decisions increases the likelihood that the student will not be successful (failure breeds failure). In all learning settings, students enter with certain attributes as to learning, personal-social, and physical and motor skills. If these abilities are not assessed prior to instruction, the probability of meeting student needs through appropriate instruction is reduced and the likelihood of student failure is increased. If a proper assessment is not made, the students, after experiencing repeated failures, begin to learn how to avoid failure. This avoidance behavior might be demonstrated in such behaviors as being late for class, continually asking off-task questions, forgetting sneakers, misbehaving in class, or complaining of frequent injuries or illnesses. Eventually, these students spend most of the instructional time learning and practicing how to avoid learning.

At the end of an instructional unit, these students have not achieved the unit objectives, leaving them even further behind. They have improved only in their ability to avoid learning situations. If this cycle is allowed to continue, eventually these students fall so far behind in their physical education skills that there is little hope of success in any physical education setting. Frequently, by the time many of them reach junior and senior high school they have experienced so much failure and their skills are so underdeveloped that they no longer have the interest or motivation to attempt physical education. Physical education becomes such a negative experience that these students are willing to accept any other alternative (punishment, failing grades, exclusion, suspension). If the cycle is allowed to reach this extreme stage it becomes extremely difficult to motivate and to remedy the accumulated deficits.

The "Failure Breeds Failure" cycle can occur in specific activities or within and across any content area. The more severe cases may withdraw from all physical education activities and are more obvious than the mild or more specific cases.

Students with some physical education skills also tend to react to failure by avoidance, but are able to cope better because they have some successful skills. These students continue to practice and further develop the skills they are successful at and receive reinforcement for and to avoid other skills they cannot accomplish. For example, a student who is good at sprinting (100 yard dash) but poor at running long distances (a mile run) frequently avoids running distances and instead continues to work on sprinting. The student is able to balance out the failure experienced in distance running by the success and reinforcement received from sprinting.

The key to reversing the "Failure Breeds Failure" cycle and creating a "Success Breeds Success" cycle (Fig. 3–1) is the assessment of student needs and the matching of appropriate instruction to meet these needs. Assessing each student's unique needs allows the teacher to adjust instruction so that the students will be successful. Success on a task reinforces the learner and provides motivation to continue practicing which eventually leads to skill mastery. The combination of success and mastering new skills motivates the learner and provides encouragement to attempt new skills.

Having established the importance of knowing student strengths and needs, the next section presents a student-centered profiling strategy to assist in making appropriate instructional decisions. To highlight the discussion and procedures presented in the following sections, one major question is posed: What student characteristics have direct implications on instruction that teachers need to address so that the student can achieve learning outcomes? Three subquestions need to be answered:

1. Does the student possess the prerequisite skills to successfully learn the instructional content specified in the target objectives?
2. Can the teacher adapt instruction to individual needs?

3. What support services are needed by the teacher to facilitate the student's achievement of specified objectives?

STUDENT NEEDS AND ABILITIES

Decision-making for programming and instruction in all learning situations should be planned and implemented according to student characteristics. Teachers need to identify significant entry characteristics considered essential to ensure that all students can progress toward achieving the objectives to be taught in the instructional program (Success Breeds Success). To accomplish this task, student characteristics should be clustered to emphasize significant characteristics that interact in instruction. These characteristics are clustered into the three major individual need areas: learning, personal-social, and physical and motor. Although primary attention is focused on student needs in these areas, student strengths in each area should also be identified and used to facilitate learning.

Tables 3–3, 3–4, and 3–5 depict needs, observable behaviors, and selected implications for instruction for each of the major need areas. The various needs presented under each area are those previously identified by teachers and therefore should not be viewed as definitive lists. Sample observable behaviors associated with each need are provided to assist the teacher in identifying student needs. Finally, selected implications for instruction are provided for each need to demonstrate how instruction can be individualized to address all students unique needs.

Profiling Individual Characteristics

If students are to be successful in physical education classes, each student must be considered as an individual with individual needs; they must not be identified by labels. This does not mean one-to-one attention. It means teachers and others must be able to address the issues pertinent to abilities and needs of students in planning instruction for the class or in making placement decisions. Each student must be seen as an individual with a range of abilities, skills, and needs to achieve desired learning outcomes.

A student needs profile form is provided in Table 3–6 to assist teachers in gathering information for making instructional decisions about students. The characteristics used in the needs profile were derived from the learning, personal-social, and physical and motor characteristics presented in Tables 3–3 through 3–5. The needs profile provides a structure to assist the teacher in screening students to:

1. Determine which characteristics have the most critical bearing on the student's ability to achieve in the instructional placement.
2. Highlight those characteristics that have implications for planning effective instruction to meet students' needs.
3. Assist in determining the ongoing appropriateness of the placement decision.

The student needs profile is provided as a model that can be modified and adapted to meet local needs. The specific characteristics used in this student needs profile were established by 25 teachers using a consensus-forming technique. Each teacher independently rated each characteristic. After the first rating, each characteristic was discussed as to the reasons why each was judged high or low on a 5-point scale for inclusion in the needs profile: 5 = extremely important; 4 = important; 3 = might be included; 2 = not important; 1 = inappropriate.

Based on the classification or new insights resulting from the discussions, each

TABLE 3–3. *Student Learning Needs, Observable Behaviors, and Selected Implications for Instruction*

LEARNING NEEDS: OBSERVABLE BEHAVIORS	SELECTED IMPLICATIONS FOR INSTRUCTION
1. Difficulty in comprehending word meaning and following directions. *Observable Behaviors* Poor vocabulary Slower rate of learning Poor sensory integration (perceptual problems in receiving and processing information)	A. Use vocabulary level appropriate for student. B. Keep the time between input and student response short. C. Vary communication modes of oral and nonverbal continuum of instruction; assisting, prompting, and fading as needed. D. Use demonstrations with verbal cueing in teaching the task. E. Use peer modeling or a "buddy system." F. Be concise, consistent, short in giving directions. G. Start with single teachable tasks, add and sequence tasks gradually. H. Use prompt positive reinforcement to provide students with knowledge of results. I. Provide structured, concrete, motor experiences for students to gain concepts of differences in time, space, color, numbers, and direction. J. Plan small group (1 to 3) and proceed to larger group discussions on a gradual basis. K. Support attempts to ask questions, seek help and assistance on tasks. L. Provide repetition and practice in a variety of instructional activities, correlating word concepts and motor skills.
2. Difficulty in attending to the task. *Observable Behaviors* Short attention span Easily distracted by sound and visual stimuli and nearness to others Hyperactive Low frustration levels Unwilling to attend to task, make decisions about tasks, follow through and complete tasks	A. Use highly structured activities to keep student attentive, make decisions about task to be accomplished, and maintain student's attention until task is completed. B. Use controlled change when shifting from one task activity to another, or when changing student's location. C. Structure success-oriented steps that are achievable by the student. D. Define the physical limits for teaching and learning activities and reduce or eliminate distractions.
3. Difficulty in memory and generalization skills. *Observable Behaviors* Poor recall and retention skill Lack of ability to transfer and generalize skills learned to other situations or for functional use	A. Use highly structured sequential instruction program. B. Deliberately plan and schedule for repetition and practice of skills learned in situations outside of the class, particularly in the home and with classroom learning. C. Use shorter and more frequent practice periods during the available time in the yearly program. D. Structure sequential tasks that build upon the initial task (chaining and shaping).
4. Difficulty in communicating (speech or other modes) with teacher and peers. *Observable Behaviors* Physical impairment (speech, hearing, orthopedic) Emotional impairment (ability to talk but does not) Delayed level or retarded intellectual functioning	A. Reinforce expressive language skills to help student develop and maintain speech quality. B. Increase intensity of cues for receiving information (verbal and nonverbal cues). C. Identify alternative communication modes (verbal and nonverbal). D. Attend to the placement of students during instruction (face-to-face visibility for speech or sign language or use of chalkboard). E. Help students keep noise level under control (hearing aids can distort sound). F. Plan coordinated experiences with the classroom teacher and/or communication specialists to acquire language base and/or alternative communication modes for input and student responses in instruction.

TABLE 3–4. *Student Personal-Social Needs, Observable Behaviors, and Selected Implications for Instruction*

PERSONAL-SOCIAL NEEDS: OBSERVABLE BEHAVIORS	SELECTED IMPLICATIONS FOR INSTRUCTION
1. Overly aggressive, inappropriate and inconsistent behaviors. *Observable Behaviors* Aggressive toward others Disruptive to others Lacks self-control, impulsive Refuses to cooperate Easily distracted Poor listening skills, interrupts Does not attend Lacks consistency of behavior with others Disrespectful and defiant Irrelevant responsiveness Low frustration level, impatient May have low self-esteem Easily angered Fights, refuses to work with others	A. Be concise, consistent, and do not give lengthy directions. B. Limit assignments and length of work periods. C. Structure success-oriented tasks in small sequential steps that are achievable by the student. D. Provide instruction in relaxation exercises. E. Minimize rules, but consistently administer those that exist. F. Reinforce appropriate behaviors promptly. G. Encourage peer reinforcement and planned ignoring of inappropriate behaviors. H. Reduce sound and visual distractions. I. Define limits of behavior, set consequences, and reinforce consistently. J. Use contracting or contingency management (reinforcers must be appropriate for age). K. Set up a reinforcement schedule and document change of behaviors over time.
2. Anxious, tense, afraid to be involved, defensive behaviors. *Observable Behaviors* Unwilling to accept assignments Lacks responsibility to complete tasks Protects self from embarrassment in front of peers, teacher Avoidance behaviors May exhibit "I don't care" attitude. Wastes time in class Misses school	A. Structure success-oriented tasks in small sequential steps that are achievable by the student. B. Identify student preferences and interests in activities and related motor skills. C. Define limits of behavior, set consequences, and reinforce consistently. D. Use planned ignoring when behavior will not cause serious problems on a short-term basis. E. Use prompt, positive reinforcement for appropriate behaviors. F. Use contracting or contingency management (something to look forward to). G. Give choices of activity participation. H. Set up a reinforcement schedule and document change of behaviors over time.
3. Withdrawn, disinterested behaviors. *Observable Behaviors* Lacks motivation Does not respond when spoken to Inconspicuous in class Fails to talk even when skill to talk is developed Plays alone majority of the time Lacks interpersonal skills with peers to play and participate in activities and games May appear confused	A. Structure success-oriented tasks in small sequential steps that are achievable by the student. B. Use group tasks requiring specific assignment such as cooperation, sharing, taking turns, and accepting responsibilities. C. Define guidelines for behaviors, and provide time and place for student to be alone. D. Identify student preferences and interests in activities and relate skill tasks to those activities. E. Encourage conversation and discussion among peers on a one-to-one or small group basis. F. Use contracting or contingency management. G. Assign a buddy to student. H. Set up a reinforcement schedule and document change of behaviors over time.
4. Delayed personal-social development. *Observable Behaviors* Lacks interpersonal skills, such as: —making and keeping friends —sharing and taking turns —accepting responsibility in group for assigned tasks —seeking help or assistance from others —maintaining self-control	A. Identify student preferences and interests in activities and use as basis for selection of activities to teach the learning task. B. Encourage parallel activities and gradually plan structured associate and cooperative play situations. C. Define guidelines for behaviors, set consequences, and reinforce promptly and consistently. D. Provide encouragement in partner and small group situations. E. Provide structured group tasks, assign roles and responsibilities that students can achieve. F. Use buddy system and peer modeling. G. Set up a reinforcement schedule and document change of behaviors.

TABLE 3–5. *Student Physical and Motor Needs, Observable Behaviors, and Selected Implications for Instruction*

PHYSICAL AND MOTOR NEEDS: OBSERVABLE BEHAVIORS	SELECTED IMPLICATIONS FOR INSTRUCTION
1. Slowed, delayed motor skill acquisition and physical development. *Observable Behaviors* Lacks physical skills to play selected activities Low levels of performance in —fundamental motor skills —low physical fitness and endurance —poor postural control Irregular physical growth patterns —height —weight —body size	A. Limit scope of objectives taught to those that are most functionally relevant. B. Modify the difficulty of objective skill levels (entry and progress). C. Vary the level of acceptable achievement on objectives for individual students. D. Structure success-oriented steps that are achievable by the student.
2. Problem in developing and maintaining adequate levels of physical fitness. *Observable Behaviors* Low levels of physical fitness —muscular strength and endurance —cardiorespiratory capacity —flexibility —cardiorespiratory endurance Weight control problem Inactive, sedentary daily life	A. Emphasize and focus on selected physical fitness objectives suited to individual learner's needs. B. Modify the difficulty of objective skill levels (entry and progress) based on fitness demands. C. Structure success-oriented steps that are achievable by the student.
3. Physical impairments that pose movement and/or safety problems. *Observable Behaviors* Low level tolerance for exercise stress Poor adaptation to environmental changes coupled with exercise stress Missing or impaired limbs Type and amount of drugs impact on exercise tolerance and/or environmental conditions during exercise Allergic conditions	A. Modify rules for individual student(s) or entire class. B. Vary the level of acceptable achievement on objectives for individual students. C. Limit scope of objectives taught to those that are most functionally relevant. D. Use periods of rest and relaxation and breathing exercises. E. Limit periods of exertion, particularly in close settings and high heat and humidity. F. Know the prior history of student's hypersensitivity to the conditions. G. Practice safe methods of falling with or without prosthetic devices. H. Use all medical resources (nurse, therapist, M.D.) available; rest and fatigue, drugs, sensitivity, type and amount of activity precautions. I. Use buddy or partner system as needed.
4. Physical impairments may limit mobility, range of motion, and varying degrees of dependence/independence. *Observable Behaviors* Limitation in range of motion Poor postural patterns Varying degrees of dependence/independence in performing tasks Inefficient traveling patterns Problems in accessibility relevant to mobility	A. Limit scope of objectives taught to those that are most functionally relevant. B. Modify the difficulty of objective skill levels (entry and progress) and/or class activities. C. Guarantee accessibility to instructional sites (for students with crutches, braces, wheelchairs, and other devices). D. Work with the physical and occupational therapist for assistance regarding: physical positioning and safety consideration for optimum learning, management of wheelchairs, braces, and crutches. E. Maximize opportunities for physical independent mobility and range of motion.

TABLE 3–6.   *Student Needs Profile*

Student Name: _____   Date: _____

Class: _____   Teacher: _____

LEARNING CHARACTERISTICS	CIRCLE RATING 1 = Low— 5 = High	COMMENTS
1. Student's ability to communicate	1 2 3 4 5	
2. Student's ability to comprehend instructions (verbal and nonverbal)	1 2 3 4 5	
3. Student's vocabulary level	1 2 3 4 5	
4. Student's memory skills	1 2 3 4 5	
5. Student's ability to follow large group instruction	1 2 3 4 5	
6. Student's ability to focus and maintain attention on tasks (not distracted or hyperactive)	1 2 3 4 5	
7. Student's ability to communicate needs, ask questions, and request assistance	1 2 3 4 5	
8. Student's learning rate	1 2 3 4 5	
9. Student's ability to follow through on assignments and learning tasks	1 2 3 4 5	
10. Student's ability to generalize and transfer skills	1 2 3 4 5	
11. Student's desire to be in class	1 2 3 4 5	

PERSONAL-SOCIAL CHARACTERISTICS	CIRCLE RATING 1 = Low— 5 = High	COMMENTS
1. Student's ability to adapt to new tasks and unanticipated changes	1 2 3 4 5	
2. Student's ability to cooperate with others—shares, takes turns, accepts responsibility	1 2 3 4 5	
3. Student's ability to follow daily time schedule	1 2 3 4 5	
4. Student's ability to work independently on assigned tasks	1 2 3 4 5	
5. Student's ability to communicate—for peer-social interaction	1 2 3 4 5	
6. Student's willingness to seek help from others on targeted learning tasks	1 2 3 4 5	
7. Student's social maturation level	1 2 3 4 5	
8. The appropriateness of the student's peer social behaviors	1 2 3 4 5	
9. Student's ability to maintain emotional self-control	1 2 3 4 5	
10. Student's motivation and interest in learning	1 2 3 4 5	

TABLE 3–6. *Student Needs Profile (Continued)*

PHYSICAL AND MOTOR CHARACTERISTICS	CIRCLE RATING 1 = Low— 5 = High	COMMENTS
1. Student's ability to maneuver in familiar locations (spatial direction orientations)	1 2 3 4 5	
2. Student's ability to manipulate equipment and materials	1 2 3 4 5	
3. Student's achievement levels on the specific skills targeted for instruction in this class	1 2 3 4 5	
4. The disparity between the student's age/interests and activity preferences in relation to the other students in the class	1 2 3 4 5	
5. Student's willingness to attempt motor tasks in the class setting	1 2 3 4 5	
6. Student's physical development/maturation in relation to the other students in the class	1 2 3 4 5	
7. Student's ability to use existing equipment without special modifications or adaptations	1 2 3 4 5	
8. Student's ability to participate safely in the class without making special health/safety modifications	1 2 3 4 5	
9. Student's ability to independently access the various instructional sites needed for instruction	1 2 3 4 5	
10. Student's ability to begin work on program objectives (prerequisite skills do not need to be developed)	1 2 3 4 5	

SCORING

Student Ratings			*Class Average Ratings*	
Sum of Learning	= _____		Learning	= _____
Sum of Personal-Social	= _____		Personal-Social	= _____
Sum of Physical and Motor	= _____		Physical and Motor	= _____
Total Sum	= _____		Total Sum	= _____

teacher independently rerated each characteristic. These reratings were then averaged and used to select the characteristics presented in the needs profile shown in Table 3–6. This process could be used by teachers to modify or develop their own needs profile instrument.

This needs profile approach carries with it the potential of addressing most of the concerns of teachers, parents, and students in regard to student achievement. In addition, the needs profile can be used to identify other concerns such as health and safety and staff and resource needs that are needed to facilitate student achievement. Specific assessment procedures related to quality programming for all students are covered in Chapter 5 (that is, student performance on the objectives to be taught).

Teachers should complete a Needs Profile on each student in a class at the beginning of the year. In large classes, profiling may have to be spread out over several classes owing to time constraints. In this situation, the students with more obvious needs should be profiled first. The information provided by the needs profile can assist teachers in recognizing what is necessary to meet the needs of all learners. The range of variability (individual differences in the regular class) should be examined from three standpoints: the diversity of individual differences, the intensity of instruction needed by individual students, and the support services available to meet teacher and student needs. Once developed, this information can be passed on from teacher to teacher as teaching tips and continuously updated to enhance student success and achievement. Such information provides teachers with teaching tips of what works and what does not work for individual students.

There are no hard and fast guidelines for interpreting the scores obtained from the student needs profile. Each student's scores must be interpreted in light of the other students' needs in the class, the ability of the teacher, resources, and support provided for the teacher to individualize instruction. Marked deviation between an individual student's score and the class average in any particular area should serve as signal for the teacher. Final decisions regarding a student's placement and instruction must be made by considering all factors, by using "holistic" judgment, or by applying locally determined weightings to each characteristic.

NEEDS PROFILING AND INSTRUCTIONAL DECISIONS

Productive accommodation of student learning needs requires more than lip service about *individual differences* for all students. Without recognizing these individual differences, the move toward a more individualized instructional program design will have little meaning for teachers, students, and the larger society.

The needs profiling approach helps the teacher become more knowledgeable about the learning needs of all students in their classes. Teachers become cognizant of what works and what does not work for their students to achieve desired learning outcomes. In addition, needs profiling can help the teacher or the team assigned to evaluate the student, answer the question of placement, and provide objective criteria for the evaluation of the appropriateness of the instructional placement prescription.

With the knowledge of student characteristics, the final question that has to be answered by the teacher or the team assigned to evaluate the student is:

> In what learning environment can the student be placed to learn and achieve desired learning outcomes?

The answer to this question is part of the Individualized Education Program (IEP).

The initial data from the needs profile can help to develop the IEP. The objective of the IEP is to develop a written plan, prescription, and placement decision that meets the needs of the unique learner. Information is obtained from the referring teacher, the parent, and the consultant specialists. Following is the type of information that may be obtained from these different sources:

Referring Teacher

1. Provide objective information on student performance in the instructional program.
2. Provide instructional and learning data—a record of what works and does not work for the student: learning needs, personal-social needs, and physical and motor needs.
3. Provide specific documentation of student needs for review and further evaluation if needed.

Parents

1. Provide descriptive information concerning the home situation.
2. Provide input for setting goals for the student.

Consultant Specialists

1. Provide comprehensive analysis of student within area of expertise.
2. Provide specific information describing the student's strengths and weaknesses in the following three need areas: learning, personal-social, and physical and motor.
3. Provide specific recommendations for related support services needed for the student to benefit from instruction.

If such student data are not available, the teacher needs to meet and observe the student in class, talk with parents, other teachers, and, if needed after assessment of objectives to be taught, refer student for more in-depth evaluation prior to making placement and/or instructional decisions to accommodate the student in the class.

Within the typical school structure, teachers often do not communicate the kinds of information needed by colleagues to ensure quality instruction for all students. There is no doubt that individualized and accountable physical education programs require new skills and competencies in teachers, as well as open communication and support systems in which professional expertise is shared with colleagues.

The student needs profile and a record of what works and does not work is an important initial step in identifying and in transmitting appropriate information to the benefit of the learner. The ABC model provides concrete data pertinent to student needs and how these can be addressed effectively in physical education.

MEDICAL CONSIDERATIONS

In addition to knowing the learning, personal-social, and physical and motor characteristics of students in their classes, teachers should be cognizant also of all medical conditions. In fact, it is the responsibility of all teachers to know the nature and implications of all medical conditions of all students in their program. Ignorance is not an acceptable excuse for negligence in this area. Failure on the part of teachers to obtain and use medical information on their students can result in unnecessary harm to both the student (injury) and/or the teacher and school (law suits).

Teachers should be aware of all medical conditions, related symptoms, treatment, associated medications, and implications for physical education that could negatively affect the students in their program. Potential conditions range from temporary impairments such as Osgood-Schlatter's disease to permanent conditions like a heart disorder. Treatments can range from daily medication for the treatment of epilepsy or diabetes to on-demand medication like antihistamine for asthma. Implications for physical education may vary from minor limitations such as no diving for a student with a middle ear condition to major restrictions in vigorous activity for a student with high blood pressure.

Ideally, medical clearance should be kept on file for all students prior to their participating in physical education. A medical release is designed to protect both the teacher and the student and to capitalize on the expertise of the medical profession to meet the needs of students. Any pertinent medical information that is obtained on students should be summarized into a usable form and discretely made available to all educators working with the students. This is

TABLE 3–7. *Sample Medical Release Form*

SCHOOL DISTRICT
Physical Education: Medical Release Form

STUDENT INFORMATION

Name _____ Date of Birth _____
Parent/Guardian _____ Home Telephone _____
Address _____
         (street)   (city)   (state)   (zip)

PROGRAM INFORMATION

Physical Educator _____ School _____ Phone _____
Physical Educators Schedule:
    Grade level _____ Number times per week _____ Class length _____
                                                                                 (minutes)
Description of Physical Education setting the student will be in: _____
_____
_____
_____

MEDICAL INFORMATION

Name/Nature of Condition _____
_____
Condition is: Permanent _____   *Temporary _____
General implications condition has for Physical Education _____
_____
Medication: Yes _____   No _____
    Name of medication _____
    When and how administered _____
    Effects on physical/motor performance _____
General warning signs or symptoms physical educator should be aware of regarding the condition and/or medication _____
_____

*If condition is temporary, the student may resume restricted activity:
_____ Only after medical review scheduled for _____ 19_____.
_____ Under the following conditions _____
_____
                                              (to be specified by physician)

particularly important in physical education where the students are more active. Many times the teacher is aware of the medical problems of his or her students but fails to record this information so that other professionals, like a substitute teacher, can have access to it. This creates a situation that is unnecessarily dangerous and libelous. A simple procedure for handling medical information on students is to put a numeric subscript next to their names in the roll book. Then on one of the last pages in the book, summarize the students' condition by the subscript numbers:

1. Asthma—should be allowed to carry and administer medication as needed. Student will remove himself from the activity if needed.
2. Diabetes—should be allowed to eat a piece of candy on demand or remove himself from the activity.
3. Grand Mal seizures—avoid heights, always have the student work with a partner. If a seizure does occur, protect the student's head and tongue and call the nurse.

This procedure allows the teacher or other staff to familiarize themselves quickly

TABLE 3–7. *Continued*

Listed below is the program the student in question will enroll in. Please review and evaluate the appropriateness of these activities for this student.

Physical Education Program Description			Physician's Evaluation	
Unit/Objective	*Instructional Setting*	*Energy Requirement*	*Physician Precautions*	*Physician Recommendations*
1. a) Move to an even beat	Gym	Mild		
b) Accent	Gym	Mild		
c) Cardiorespiratory Endurance	Gym/Outside	Vigorous		
d) Abdominal Strength	Gym	Vigorous		
2. a) Kick	Gym/Outside	Moderate		
b) Inverted Balance	Gym	Mild		
c) Cardiorespiratory Endurance	Gym/Outside	Vigorous		
d) Abdominal Strength	Gym	Vigorous		
3. a) Catch	Gym/Outside	Moderate		
b) Cardiorespiratory Endurance	Gym/Outside	Vigorous		
c) Abdominal Strength	Gym	Vigorous		
4. Basketball	Gym			
a) Chest Pass	Gym	Mild		
b) Dribbling	Gym	Moderate		
c) Cardiorespiratory Endurance	Gym/Outside	Vigorous		
d) Abdominal Strength	Gym	Vigorous		
5. Softball	Gym/Outside			
a) Running Bases	Gym/Outside	Moderate		
b) Fielding	Gym/Outside	Moderate		
c) Cardiorespiratory Endurance	Gym/Outside	Vigorous		
d) Abdominal Strength	Gym/Outside	Vigorous		

Physicians Summary Recommendation

_____ *Student may participate in the described program assuming the physician precautions and recommendations are followed.*

_____ *A specialized program will have to be designed to meet this student's unique physical and motor needs. The program described here is inappropriate for this student.*

Comments: _____

_____

Physician _____ *Date* _____

Phone _____ *Address* _____

with any medical information they need to safely work with the class in a physical education setting.

Requesting medical information on students requires both tact and professionalism. The teacher needs first to know the school system procedures and to establish a rapport with the various physicians in the community. Many physicians may not fully understand the benefits of physical education and therefore frequently excuse students because of their misconceptions regarding the program and/or because of a request from the student's parents. Unfortunately, these inappropriate exemptions may be encouraged by requesting blanket medical releases on students from physicians. A physician is unlikely to approve unrestricted participation in physical education for a student with a medical condition when they are unaware of the nature of the physical education program. Remember that whenever a physician signs a medical release, he or she assumes a certain degree of responsibility for that student's health and safety.

The first step in obtaining medical releases is to inform the physicians in the community of the purpose and rationale behind requesting this information. The goals of the physical education program and the objectives that are targeted for instruction for a given student should be highlighted. This process can be done with a simple cover letter and a medical release form like the example shown in Table 3–7. The physician should understand that the goal of the release is to provide the student with the most appropriate physical education program possible within the student's capability. The physician should perceive his or her role in this process as a contributing member of a team and not just as a scapegoat to protect the physical education teacher. To receive full cooperation, the physician must be convinced that their recommendations will be used.

The sample medical release form in Table 3–7 includes several key components that require a brief explanation. First, the form clearly identifies what instructional content will be worked on. This information informs the physician of the nature of the program and how well planned and organized it is. Second, the form tells the physician of the relative energy capacity needed to participate in the program. This information allows the physician to make more accurate decisions and recommendations regarding the appropriateness of the activities for the student in question. Third, the form allows the physician an opportunity to express his or her concerns (precautions) and/or make modifications to the proposed program (recommendations) to accommodate the medical needs of the student. Finally, the form is relatively short and concise and can be completed quickly by the physician. The teacher should complete all parts of the form except the medical sections before sending it to the physician. Too great a demand on the physician's time might result in an inappropriate decision (exclusion from physical education) because it is a more expedient option than completing the form. When the physician does not provide all the information requested, the physical educator should follow-up the application with a personal call to the physician explaining the purpose of the release form. If the physician's recommendations cannot be accommodated in the regular physical education program, the student should be referred for administrative action at the school level.

In addition to facilitating the physician response, the medical release form (Table 3–7) is designed also to assist the physical education teacher. The form provides six basic forms of information needed to accommodate students with medical conditions:

—Name or nature of the condition
—Implications for physical education
—Medication
—When and how medication is administered
—Effects of the medication on physical and motor performance
—Warning signs or symptoms associated with the condition or medication that may be observed in physical education

Although the procedures associated with requesting and managing student medical information may appear initially as a major task, it need not be that way. In many schools the necessary medical information may already be on file in the nurses' office. In schools where the physical education teacher must initiate this process, it can be implemented slowly and systematically over a period of time. The teacher may elect to start with requiring medical forms on all students with known medical conditions. When this phase is completed the teacher begins to systematically require medical forms for students in different grades each year. Eventually there will be completed forms on all students and the only students that will need to complete forms in subsequent years will be new students entering the school. When initiating any large scale medical release request, the demands being placed on physicians and parents must be considered. Physicians will probably be receptive to completing a small number of medical forms periodically, but probably would not be pleased with receiving 100 requests in the period of a few weeks. Accommodations also have to be made for parents who do not have a family physician or who are unable to pay for a medical examination. The school nurse may be able to assist in locating a physician or clinic to accommodate these families.

After establishing a medical release system, these records must be kept up-to-date. How frequently the system is updated can be decided by each school district. Students with no medical problems may be required to get a medical release at the start of each program level (kindergarten, grade 7, and grade 10). Students with serious medical problems may be required to get a medical release at the start of each year.

To facilitate rapport with physicians, teachers should periodically follow-up with a report to the physician regarding their recommendations and the students' performance in physical education. Reports of this nature can serve to increase the physician's understanding and confidence in the physical education program, which may result in greater communication and cooperation on future medical referrals.

SYNOPSIS

Our professional commitment is to provide all students with the opportunity to reach their maximum potential as "physically educated" individuals. A quality program is individualized and accountable, enabling all students to achieve success in physical education. Instruction should be delivered in a systematic and effective way that guarantees that the objectives targeted for instruction will be achieved.

Students' characteristics and implications for instruction were discussed in this chapter from the perspective of students' abilities and needs, not labels. Key student characteristics and their implications for planning instruction for each student to achieve were identified. The degree to which a teacher can accommodate individual differences and the range of skills and abilities in the class, rests on a decision as to what is judged to be the range of variability that can be productively accommodated for all students to achieve desired learning outcomes. The needs profiling method was presented to assist teachers and others to identify significant student characteristics crucial to making appropriate instructional and placement decisions.

The final section of the chapter highlighted the need for teachers to obtain and understand all medical information related to their students. They must know the procedures required to design medical release forms, communicate with physicians, and manage medical information on their students.

RESOURCES FOR TEACHERS

Adams, R.C., Daniel, A.N., McCubbin, J.A., and Rullman, L.: Games, Sports, and Exercises for the Physically Handicapped. Rev. Ed. Philadelphia, Lea & Febiger, 1980.
Auxter, D., and Pyfer, J.: Principles and Methods of Adopted Physical Education and Recreation. 5th Ed. St. Louis, Time Mirror/Mosby, 1985.
Bleck, E.E., and Nagel, D.A.: Physically Handicapped Children: A Medical Atlas for Teachers. 2nd Ed. New York, Grune & Stratton, 1982.
Cratty, B.J.: Adapted Physical Education for Handicapped Children and Youth. Denver, Love Publishing, 1980.
Crowe, W.C., Auxter, D., and Pyfer, J.: Adapted Physical Education and Recreation. 4th Ed. St. Louis, C.V. Mosby, 1981.

Fait, H.F., and Dunn, J.: Special Physical Education: Adapted, Corrective, Developmental. 5th Ed. Philadelphia, W.B. Saunders, 1983.

French, R., and Jansma, P.: Special Physical Education. Columbus, OH, Charles E. Merrill, 1982.

Kalakian, L.H., and Eichstaedt, C.B.: Developmental/Adapted Physical Education. Minneapolis, Burgess, 1982.

Seaman, J.A., and DePauw, K.P.: The New Adapted Physical Education: A Developmental Approach. Palo Alto, CA, Mayfield Publishing, 1982.

Sherrill, C.: Adapted Physical Education and Recreation. 2nd Ed. Dubuque, Iowa, Wm. C. Brown, 1981.

Weisman, D.C.: A Practical Approach to Adapted Physical Education. Reading, MA, Addison-Wesley, 1982.

Winnick, J.P.: Early Movement Experiences and Development: Habilitation and Remediation. Philadelphia, W.B. Saunders, 1979.

ACTIVITY 3–1.	Developing a student needs profiling instrument.

Objective:	To develop a student needs profiling instrument that is specific to an individual's student population.
Materials:	A copy of the student needs profile presented in Table 3–6. Worksheet 3–1 provided

WORKSHEET 3–1

Directions:	**1.** Have the group independently review and evaluate the characteristics included in the student needs profile instrument and add or delete items as they deem necessary.
	2. Apply a consensus-forming technique to the list of characteristics that were identified in step 1 to identify the final items to be used in the needs profile.

—Have each person independently rate each item using the following scale:

     1 = inappropriate

     2 = not important

     3 = might be included

     4 = important

     5 = extremely important

—Summarize the group ratings and discuss why each characteristic was rated high or low.

—Based on clarification and/or new thoughts resulting from the discussion, have each person rerate each item.

—Develop the final version of the checklist using all evaluation items that receive an average rating of 3.0 (the actual cut off value can be locally determined) or better.

Variation:	Divide the group into subgroups and perform the activity as previously described. Then have each subgroup present their profile and have the group compare and evaluate them.

WORKSHEET 3–1. *Student Needs Profile*

CIRCLE RATING: 1 = Low
                5 = High

LEARNING CHARACTERISTICS	FIRST RATING	SECOND RATING	AVERAGE RATING
1. Student's ability to communicate	1 2 3 4 5	1 2 3 4 5	
2. Student's ability to comprehend instructions (verbal and nonverbal)	1 2 3 4 5	1 2 3 4 5	
3. Student's vocabulary level	1 2 3 4 5	1 2 3 4 5	
4. Student's memory skills	1 2 3 4 5	1 2 3 4 5	
5. Student's ability to follow large group instruction	1 2 3 4 5	1 2 3 4 5	
6. Student's ability to focus and maintain attention on tasks (not distracted or hyperactive)	1 2 3 4 5	1 2 3 4 5	
7. Student's ability to communicate needs, ask questions, and request assistance	1 2 3 4 5	1 2 3 4 5	
8. Student's learning rate	1 2 3 4 5	1 2 3 4 5	
9. Student's ability to follow through on assignments and learning tasks	1 2 3 4 5	1 2 3 4 5	
10. Student's ability to generalize and transfer skills	1 2 3 4 5	1 2 3 4 5	
11. Student's desire to be in class	1 2 3 4 5	1 2 3 4 5	

PERSONAL-SOCIAL CHARACTERISTICS			
1. Student's ability to adapt to new tasks and unanticipated changes	1 2 3 4 5	1 2 3 4 5	
2. Student's ability to cooperate with others—shares, takes turns, accepts responsibility	1 2 3 4 5	1 2 3 4 5	
3. Student's ability to follow daily time schedule	1 2 3 4 5	1 2 3 4 5	
4. Student's ability to work independently on assigned tasks	1 2 3 4 5	1 2 3 4 5	
5. Student's ability to communicate—for peer-social interaction	1 2 3 4 5	1 2 3 4 5	
6. Student's willingness to seek help from others on targeted learning tasks	1 2 3 4 5	1 2 3 4 5	
7. Student's social maturation level	1 2 3 4 5	1 2 3 4 5	
8. The appropriateness of the student's peer social behaviors	1 2 3 4 5	1 2 3 4 5	
9. Student's ability to maintain emotional self-control	1 2 3 4 5	1 2 3 4 5	
10. Student's motivation and interest in learning	1 2 3 4 5	1 2 3 4 5	

PHYSICAL AND MOTOR CHARACTERISTICS			
1. Student's ability to maneuver in familiar locations (spatial direction orientations)	1 2 3 4 5	1 2 3 4 5	
2. Student's ability to manipulate equipment and materials	1 2 3 4 5	1 2 3 4 5	
3. Student's achievement levels on the specific skills targeted for instruction in this class	1 2 3 4 5	1 2 3 4 5	
4. The disparity between the student's age/interests and activity preferences in relation to the other students in the class	1 2 3 4 5	1 2 3 4 5	
5. Student's willingness to attempt motor tasks in the class setting	1 2 3 4 5	1 2 3 4 5	
6. Student's physical development/maturation in relation to the other students in the class	1 2 3 4 5	1 2 3 4 5	
7. Student's ability to use existing equipment without special modifications or adaptations	1 2 3 4 5	1 2 3 4 5	
8. Student's ability to participate safely in the class without making special health/safety modifications	1 2 3 4 5	1 2 3 4 5	
9. Student's ability to independently access the various instructional sites needed for instruction	1 2 3 4 5	1 2 3 4 5	
10. Student's ability to begin work on program objectives (prerequisite skills do not need to be developed)	1 2 3 4 5	1 2 3 4 5	

ACTIVITY 3–2. Identifying and categorizing common characteristics of handicapping conditions.

Objective: To identify and contrast the common characteristics associated with common handicapping conditions found in the public schools.

Materials: Access to the adapted physical education textbooks listed in the Resources for Teachers section at the end of Chapter 3. Several copies of Worksheet 3–2 included with this activity. Worksheet 3–2 provided.

WORKSHEET 3–2

Directions:
1. Identify the handicapping conditions the group is most likely to encounter in their physical education classes. This list can include any of the traditional handicapping conditions defined in PL 94-142 as well as normal conditions such as posture deviations, low physical vitality, obesity, pregnancy, or other special needs.
2. Have the group review Worksheet 3–2 and operationally define the three categories (learning, personal and social, physical and motor).
3. Have the group members individually review several of the adapted physical education books and complete a copy of Worksheet 3–2 for each condition.
4. Using the chalk board, summarize what the group has identified as characteristics for each handicapping condition under each of the three categories.
5. Have the group rank within each condition which characteristics have the greatest effect on students' performance in physical education.
6. Have the group analyze the summary produced in step 4 and discuss the commonality and differences observed between the various conditions.
7. Have the group discuss how each of the various characteristics identified interact with instruction and can be accommodated in physical education with or without teacher or student support services. If support is needed, have the group identify the type of support needed.
8. Have the group compare the summary produced in step 6 with the student need profile final version in Activity 3–1.

Variation: Divide the group into smaller subgroups. Have each subgroup investigate one of the identified conditions. Then have the subgroups report their findings and continue the activity as described from step 4.

WORKSHEET 3–2. *Identification of General Characteristics Associated with Specific Handicapping Conditions*

Student Name _____   Date _____

Handicapping Conditions _____

LEARNING	PERSONAL AND SOCIAL	PHYSICAL AND MOTOR

ACTIVITY 3–3. Administration and interpretation of data collected with a student needs profiling instrument.

Objective:	To administer and interpret the data collected using a student needs profiling instrument.
Materials:	A student needs profiling instrument. The version presented in Table 3–6 or the revised form created in Activity 3–1 can be used.
	Access to a class of students to observe and assess.

WORKSHEET 3–3: Use Activity 3–1 or Table 3–6 Version

Directions:
1. Have the group review the characteristics in the instrument and clarify any questions related to the characteristics.
2. Divide the group into small subgroups of 2 or 3 members. Assign each subgroup a child to observe and assess.
3. Have each subgroup arrange to observe their student. Time will have to be scheduled also to discuss the student with the physical education teacher since it is not possible to complete several of the items based solely on one observation.
4. Have the subgroups compare their assessments within the subgroups and discuss any discrepancies in their ratings.
5. Have the entire group share their experiences and findings using the needs profiling instrument. Identify any common problems that were encountered using the instrument and discuss how these could be corrected. If necessary, have the group discuss how the instrument should be modified.

Variation:
Have each member of the group explain the needs profiling instrument to a different physical educator. The physical educator should be asked to use the instrument and evaluate its effectiveness. After interviewing his or her physical educator each member should report his or her findings to the group. Then complete step 5 as described.

Have each member of the group identify what kind of data he or she would like to have on the student before placement in the class related to the characteristics on the final needs profiling instrument. Then complete step 4 as described. This activity results in a teacher's tip sheet—what works well and what does not—that can structure a cumulative record for the student to help plan instruction.

Example of a checklist of the type of data teachers identified that they would like to have about the student placed in their class is provided.

WORKSHEET 3–3. *Sample Checklist: Prior Student Data*

Name of Student _____ Grade Level _____
Age _____ School _____
Teacher _____

1. What is the student's level of achievement in the instructional objectives of the unit/time interval in the schedule where he or she will be entering?

   _____ _____
   _____ _____

2. To what extent can the student interact successfully with other students?

	Great deal	Little	Not at all
Large group games	_____	_____	_____
Small group work	_____	_____	_____
One-to-one	_____	_____	_____
Station/Centers	_____	_____	_____
Team sports	_____	_____	_____

3. To what extent will the student accept/respond to:

	OK	Poor	Not at all
Distractions	_____	_____	_____
Waiting	_____	_____	_____
Praise	_____	_____	_____
Responsibility	_____	_____	_____
Peer-directed on-task work	_____	_____	_____
Self-directed on-task work	_____	_____	_____
Adult-directed on-task work	_____	_____	_____
Contracts	_____	_____	_____
Auditory Directions	_____	_____	_____
Visual Directions	_____	_____	_____
Demonstration	_____	_____	_____

4. How can the student be tested:

Verbal	_____	Small group	_____
Nonverbal	_____	Large group	_____
Need aide	_____	Partner	_____

5. Does the student respond easily/quickly with (Answer yes or no)

Anger	_____	Embarrassment	_____
Laughter	_____	Withdrawal	_____
Hostility	_____	Aggressiveness	_____

6. Does the student need physical equipment devices in performing the tasks? (Answer yes or no)

Crutches	_____	Other	_____
Wheelchair	_____	_____	

7. Does the student have a physical or health condition that requires special safety procedures. (Yes or No)
   Fatigue Factor:
   Tires easily _____
   Requires more time to complete task _____
   Needs rest periods _____
   Relaxation skills _____

8. Does the student have speech problems (communication skills) or atypical mannerisms? (Yes or No) What?

   _____
   _____

   What procedure do you use?
   _____
   _____

9. What social skills should be stressed with this student?

   _____
   _____

ACTIVITY 3–4. Identifying key personnel who provide support services for teachers in regular education in the school program and what placement options are available for students with special needs in physical education programs.

Objective: To understand how local or intermediate school districts provide support services for regular physical education teachers and typical placement options for physical education.

Materials: Contact local school or school district administrative personnel or State Department personnel or the State Director of Physical Education.

Obtain a copy of a school district's plan for providing services to special education students and placement options for students in special education. Obtain a copy of the total number of students served in the district by program level and special education groups.

Worksheet 3–4 or redesign as needed using "feeder" schools to your school and program level.

WORKSHEET 3–4

Directions:
1. Using the worksheet provided, check your findings related to support services available for the regular physical education teacher who has special education students assigned to the class full- or part-time.
2. Using the worksheet provided, check your findings related to placement options available for students in special education to receive appropriate physical education services.

Variations:
1. Use Worksheet 3–4 or redesign.
2. Interview professional personnel at the local or intermediate school district level. Record answers on the worksheet.

School District _____

Total Number of Students in District

	Regular	Special Education	Special Education Students % in Regular Classes	% in Physical Ed. Classes
Elementary	_____	_____	_____	_____
Middle	_____	_____	_____	_____
Secondary	_____	_____	_____	_____

	PLACEMENT OPTIONS AVAILABLE IN PHYSICAL EDUCATION			
PLACEMENT	ELEMENTARY NO. OF SCHOOLS	MIDDLE NO. OF SCHOOLS	SECONDARY NO. OF SCHOOLS	OTHER
Regular physical education classes	_____	_____	_____	_____
Regular physical education classes with support services	_____	_____	_____	_____
Adapted physical education classes in regular schools	_____	_____	_____	_____
Adapted physical education classes special day centers	_____	_____	_____	_____

What type of support services are available for the physical education teachers with special education students assigned to their classes?

TYPE OF SUPPORT SERVICES MOST COMMON. LIST BELOW	ELEMENTARY	MIDDLE	SECONDARY	OTHER
_____	_____	_____	_____	_____
_____	_____	_____	_____	_____
_____	_____	_____	_____	_____
_____	_____	_____	_____	_____

ACTIVITY 3–5. Identifying and evaluating the program and building accessibility for students with special needs.

Objective: To gain understanding of the building structures—barriers and facilitators—to enhance the mobility and ease of moving from place to place when participating in physical education activities—instructional and recreational.

Materials: Obtain a copy of the Accessibility Checklist to facilitate evaluating a facility in terms of freedom from barriers and ease of access by handicapped persons. There are also available copies of Recommended Building Specifications for Wheelchair Use.

Use these references and design a checklist to conduct a survey of a local school building. One example checklist is provided. To use this checklist, you will need the specifications assigned to each item.

WORKSHEET 3–5

Directions:
1. With the specifications checklist, survey a school building and playgrounds. Be sure to include the physical education facilities for teaching and nonacademic services (athletics, intramurals, recreational playgrounds, or special interest groups such as art, science, computers, chess, band, and so forth).
2. Record your findings on Worksheet 3–5 or redesign the worksheet adapting it to a particular school setting.
3. Conduct the survey. Draw conclusions and make recommendations.

Variations:
1. Conduct the survey and have members of the group in wheelchairs, blindfolded, and limit their hearing.
2. Have special education students work with members of the group conducting the survey.

Additional Resources:

Accessibility Checklist. NASDSE Publications, 1201 16th Street, N.W., Washington, D.C. $7.00 per copy; $2.00 each with orders over 5 or more.

A World of Options. Mobility International USA, P.O. Box 3551, Eugene, OR 97403. $3.50 per copy.

SAMPLE WORKSHEET 3–5. *Accessibility*

CHECKLIST FOR ACCESSIBILITY

All Acceptable	Some Acceptable	None Acceptable	
			I. Walks
————	————	————	a. Grade
————	————	————	b. Width
————	————	————	c. Surface
			II. Curb Cuts
————	————	————	a. Grade
————	————	————	b. Width
————	————	————	c. Surface
			III. Ramps
————	————	————	a. Grade
————	————	————	b. Width
————	————	————	c. Surface
————	————	————	d. Rails
			IV. Parking
————	————	————	a. Location
————	————	————	b. Transfer area
————	————	————	c. Signage
————	————	————	d. Number of spaces
			V. Doors
————	————	————	a. Width
————	————	————	b. Threshold height
————	————	————	c. Hardware (door knobs, handles, and kickplates)
————	————	————	d. Floor area
			VI. Rest Rooms
————	————	————	a. Lavatories
————	————	————	b. Mirrors
————	————	————	c. Dispensers
————	————	————	d. Toilets
————	————	————	e. Stalls
			VII. Cafeteria
————	————	————	a. Foodlines
————	————	————	b. Dining area
			VIII. Drinking fountain
————	————	————	a. Height
————	————	————	b. Controls
			IX. Library
————	————	————	a. Aisle width
————	————	————	b. Index and reference tables
			X. Gymnasium facilities
————	————	————	a. Lockers
————	————	————	b. Dressing tables
————	————	————	c. Showers
————	————	————	d. Pools
————	————	————	e. Spectator areas
			XI. Performing arts
————	————	————	a. Aisles
————	————	————	b. Seating
			XII. Classrooms/Laboratories/Kitchens
————	————	————	a. Aisles
————	————	————	b. Seating
————	————	————	c. Counter/desk tops
————	————	————	d. Sinks
			XIII. Determine whether the following routes can be negotiated in a wheelchair:
————	————	————	a. Parking lot to school
————	————	————	b. Entrance to any student area (classroom, office, gymnasium, cafeteria, bathroom, etc.)
————	————	————	c. Movement within all school rooms

ACTIVITY 3–6. Identifying and evaluating medical forms and procedures for collecting and managing student medical data.

Objective: To identify and evaluate the medical release forms and procedures used to obtain and manage medical information in local schools.

Materials: Worksheet 3–6 provided

WORKSHEET 3–6

Directions:
1. Based upon the content presented in Chapter 3, have the group identify evaluative criteria they feel should exist in schools in each of the following areas:
   —content of a medical release form
   —data collection procedures
   —data management procedures
2. Divide the group into subgroups of 2 or 3 members. Assign each subgroup a local school to evaluate.
3. Using the criteria identified in step 1, have each subgroup evaluate the medical procedures used in the school they were assigned. Encourage the subgroups to collect sample copies of any forms the school is willing to give them.
4. Have the subgroups report their findings to the total group. Have the total group evaluate the material presented from each subgroup and identify exemplary procedures in each area that are being used in the various schools. Also have the group identify procedures that they feel are inadequate and ways these procedures can be improved.
5. Have each subgroup summarize the recommendations the total group has made for their school and then share this information with the staff of the school they evaluated.

WORKSHEET 3–6. *Medical Form Content and Procedures*

EVALUATIVE CRITERIA		
MEDICAL FORM CONTENT	DATA COLLECTION PROCEDURES	DATA MANAGEMENT PROCEDURES

PART II

Implementation

The chapters in this section provide information and procedures that help teachers and administrators plan and implement effective instructional programs.

Chapter 4 presents the "how-to" procedures to define program goals and objectives, identify essential objectives, and structure sequential learnings at all levels: for multi-year, yearly, by unit, or lesson.

In Chapter 5, assessment of students' status on what is to be learned is discussed. The advantages and disadvantages of both criterion-referenced and norm-referenced tests are discussed. The achievement-based curriculum model focuses on criterion-referenced tests, criterion-referenced evaluation procedures for individualizing instruction and evaluating desired learning outcome. Criteria for appropriate placement and classification decisions are provided.

Chapter 6 provides the instructional planning processes to help teachers make and implement instructional decisions before, during, and after instruction based on three key student behaviors impacting on achievement: success, objectives taught and tested, and student involvement (active learning time). Five teacher behaviors related to student achievement are discussed: clarity of presentation; feedback and corrective procedures; practice, guided and independent; and use of instructional time and staff.

Chapter 7 presents more in-depth coverage of practices that promise to foster students' motivation in learning and effective class management.

CHAPTER 4

Program Planning

What is a Comprehensive Program Plan?

A comprehensive program plan identifies program goals and objectives and sequentially organizes these goals by program levels that can be taught effectively, thus enabling students to achieve desired learning outcomes from Kindergarten through Grade 12. This program plan is sometimes called a long-term plan.

How is it Developed?	*Decision Aids*
1. Identify appropriate program goals and objectives for each goal.	Contributions of physical activity Student needs Community values Objectives operationalizing goals
2. Place program objectives in appropriate program levels.	School program levels Growth and development characteristics Sequential motor skill actions Enabling skills Relative goal emphasis

3. Determine the amount of time needed for effective instruction.	Amount of instructional time available
	Estimations of time needed for meaningful performance gains:
	    Student expectancies
	    Group expectancies

4. Determine the total number of program objectives that can be included.	Time available Time needed for meaningful performance gain
5. Develop a comprehensive program plan.	Prioritized list of objectives for each goal Criteria for selection of essential objectives
6. Develop a yearly program plan of sequential instructional units.	Compatibility of objectives Time allotments for each unit Time allotment for program objectives School calendar
7. Construct unit lesson plans.	Daily time allotments Time for assessment, reassessment, and teaching Compatibility of objectives Enabling skills

A quality program has a clearly developed mission, which is focused and clear for teachers, students, parents, and other school-community members. Mager (1975) summarized the importance of specifying the intent of instruction as follows: "You cannot concern yourself with the problem of selecting the most efficient route to your destination until you know what your destination is . . ."

Relevant and defensible program goals and objectives clearly describe instructional intent and direction of physical education programs. Program objectives organized over students' school years operationally define the long-term program goals on a continuum of essential skills for all students to achieve. These objectives, subdivided into instructional skill levels, become specific instructional objectives—that type of instructional objective that requires specification of student learning in terms of observable, measurable behavior.

This chapter focuses attention on the first component of the Achievement-Based Curriculum (ABC) Model—planning the program. First, the nature and function of program goals and objectives are examined with respect to specificity, purpose, and appropriateness. Second, procedures are offered for: (1) selecting appropriate program goals and objectives; (2) organizing an objective-based instructional program for kindergarten through Grade 12; and (3) designing yearly objective-based instructional units and lesson plans. A consensus-forming planning process is presented to help reduce or eliminate many difficulties generally encountered in specification of goals and objectives by school districts.

PROGRAM GOALS AND OBJECTIVES

A Continuum of Objectives: Specificity and Purpose

Educational objectives are stated at various levels of specificity and for different purposes. At one end of the continuum of objectives are the broad general goals

TABLE 4–1. *Example Goal and Its Array of Program Objectives*

Goal Area: Fundamental Motor Skills
Goal: TO DEMONSTRATE FUNCTIONAL COMPETENCE ON SELECTED
FUNDAMENTAL MOTOR SKILLS
Program Objectives (PO's)

LOCOMOTOR	OBJECT CONTROL	RHYTHM
1. Gallop	1. Bounce	1. Even beat
2. Hop	2. Catch	2. Uneven beat
3. Horizontal jump	3. Kick	3. Communication
4. Leap	4. Overhand throw	4. Accent
5. Run	5. Punt	
6. Skip	6. Backhand strike	
7. Slide	7. Forehand strike	
8. Vertical jump	8. Two-hand sidearm strike	
	9. Underhand roll	
	10. Underhand throw	

of the program. These program goals relate to the educational needs, expectations, and social values of society. They provide the philosophical guidance necessary for determining content—what objectives should be included in the curriculum. As a broad general statement of intent, goals represent large unique "chunks" of content. Cumulatively, the goal statements represent the content of the entire physical education instructional program plan. For example, goal statements represent content areas in the effective, cognitive, and psychomotor domains based on the contribution of physical education.

Program objectives, the next level of specificity, define the program's content. The specific meaning of each goal is operationally defined by the program objectives that comprise its content. Program objectives are short, descriptive statements of a desirable level of skill that learners will attain as a result of participating in the program. Table 4–1 presents an example goal and an array of program objectives that comprise its content.

At the other end of the continuum are specific instructional objectives. These instructional objectives are derived from program objectives. Each program objective may be divided into two or more instructional teaching or skill levels. These skill levels represent student performance abilities that range from near zero to some defined level of functional competence. The number of skill levels, learning steps, depend on student needs, teacher preference, and reporting requirements. Each instructional objective requires specification of student learning in observable, measurable behavior. These objectives clearly and completely prescribe the behaviors students are to acquire as a result of completing instruction.

In the selection and/or the development of instructional objectives to implement the ABC model, three important criteria must be used. Each instructional objective must clearly identify:
- observable, measurable behaviors that students will be asked to perform to demonstrate mastery of the objectives;
- important conditions under which students are expected to demonstrate achievement of the objective: time limits, cues, equipment, and special instruction; and
- the criterion used to evaluate the success of the student's performance: qualitative, quantitative, percent correct, number of trials, or time to complete the task.

TABLE 4–2.   *A Continuum of Educational Objectives: Example of Goal, Program Objectives, and Instructional Objectives with the Number of Learning Tasks*

Program Goal: Demonstrate functional competence on selected fundamental motor skills
Program Objective: Demonstrate a functional overhand throw

	INSTRUCTIONAL OBJECTIVES			
	CONDITIONS			NUMBER OF LEARNING TASKS
SKILL LEVEL	DIRECTIONS	EQUIPMENT	OBSERVABLE, MEASURABLE STUDENT BEHAVIORS STANDARD(S): CRITERION USED TO EVALUATE PERFORMANCE	
I	Given a verbal request and a demonstration, the student will, with one practice	2 or 3 inch (tennis) ball	Throw a ball at least 40 feet three consecutive times in the following manner: —side orientation with weight on the rear leg to initiate the throw; —nearly complete extension of throwing arm to initiate the throw; —weight transfer to the foot opposite the throwing arm, with marked hip and spine rotation during the throwing motion; —a follow-through well beyond ball release; —smooth (not mechanical or jerky) integration of the above.	6
II	Given a verbal request and a demonstration, the student will, with one practice trial	2 or 3 inch (tennis) ball	Throw a ball 10 consecutive times using Level I standards and —hit a 6 foot square target located 1 foot off the ground with number recorded; —hit the target 10 out of 10 times.	2
			Total	8

Table 4–2 provides an example statement of a goal, program objective, and its instructional objectives. The goal area is fundamental motor skills, the program objective is overhand throw, and the instructional objectives represent: (1) a quality (biomechanically correct) throwing pattern and (2) an example of functional competence.

Prior to a unit of instruction, instructional objectives are used to assess students to determine: (1) their level of skill, (2) whether they need to omit any objective or have the necessary prerequisite skills for instruction, and (3) what instructional activities should be prescribed to move student(s) from lower to higher levels within each program objective. When students complete the unit, instructional objectives are used to evaluate whether instruction was successful as well as the progress of the students on the unit objectives.

APPROPRIATENESS OF PROGRAM GOALS AND OBJECTIVES

Program goals and objectives provide the structure for quality programming—the design, implementation, and evaluation of the achievement-based curriculum model. They provide the basis for:

1. Communication of "what" is included in the curriculum as well as "why" and "when" it is included.
2. Organization of sequential program objectives that can be effectively taught in instruction: lesson, yearly, multiyear, long-term.
3. Instructional objectives for evaluating student status and progress.

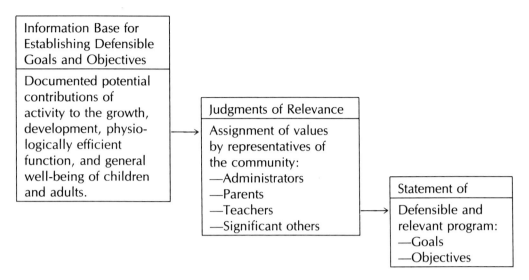

Figure 4–1. *Selecting defensible and relevant program goals and objectives.*

4. Selection and development of instructional activities that are directly linked to stated instructional objectives.
5. Program strengths and weaknesses that are easily identified through evaluation of the degree to which stated instructional objectives are being achieved by a given student population.

The use of program goals and objectives in and of themselves does not result in quality programming. Their selection, statement, and purpose must be appropriate. To determine the appropriateness of a set of program goals and objectives, four criteria are recommended:
1. The goals and objectives must be defensible in terms of the potential outcome they represent.
2. They should be stated in output terminology and specify performance level.
3. They should reflect the values of the community program they represent.
4. They should represent the unique needs of all individuals in the program.

Procedures to identify appropriate, selected goals and objectives are presented in the next section.

IDENTIFYING PROGRAM GOALS AND OBJECTIVES

Program goals and objectives are a written description of the instructional content—"what" each student is to learn as a result of participating in the program. They are defensible and relevant—"why" were they included in the program? Program goals and objectives are defensible and relevant when they:
- maintain a direct relationship to documented potential contributions of activity to the quality of life;
- are appropriately matched to the target population group.

The process for attaining defensibility and relevancy is portrayed in Figure 4–1.

The information base describes the potential contributions of the physical activity on growth, development, and general well-being of children and adults. Relevancy is claimed by the degree that program goals and objectives match the student's needs and the potential contribution judged important by the community.

TABLE 4–3.   *Steps for Building a Working Consensus*

Consensus-Building Technique
1. Selected representatives of the community (administrators, teachers, parents, appropriate others) independently rate each goal statement using the criteria to measure the importance of each possible goal and program objective for instruction.
1   = should be included
2   = important
3   = extremely important
blank = inappropriate
2. For each statement, team members discuss the reasons why each goal was judged appropriate or inappropriate for inclusion in the program.
3. Based on clarifications and/or new insights resulting from the discussions, each team member independently rerates each statement.
4. Reratings are then averaged with the average rating reflecting group consensus.

Developing a program plan that includes functional and attainable program goals and objectives sometimes changes what should be a cooperative process into a battle of "wills." To improve the effectiveness and efficiency of communication among team members, including the parents and students, requires a planning process that provides:

- equal consideration of the views of each member and equal weight to their opinions;
- a framework whereby disagreements among team members may be worked out;
- documentation of this process in an efficient way.

A four-step, consensus-building technique as shown in Table 4–3 uses these criteria. This technique is a systematic procedure for prioritizing goals and objectives.

The consensus-building process helps the team achieve a productive and highly functional relationship to systematically develop a program plan of essential objectives to be taught from kindergarten through Grade 12. First, the team selects a person who will facilitate and monitor the process. Second, to expedite the process, a list of goal statements and their supporting rationale (criteria) is presented and discussed.

SELECTING DEFENSIBLE AND RELEVANT PROGRAM GOALS

The group reviews potential goal statements and their supporting rationale. To accomplish this task, a list of statements that represent the effect of activity on individuals when administered in appropriate durations, frequencies, and intensities is required. A partial list of potential contributions of activity is presented in Table 4–4.

It is important to note that these results do not occur automatically as a result of general participation in physical education activities, or by simply maintaining an active life while growing up. The literature is clear; activity effects are very specific. Activities are specifically selected and structured for children to develop fundamental movement skills and related sport, dance, and daily-living skills.

The next procedure is to write goal statements with supporting rationale reflecting these activity contributions. Table 4–5 gives an example of a goal statement with supporting rationale.

Working with local school districts, we have found similarity of program goals

TABLE 4–4. *A Partial List of Potential Contributions Obtained from Physical Activity Derived from the Literature*

What Participation in Appropriate Kinds and Amounts of Physical Activity Can Do:

1. Promote healthy growth and development.
2. Reduce and prevent the occurrence of injury.
3. Provide for the development and maintenance of efficient posture.
4. Increase adaptability to stress.
5. Improve physiologic and anatomic function.
6. Enhance emotional well-being.
7. Promote the release of tension and stress.
8. Improve motor skills.
9. Promote body awareness and concept formation.
10. Provide weight control measures.
11. Provide for social development and interactions.
12. Provide for effective use of active-social leisure sports.
13. Improve health-related life styles.
14. Improve muscular strength and endurance; cardiorespiratory efficiency.
15. Delay the aging process.

in special and regular education in a wide variety of communities. What is always different is the relative emphasis given to these goals at different program levels and the program objectives selected to put each goal into operation. Typically, rationale derived from the activity contributions supported six common program goals. Four of the six common goal statements are unique to the physical and motor skills content of physical education. The six goal statements include:

1. Demonstrate functional competence in selected physical fitness skills.
2. Demonstrate functional competence in selected body management skills.
3. Demonstrate functional competence in selected fundamental motor skills.
4. Demonstrate functional competence in selected dance, sport, and leisure skills.

TABLE 4–5. *Example Program Goal with Supporting Rationale Based on Potential Activity Contribution*

Goal Statement:
TO DEMONSTRATE FUNCTIONAL COMPETENCE ON SELECTED PHYSICAL FITNESS SKILLS.

Consensus ☐   Initial Rating ( )
                           Second Rating ( )

Rationale:
• Physical fitness capabilities are necessary to meet man's biologic needs for activity (normal growth and development).
• Physiologic adaptations to stressors promote the ability to adapt to stress.
• Physical fitness capabilities are necessary to provide sufficient strength, endurance, and flexibility necessary to meet the demands of daily living and to have a residual for extra needs.
• Fitness capabilities provide the base (necessary prerequisites) for the efficient acquisition of skill (delay aging, self-concept) and other stated objectives.
• Physical fitness capabilities play a role in effective weight control.
• Injury and problems can be reduced and/or prevented because of physical fitness capabilities.

5. Demonstrate functional competence in selected personal and social skills.
6. Demonstrate functional competence in selected knowledge concepts.

SELECTING APPROPRIATE PROGRAM OBJECTIVES

Program goals provide an excellent description of "what" the results of instruction are intended to be and "why" they are important for a quality physical education program. Instructional content to operationalize each goal in terms of student learnings is provided by program objectives. Objectives identify the specific results of participation in the program. They provide an effective procedure to organize and sequence instructional content.

To select program objectives for each program goal identified, selection criteria are stated. Examples of selection criteria for health-fitness, fundamental motor skills, body management, and sport-dance and active-leisure goals are provided below.

Objectives selected must provide:
- a balance of physical fitness skills that accommodate all ages and individuals;
- healthy growth and development commensurate with the individual's potential;
- sport and dance-leisure capabilities for a high level of wellness—high, moderate, and low intensity of energy output at all ages;
- sport and dance-leisure skills that accommodate individual, partner, and team activities with appropriate balance for seasons;
- competitive and noncompetitive activities;
- skills that may be developed and maintained without excessive costs, such as using community resources;
- sports and dance skills that can accommodate special needs;
- high interest sports that also meet other selection criteria;
- enabling skills to progress to the more complex skills required in sports, dance, and physical fitness activities included in the program, or complex skills that are important but not offered in the regular program;
- enabling skills for efficient movement in daily-living activities and prevention of injuries;
- physical fitness, sport, dance, and leisure skills that are durable, usable over time, and essential (basic) for all students to progress toward mastery and achievement.

Table 4–6 presents an example goal statement with selection criteria and potential program objectives selected to put the goal into operation.

The list of potential objectives is developed without consideration of the total number of objectives that can be included in the program. Reduction in the total number of objectives and selection of essential objectives are considered later in the planning process. For effective instruction, these decisions require knowledge of available instruction time and expected student achievement gains. Placing the selected program objectives by program level, the "when" of instruction is the next step in program planning.

DEVELOPING AN ACHIEVEMENT-BASED CURRICULUM PLAN

The term "program" implies the "what," "why," and "when" of preschool through secondary school instruction. Specification of program goals and objectives, the "what" and "why" of instruction, is completed before the "when," the program organization, is considered. Program organization is a term referring to placement of program objectives to promote continuous student learnings. The organization of the program provides the sequential basis for contin-

TABLE 4–6. *Example Program Goal; Selection Criteria and a List of Potential Program Objectives*

Goal Statement:
TO DEMONSTRATE FUNCTIONAL COMPETENCE ON SELECTED PHYSICAL FITNESS SKILLS.

Selection Criteria:
• Consider the cost of special facilities and equipment.
• Skills that may be developed and maintained without excessive equipment: school and/or home situation.
• Skills that provide a balance of health-related physical fitness capabilities.
• Skills that relate most closely to health or high-level wellness.
• Skills that are enabling to more complex activities, daily living, dance, sports, and leisure.

Potential Program Objectives

Muscular Strength and Endurance	*Cardiorespiratory Endurance*
Arms/Chest/Shoulders	*Relaxation*
Abdominal	*Personal Conditioning*
Back	*Weight Control/Body Composition*
Legs	
Flexibility	
Arms/Shoulders	
Trunk/Legs	
Ankles	

uous learning of students as they advance from grade to grade or from level to level.

Achievement is the key word in considering sequential placement of objectives. Instruction at each level or grade of the school's program is focused on supporting student achievement of the objectives included. For example, a sequential program results in a high proportion of students achieving functional competence on program objectives such as "run," "catch," and "throw" (enabling skills) prior to expecting them to achieve a program objective such as "fielding" in softball.

Achieving functional competence of essential physical and motor objectives is of critical importance. Teaching too many objectives for too little time for students to achieve mastery is a common problem. Students move from level to level or from grade to grade without ever mastering needed prerequisites for continuous learning to progress toward achieving program goals. No matter how well the program is sequenced, if students do not master prerequisites, progressive achievement is not possible.

Program objectives, appropriately sequenced, are key ingredients of quality programming—individualized and accountable. They provide a structure for:
• optimum placement of students into all or portions of the regular program in accordance with their capabilities—prerequisite skills and learning needs;
• modification and adaptation of program objectives and instructional activities to accommodate students;
• monitoring and evaulating student progress and results of instruction.

Verification of the appropriateness of selected program objectives by level or grade to accommodate student needs is depicted in Figure 4–2. This process is highlighted to emphasize the individualization and personalization of program goals and objectives in the Achievement-Based Curriculum Model.

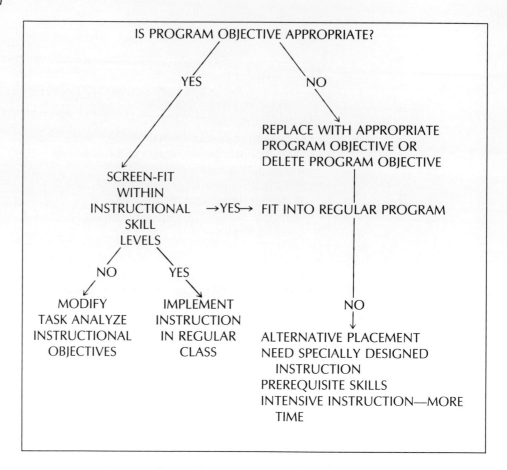

Figure 4–2. *Verification of the appropriateness of program objectives to meet students' instructional needs.*

PLACING PROGRAM OBJECTIVES IN APPROPRIATE PROGRAM LEVELS

Program objectives selected for inclusion are placed in the program where they are most likely to be worked on and achieved by the students. Program levels are unique to each school district. Typically, they are dependent on current or future facilities and/or district-wide school schedules and staffing patterns. Table 4–7 presents two common examples of program levels.

Other possibilities exist for organizing a program into logical levels or breakpoints. A multiplicity of breakpoints might be identified by reviewing content dependencies and growth and development needs of students. This procedure is very time-consuming, and in our experience these breaks do not markedly change placement decisions. Too many breaks make it difficult to clearly communicate the intent and purpose of the program.

Ideally, three to five program levels are recommended for the initial model implementation years. Using fewer program levels facilitates completing program organization without time-consuming placement decisions which often get

TABLE 4–7. *Two Common Program Level Patterns*

EXAMPLE	K	1	2	3	4	5	6	7	8	9	10	11	12
1	(	K – 2		)(	3 – 5		)(	6 – 8		)(	9 – 12		)
2	(	K – 3			)(	4 – 6		)(	7 – 10			)	

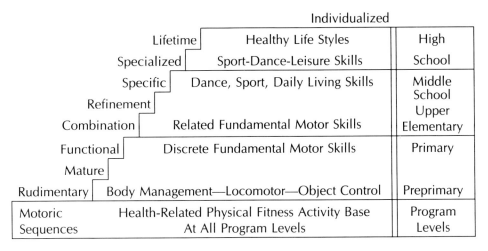

Figure 4–3. *Overview of sequential motor skill sequences by program levels.*

changed. As the model is implemented, program objective placements are modified based on the student's progress and results of instruction. Using evaluative data is an ongoing recycling process of the Achievement-Based Curriculum Model.

Placement of program objectives is completed by physical education staff members. These members represent all levels of the school program. They know the program levels and are familiar with the characteristics and achievement expectancies of students. Their knowledges and experiences are supplemented by selected resource personnel and information drawn from the literature. Later, with the ABC program plan in place, student data provide needed documentation on the determination of expectancies.

With information on growth and development characteristics described for program levels, the next step is to identify sequential skill acquisition of the selected program objectives. Figure 4–3 illustrates general sequences of motor skills in program levels.

These progressions, along with specification of enabling skills to the more complex dance, sport, and leisure skills and relative goal emphasis, provide decision-making criteria for initial placement of program objectives in program levels. Figure 4–4 presents an overview to assist in specifying enabling skills.

Relative goal emphasis refers to the importance of each program goal at a program level as students progress toward achieving desired learning outcomes. To help the group make these decisions, points (100%) are distributed across all goals. The percent value assigned to each goal represents the relative importance, weighting, assigned to each goal. Table 4–8 illustrates this procedure.

At this step in the planning process, the ABC program plan is considered "ideal." Program objectives, prioritized and selected, are not restricted to school-related factors, such as instructional time, equipment, facilities, or staffing patterns. Formulation of an "ideal" program plan is not a limitation. It is a strength in the planning process. Table 4–9 is an example of such an ABC program plan.

The next step in the planning process is to determine the total number of objectives that can be effectively taught in a specific school program K through Grade 12.

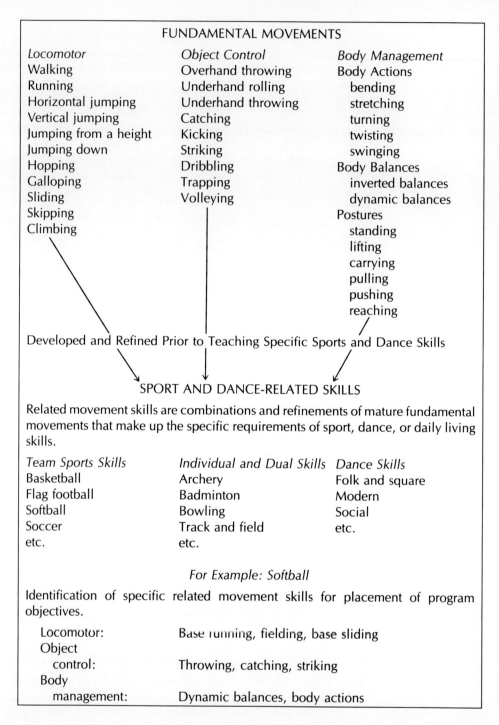

Figure 4–4. *Example of enabling skills related to dance, sport, and leisure skills.*

DETERMINING TIME NEEDED FOR EFFECTIVE INSTRUCTION

Discriminating use of available instruction time is an essential condition for quality programming. Quality is directly related to the number of objectives that can be effectively taught in the instructional program. Students need sufficient amounts of time to allow for improvement gains on the objectives selected for the program. The amount of instructional time allotted to each program objective is crucial to student achievement. Two instructional time factors of effective

TABLE 4–8. *Relative Importance (Percentage) of Each Goal by Program Level*

GOAL AREAS	REGULAR EDUCATION GRADE LEVELS[1] %			SPECIAL EDUCATION AGE LEVELS[2] %		
	K–3	4–6	7–10	3–8	9–14	15–25
1. Demonstrate functional competence on play, sport, and leisure skills	10	35	60	10	20	45
2. Demonstrate functional competence on fundamental motor skills	50	35	10	50	40	25
3. Demonstrate functional competence on body management skills	20	10	10	20	20	10
4. Demonstrate functional competence on physical fitness skills	20	20	20	20	20	20
TOTAL (%)	100	100	100	100	100	100

[1]Regular education emphasis is divided by the grade levels used in schools.
[2]Special education emphasis is divided by age levels since many special education students are assigned by age and not by grade level.

instruction need to be considered to determine the total number of program objectives to be included: instructional time available and time needed for students to achieve meaningful performance gain.

Time Available for Instruction. To determine available instructional time is a fairly simple procedure. Count the number of days available in the school year for instruction. Multiply this number by the length of each instructional period. The answer represents how much time in minutes or hours a teacher has available to teach. The calculation is adjusted to account for lost instructional days that occur because of fire drills, assemblies, field trips, snow/storm/spring days, and other situations. An example of available instructional time is presented below:

School District: Pine Tree	*Class/Level:* K–3	*Teacher:* J. Walkley
Instructional weeks	6 units of 6 weeks	= 36 weeks
Three times per week	3 × 30 min	= 90 min
Available instructional time	3 × 30 min × 36 weeks	= 3,240 min
Adjustments for "lost" instructional days		
Experience shows that this "lost" time is		
approximately 10% of available time: 3,240 × .90 = 2,916 min or 48¼ hours yearly		

Meaningful Performance Gain. To determine needed instructional time for meaningful student gain on program objectives is more complex. The term "meaningful gain" refers to the amount of performance gain that is judged to make a difference in the student's ability to demonstrate a significantly higher level of competence on the objective. It is linked to exit competency. Gains need to be large enough to accumulate, within the total allotment of instructional time over the school years, to a standard performance level upon exit from the school program. For example, if students require 360 minutes (6 hours) of instruction

TABLE 4–9.   *Achievement-Based Curriculum Program Plan for K through 10*

| Goals | PROGRAM LEVELS/GRADES | | |
	EARLY ELEMENTARY K–3	LATER ELEMENTARY 4–6	MIDDLE AND HIGH SCHOOL 7–10

1. Fundamental motor skills	Run
	Horizontal jump
	Vertical jump
	Hopping
	Skipping
	Sliding
	Climbing
	Overhand throw
	Underhand roll
	Underhand throw
	Catching
	Kicking
	Striking
	  Sidearm
	  Underarm
	  Overarm
	Bowling ball
	Rhythms
	  Move to even beat
	  Move to uneven beat
	  Accent
	  Communication
		Overhand throw
		Catching
		Striking
		Volleying
		Dribbling
		Taught singly and in combinations
		Others taught in specific sports
		Rhythms
		  Creative
			Taught as needed for sport, leisure, dance, or leisure skills

2. Body management	*Body awareness*
	  Body parts
	  Body actions
	  Body planes
	Body control
	  Log roll
	  Forward roll
	  Backward roll
	  Balances
	  Stunts
	Spatial awareness
	  Size and shapes
	  Directions in space
	  Personal space
		Body control
		  Taught in gymnastics
		Body Awareness
		Spatial Awareness
		Taught with motor skills
		Positive daily living
		  Holding
		  Lifting
		  Carrying
		  Pushing
		  Pulling
		  Standing
		  Sitting
		  Walking
			See Gymnastics
			Positive daily living
			  Holding
			  Lifting
			  Carrying
			  Pushing
			  Pulling
			  Standing
			  Sitting
			  Walking

to achieve a mastery level of performance on an objective in the program plan, on-task, active learning time, must be allocated accordingly. In this instance it may be 60 minutes per year for 6 years.

Time estimates for students to achieve meaningful performance gain requires three decisions. The first requires a decision regarding how much individual student gain is enough to be identified as meaningful. The second requires a decision regarding the number of students (percent) within a class or program level who achieve the meaningful gain to claim that instruction is effective. These estimates change as they are applied to different student population groups or

TABLE 4–9. *Achievement-Based Curriculum Program Plan for K through 10 (Continued)*

	PROGRAM LEVELS/GRADES		
GOALS	EARLY ELEMENTARY K–3	LATER ELEMENTARY 4–6	MIDDLE AND HIGH SCHOOL 7–10

3. Health and Fitness	Cardiorespiratory endurance
	Strength muscular endurance
	  Arms, chest, shoulders
	  Abdominal
	Flexibility
	  Trunk and legs
	  Arms and shoulders
	  Ankle
	Relaxation
		Strength muscular endurance
		  Arms, chest, shoulders
		  Abdominal
		Flexibility
		  Trunk and legs
		  Arms and Shoulders
		  Ankle
		Relaxation
			Personal conditioning
			  Muscular strength endurance
			  Flexibility
			  Cardiorespiratory endurance
			  Relaxation
			  Weight/body composition

4. Dance, sport, leisure and active leisure skills	*Free play*
	Organized games
	  Partner
	  Small group
	  Large group
		Team sports
		  Basketball
		  Soccer/speedball
		  Softball
		Gymnastics
		  Stunts combination
		  Apparatus
		  Inverted balance
		  Free exercise
		Dance
		  Folk
		  Square
		  Aerobics
		Track and field
		  Sprints
		  Distances
		  Field events
		Aquatics
		  Diving
		  Swimming
		  Survival
			Team sports
			  Basketball
			  Football
			  Hockey
			  Soccer/speedball
			  Softball
			  Volleyball
			Individual and dual
			  Archery
			  Badminton
			  Bowling
			  Golf
			  Gymnastics
			  Tennis
			  Skiing cross-country
			  Track and field
			  Wrestling
			Aquatics
			  Diving
			  Swimming
			  Survival
			Dance
			  Aerobics
			  Social

individual students. The third decision requires time estimates for students to achieve meaningful gain on program objectives in program levels.

    Student Expectancies. The amount of meaningful student gain involves a subjective and an objective element. The objective element requires that the performance gain be the direct result of instruction—not chance. The teacher knows the entry status of the student on objectives to be taught, plans and implements instruction to support student's learning, and evaluates each student's performance achievement as a result of instruction.

    The subjective element relates to the following considerations by the teacher:

1. Skill level necessary to be considered functional (mastery level) for the individual student or student group.
2. Instructional time and resources needed to achieve desired performance gain.

3. Entry status of student on the particular instructional objective or set of objectives.
4. Capability of student to learn.

Prior to determining the size of student gain to be considered meaningful, the amount of gain for functional competence must be established. Functional competence is the achievement of a performance level that allows the student to gainfully participate in active play-leisure activities and/or enables the student to achieve higher levels of skills consistent with innate abilities. Gainful participation means that the student's participation capability results in the attainment of activity benefits that the particular activity offers for quality of life.

The determination of functional competence varies across individuals and skills. To help in this determination, the concept of mastery stabilizes functional competence. Mastery is defined as the amount of performance. The level of performance is limited only by the individual's ability, interest, and practice time. For example, the results of instruction designed to develop abdominal strength can be estimated by the number of sit-ups students can perform. In a class of 40 students, it is common to have students achieve 35 different levels of performance. The objective of instruction is to attain a functional competence specified at the seventy-fifth percentile level for age and sex. This level of abdominal strength facilitates, or at least does not limit, participation. It is enabling to further development of this ability. With such a criterion, a high percentage of students can achieve a "functional" mastery level.

Teachers experienced with content of physical education and abilities of students can identify the amount of a given skill that would be usable by the student. Parent involvement in these determinations provides another source in establishing functional competence. If, together, parents and teachers decide that the performance level necessary to be useful for a child is beyond the capabilities of a given student to achieve within available instructional time, they need to target alternative program objective(s) or additional instructional time needs to be available for more intensive instruction.

With functional competence, entry performance level status, knowledge of the individual's or given student population's learning characteristics, and known amount of time available for instruction, the teacher establishes the size of performance increments necessary for the student to achieve "meaningful gains." For example, in teaching the fundamental skill "overhand throw," the instructional objective could be viewed across 2 skill levels comprising 8 learning tasks. Learning tasks are the criteria specified to determine mastery of each skill level comprising the instructional objective. For fundamental motor, health-fitness, and body management skills, learning tasks may range from 6 to 8. For a student having difficulty learning, these instructional objectives are broken down (task-analyzed) into 10 to 15 learning tasks. These tasks begin with total assistance in grasping a ball and throwing overhand through some specified level of functional throwing ability. With the number of learning tasks (units of gain) for functional competence established, teachers can estimate how much instructional time (on the average) is required for students to achieve a meaningful gain.

Class Group Expectancies.   With functional competence criterion specified on program objectives for a given population, teachers estimate the total amount of instructional time required for a high proportion (90%) to achieve criterion at each program level. For example, if a program objective is included in the last year (grade 3) of the early elementary program and in later elementary program (grade 4), the objective is taught in 2 units of instruction. With this time period, students (90% of the class) are expected to achieve functional competence. Instructional time needs to be allotted to a program objective to take the students from entry-skill level to functional competence. Achievement is not deferred to other program levels. Each program level has allotted time for essential objectives.

Several options are available if expectations for the class or individual students are not achieved as specified. The program plan and expectancies are not etched in stone. They are modified for class or an individual student based on evaluative data. These options provide individualization as well as accountability, such as

- redefining the program plan for the end of the year or the following year on objectives to be taught, deleting lower priority objectives and allowing more time on higher priority objectives;
- modifying expectations for class or student—to low or high criterion set for functional competence on a given objective;
- increasing instructional time available—home training programs for parents and peer tutoring; and
- examining instructional activities, class management procedures, methods, and time on tasks.

Procedures described in later chapters help teachers make these decisions once the program plan is implemented and results evaluated.

Time Estimates for Achieving Meaningful Gain. The amount of time needed is an estimate of how much time is required to teach program objective(s) taught within each year of the program for the class (90%) or an individual student to make a meaningful gain on learning tasks identified for each instructional objective. Time estimates vary, depending on the speed at which students learn, the amount of skill that is needed for meaningful gain, and the instructional setting. Based on experiences of teachers who have implemented the model in special education or regular education classes, guidelines for achieving meaningful gain are presented on the following page.

Program Level	Special Education (minutes)	Regular Education (minutes)
Preschool	270	210
Elementary	210	180
Secondary	180	120

Expected Meaningful Gain	1–2 Learning Tasks	2–4 Learning Tasks
Expected Mastery Level Performance on Program Objective	10–15 Learning Tasks	6–8 Learning Tasks

Time estimates per objective will increase and the number of objectives decrease when mastery level of performance for a high proportion of the students is the expected outcome. Table 4–10 presents guidelines for initial time estimates for determining total number of objectives. Many factors will influence student achievement. The impact of class size and staffing may influence the effectiveness of instruction.

These time estimates indicate the approximate number of minutes needed for a high proportion of students (90%) to achieve expected student gain on selected program objective. The allotments include time needed for assessing, teaching, and reassessing. Some program objectives require more time, while others require less. It is not critical that the estimates are exactly on target. It is critical that an estimate be made. These initial estimates are modified during

TABLE 4–10. *Guidelines to Estimate Time Needed for Students to Achieve Meaningful Gain and Mastery Level Performance: Regular Class Setting*

1.

CASE STUDY PROGRAM PLAN	TEACHING TIME		PROGRAM OBJECTIVE MEANINGFUL GAIN	PROGRAM OBJECTIVE MASTERY MEANINGFUL GAIN ÷ 2
K–3	33 wk × 2 days = 66 days 66 days × 20 min = 1,320 min 1,320 min × 4 grades = 5,280 min		24 210)5,280	12 2)24
4–6	33 wk × 2 days = 66 days 66 days × 30 min = 1,980 min 1,980 min × 3 grades = 5,940 min		33 180)5,940	17 2)33
7–10	30 wk × 2 days = 60 days 60 days × 40 min = 2,400 min 2,400 min × 4 grades = 9,600 min		80 120)9,600	40 2)80
Total Program Objective	K–10		137	69

2.

CASE STUDY PROGRAM PLAN	K 1 2 3	4 5 6	7 8 9 10	GRAND TOTAL
Meaningful Gain	6 6 6 6	11 11 11	20 20 20 20	137
Student Expectancies Meaningful Gain	Grade 3 24	Grade 6 33	Grade 10 80	
Mastery Level	3 3 3 3	5 6 6	10 10 10 10	69
Student Expectancies Mastery Level	Grade 3 12	Grade 6 17	Grade 10 40	

Factors: Size of Regular Class

3.

CLASS SIZE	UNDER 35	35–40	40–50	50–60	
Percent Program Objectives	100%	85%	70%	50%	

implementation and evaluation of the program. The estimates are targets to aid teachers in implementing and evaluating the effectiveness of instruction. With instructional time available, the estimates are used to project the total number of program objectives to be included at program levels and for a yearly program plan.

DETERMINING TOTAL NUMBER OF PROGRAM OBJECTIVES TO BE INCLUDED

To determine how many program objectives to include in the program plan, divide the average amount of time needed for effective instruction into the amount of time available. These determinations are completed for each level of the program as shown in the following tabulations.

TABLE 4–11. *Total Number of Essential Program Objectives (POs) for Meaningful Gain per Year K through 12*

CASE STUDY REGULAR CLASS SETTING	PROGRAM LEVELS/GRADES		
	LOWER ELEMENTARY K–3	UPPER ELEMENTARY 4–6	INTERMEDIATE AND SECONDARY 7–10
1. Yearly instructional time available in minutes	1,320 min	1,980 min	2,400 min
2. Instructional time requirements for meaningful student gains on program objectives, using average minutes for program level	210	180	120
3. Total number of program objectives that can be effectively taught per year	1,320 ÷ 210 = 6 +	1,980 ÷ 180 = 11	2,340 ÷ 120 = 20
4. Relative emphasis by goal area and number of program objectives	Per Year	Per Year	Per Year
	% — No. POs	% — No. POs	% — No. POs
Dance, sport, and lesisure skills	10 — 1	35 — 4	60 — 12
Fundamental motor skills	50 — 3	35 — 4	10 — 2
Body management skills	20 — 1	10 — 1	10 — 2
Physical fitness skills	20 — 1	20 — 2	20 — 4
TOTALS	100 — 6	100 — 11	100 — 20

Level/ Grades					*Yearly*		*Years*		*Total*
K–3	1,320	÷	210	=	6	×	4	=	24
	Total time available in minutes		Minutes/program objectives meaningful gain		Total program objectives				
4–6	1,980	÷	180	=	11	×	3	=	33
7–10	2,340	÷	120	=	20	×	4	=	80

Grand Total 137

Knowing the total number of objectives that can be taught effectively by program level and relative goal emphasis, the total of objectives for each goal can be determined. Table 4–11 presents a case study for one school program based on all foregoing time determinations and relative goal emphasis.

DEVELOPING A COMPREHENSIVE PROGRAM PLAN: GOALS AND ESSENTIAL OBJECTIVES

Knowing the total number of program objectives to be included, the consensus-forming technique is used to select essential program objectives for each goal and program level. It is this long-term program plan that clearly communicates the purpose of the program and specifies the essential objectives (content) to be achieved by all students.

What are essential objectives? They are objectives that broadly define skills that a community wishes their children to achieve as a result of schooling. They are objectives identified and accepted by all concerned with the school program:

TABLE 4–12. *Essential Objectives Selected for Mastery by Program Level K through 10*

PROGRAM GOAL AREAS	PROGRAM LEVELS/GRADES			
	K–3	4–6	7–10	TOTAL
Fundamental motor skills	Run 6 Jump (horizontal) Underhand roll Overhand throw Bouncing ball Move to even beat	Kick 6 Catch Forehand strike Communication Accent Move to uneven beat	Backhand strike 4 Underhand strike Horizontal jump High jump	16

Body management	Log roll 2
	Forward roll
	Backward roll
	Body parts
	Body actions
	Shapes/Sizes
	Posture
		Gymnastics 2
		  apparatus
		  inverted balance
		  stunts
		  tumbling
			Gymnastics 4
			  free exercise
			  apparatus
			  inverted balance
				8

Health/physical fitness	2
	Cardiorespiratory
	  endurance
	Abdominal strength/
	  endurance
		3
		Cardiorespiratory
		  endurance
		Abdominal strength
		  endurance
		Trunk/leg flexibility
			6
			Personal conditioning
			Posture-body mechanics
			                                    2
				13

Dance, sports, leisure	2
	Free play (handing/
	  climbing, rolling,
	  scooter)
	Organized games
	  running
		6
		Basketball (2)*
		Softball (2)
			24
			Basketball (3)
			Tennis (3)
			Soccer (3)
			Bowling (2)
			Orienteering (2)
			Volleyball (3)
			Cross country
			Skiing (2)
			Badminton (3)
			Social dance (3)
				32

Mastery level Total Number	12	17	40	69

*Represents number of objectives selected for each sport.

parents, students, teachers, administrators, and other members of the community. These objectives are to be acquired by all the students for whom instruction is planned, implemented, documented, and evaluated as to effectiveness.

Two criteria are emphasized in the selection of essential objectives: durability and utility. Durability over time refers to those skills and concepts that have long-range benefits for each student. These objectives have extended utility during maturation and for all ages. Their contributions are focused on healthy life styles, efficiency in daily living activities, and joy of participation in active sports, dance, and leisure pursuits for all ages. Table 4–12 is an example of a school program plan of essential objectives selected by the foregoing processes.

What about objectives that are considered important but are eliminated? Typically, teachers resist deleting objectives from the program. They feel that students are short-changed; however, putting the objectives back in is not the answer. If estimates are on target, instruction is effective: students achieve essential objectives. Putting objectives back in, without increasing instructional time, decreases the effectiveness of the program.

Another way to look at the program objectives that are important but did not find their way into the program is to consider the rationale for requesting an increase in resources: time, equipment, facilities, and staffing. With a program plan focused on quality—achievement on objectives taught by a high proportion of students—the school can demonstrate effectiveness of instruction. These results can be communicated to all members of the school and the community at large. Teachers identify objectives eliminated due to limited resources. In this way, a direct link exists between results of the program and resources allotted to it. Reductions in staff, time, equipment, and facilities reduce program output, student achievements. Increases in these same resources will provide additions to output objectives. Administrators and others know exactly what the impact of resource decisions is on the program.

DESIGNING YEARLY INSTRUCTIONAL UNITS AND UNIT LESSON PLANS

ARRANGING PROGRAM OBJECTIVES INTO INSTRUCTIONAL UNITS

Essential program objectives identified are organized into a teaching sequence. This is a September-to-June sequence of objective-based instructional units. Each unit is made up of clusters of objectives that are grouped together for teaching purposes. The amount of time allotted to instruction on each objective and for the total unit is specified. Table 4–13 illustrates ABC instructional units in a yearly program plan.

Several points to consider in developing a yearly program plan exist. These are:

- instructional compatibility of objectives;
- sequencing of units;
- time allotments for units;
- time allotments for each objective in the unit.

Instructional Compatibility of Objectives.   Three types of units to consider in grouping objectives for a yearly program plan are: traditional, continuous, and long-term. Traditional units are those that cluster program objectives together within a sport of "like content" unit. These units are taught over a period of approximately three to six weeks. An example is a volleyball unit. Seasonal activities may also influence the grouping of program objectives. For example, program objectives such as overhand throw, horizontal jump, and run may be grouped as a Track and Field Unit or Special Olympics Unit in the spring. At the elementary level, the objectives are clustered according to enabling skills, similarities in use of equipment and facilities, and season of the year.

Long-term units are those clusters of program objectives that are taught periodically across all units. These objectives are taught simultaneously with all other units and consume a small amount of time within each unit lesson. A typical example is a fitness unit. A cluster of fitness program objectives is taught within a warm-up period preceding the teaching of program objectives of another unit such as volleyball.

A continuous unit is the intermittent teaching of program objectives that are not specifically scheduled. These program objectives are taught when appropriate circumstances occur and are an integral component of class management procedures. This type of unit is typified by program objectives arranged in clusters representative of effective, personal-social learnings. Sharing, self-control, responsibility, and respect for others are examples. Situations to facilitate

TABLE 4–13. *A Yearly Program Plan: Achievement-Based Curriculum Instructional Units*

Class/Level Upper Elementary: Grade 5 Regular Class

SEQUENTIAL UNITS	TIME (min)	TOTAL TIME (min)	WEEKS
1. a. Overhand throw	180		
b. Catch	180		
c. Cardiorespiratory	30		
d. Abdominal strength	30	420	7
2. a. Move to uneven beat	180		
b. Accent	180		
c. Cardiorespiratory	30		
d. Abdominal strength	30	420	7
3. a. Accent	180		
b. Cardiorespiratory	60		
c. Abdominal strength	30	270	4.5
4. Basketball			
a. Chest pass	180		
b. Dribbling	180		
c. Cardiorespiratory	45		
d. Abdominal strength	45	450	7.5
5. Softball			
a. Running bases	180		
b. Fielding	180		
c. Cardiorespiratory	15		
d. Abdominal strength	45	420	7
		1,980	33 wks.

instruction in these program objectives constantly occur in competitive and interactive game activities and merit specific instruction at that time.

Sequencing Unit Objectives. With objectives clustered, the instructional sequence of units needs to be decided. This decision is based on scheduling, such as

- outdoor units and time of year;
- seasonal activities;
- availability of facilities;
- enabling or prerequisite skills: teaching hop before skip.

Time Allotment for Each Unit. The length of time for instruction for each unit varies. It is indicated by weeks, days, or minutes. Some units require much more time than others. This variation may be due to the difficulty of the objectives or to the number of objectives that make up the unit. The units that require less time of instruction may be review units or those that check on retention of what was learned rather than on initial skill development. Each unit is assigned an estimated time allotment in weeks or days. For example, multiply the number of weeks or days for each unit by the number of minutes available for class instruction by the week or day:

$$
\text{unit length} = \begin{array}{r} 12 \text{ days} \\ \times\ \underline{45 \text{ min gym/day}} \\ 540 \text{ total min/unit} \end{array}
$$

$$\text{unit length} = \frac{4 \text{ weeks}}{540 \text{ total min/unit}} \times \frac{135 \text{ min gym/week}}{} \begin{array}{l} (45 \text{ min/day} \\ 3 \text{ days/week}) \end{array}$$

Time Allotment for Program Objectives. Time allotment is based on the estimate of minutes needed for each program objective computed previously. When assigning minutes for each objective in the yearly program plan, these points are considered. Some objectives may require less time per unit. These objectives are repeated across two or more units—fitness objectives or objectives for review. Other objectives require more time because they are more difficult to learn. For example, assigning minutes to basketball with three objectives listed may be preferable if these objectives are taught simultaneously. Table 4–13 illustrates a yearly program plan.

DEVELOPING UNIT LESSON PLANS

Unit lesson plans are smaller "chunks" of content to be taught. They are developed from the yearly program unit plan. Each unit lesson plan describes instruction on a daily schedule as to the
- organization and sequence of objectives within each unit;
- daily time allotment for each objective taught;
- actual time taught on each objective;
- actual length of the total unit in number of days;
- activities within each unit.

Table 4–14 illustrates unit lesson plans for one unit of the previously described yearly program plan.

Each box represents one daily lesson within the unit. Each objective to be assessed, taught, and reassessed during a class period is identified. The estimated time allotment for instruction on each objective is specified. A date is entered into *each box* upon completion of that day's lesson. At the completion of the unit lesson plans, any changes are noted: objectives, time allotment, activities, or sequences.

The development of yearly unit programs and lesson plans by clustering program objectives for effective instruction is a creative act of teachers. There is an infinite number of combinations. The key criterion of effectiveness of the unit is the result of instruction—student achievement. Did its implementation result in a high proportion of students achieving meaningful gains on objectives taught? The other key criterion is: Can the unit be described sufficiently so that it can be replicated for a like population and result in important student gains?

SYNOPSIS

Identifying "where you are going" prior to determining "how to get there" is the focus of this chapter. The term *program* refers to the "what," "why," and "when" of instruction. Program goals and objectives—defensible and relevant—provide the "what" and "why" of instruction. Program goals and objectives organized and sequenced in program levels and arranged into yearly, sequential, ABC instructional units are the "when." The individualization, personalization, and appropriateness, of these goals and objectives were highlighted. A systematic planning process was presented to develp an ABC sequential program plan of essential objectives that could be effectively taught and achieved by all students. The planning process culminates in a school program plan, yearly instructional units, and unit lesson plans that can be replicated and systematically changed to indicate revision recommendations to be implemented and re-evaluated.

TABLE 4–14. *Unit Lesson Plans*

	Days/Weeks		PO's	Min		PO's	Min
Gym:	# _2/7_ Min/Days		Overhand throw	180		Cardiorespiratory (CR)	30
	# _30_		Catch	180		Abdominal Strength (AS)	30

Projected Time: ___10/31___ to ___12/19___

CLASS LEVEL __Upper Elementary, Grade 5 Regular__ NAME _____Smith_____ UNIT _____#1_____

Overhand throw 13 Catch 12 Assess both CR 2 AS 3 10/31	Overhand throw 13 Catch 13 Assess both CR 2 AS 2 11/2	Overhand throw 12 Catch 13 CR 3 AS 2 11/7	Overhand throw 15 Catch 10 CR 2 AS 3 11/9	Overhand throw 12 Catch 13 CR 3 AS 2 11/14
Overhand throw 13 Catch 13 CR 2 AS 2 11/16	Overhand throw 10 Catch 15 CR 2 AS 2 11/21	Overhand throw 15 Catch 15 Reassess both CR 2 AS 2 11/23	Overhand throw 12 Catch 12 CR 2 AS 2 11/28	Overhand throw 13 Catch 13 CR 2 AS 2 12/5
Overhand throw 12 Catch 13 CR 2 AS 2 12/7	Overhand throw 13 Catch 12 CR 2 AS 2 12/12	Overhand throw 13 Catch 13 Reassess both CR 2 AS 2 12/14	Overhand throw 13 Catch 13 Reassess both CR 2 AS 2 12/19	

A consensus-forming technique involves team members representing parents, students, teachers, administrators, and other school/community personnel. This technique reduces or eliminates many difficulties encountered in specification of program goals and objectives, structuring and sequencing objectives, and providing effective articulation with all program elements. Using this technique, the following procedures describe how to . . .

1. Identify documentable potential contributions of physical activity to the quality of life.
2. Communicate the intent and purpose of the program by compiling the "valued" statements and reflecting them in program goal statements.
3. Identify "valued" content (skills and concepts) in terms of program objectives for each goal according to stated selection criteria.
4. Place program objectives by school program levels for each goal according to sequential progressions, enabling skills, and relative goal emphases.
5. Determine total number of program objectives to be included in the program plan using time available for instruction and estimate of time needed for students to achieve meaningful performance gains by program levels.
6. Develop a school program plan representing essential objectives for each goal that can be effectively taught and achieved by students at each program level K through 12.
7. Design yearly instructional units sequencing essential objectives and allocating instructional time for each objective.
8. Develop unit lesson plans, daily schedules specifying essential objectives

(taught and sequenced) within and between lessons, time allotments for each objective for assessing, teaching, and reassessing activities.

RESOURCES FOR TEACHERS

American Alliance for Health, Physical Education, Recreation and Dance: Knowledge and Understanding in Physical Education. Reston, VA, 1973.
————: Health-related fitness. J. Phys. Educ. *52*:(1) 26–39, 1981.
————: Elementary Curriculum: Theory and Practice. Reston, VA, 1982.
————: Physical Education and Sport for the Secondary School Student. Reston, VA, 1983.
Annarino, A.A., Cowell, C.C., and Hazelton, H.: Curriculum Theory and Design in Physical Education. 2nd Ed. St. Louis, C.V. Mosby, 1980.
Bank, A., Henerson, E., and Eu, L.: A Practical Guide to Program Planning: A Teaching Models Approach. New York, Teachers College Press, 1981.
Gallahue, D.L.: Developmental Movement Experienced for Children. New York, Wiley, 1982.
————: Understanding Motor Development in Children. New York, Wiley, 1982.
Godfrey, B., and Kephard, N.C.: Movement Patterns and Motor Education. New York, Appleton Century Crofts, 1969.
I CAN Resource Materials: Criterion-Referenced Instruction
    I CAN Preprimary Motor and Play Skills. East Lansing, MI, Instructional Media Center Marketing Division, Michigan State University, 1980.
    I CAN Primary Skills. Northbrook, IL, Hubbard, 1976.
    I CAN Sport, Leisure and Recreation Skills. Northbrook, IL, Hubbard, 1979.
Lawther, J.: The Learning and Performance of Physical Skills. Englewood Cliffs, NJ, Prentice-Hall, 1977.
Logsdon, B., et al.: Physical Education for Children: A Focus on the Teaching Process. 2nd Ed. Philadelphia, Lea & Febiger, 1984.
Mager, R.F.: Preparing Instructional Objectives. 2nd Ed. Belmont, CA, Fearon Publishers, 1975.
Popham, W.J.: Criterion-Referenced Instruction. Belmont, CA, Fearon Publishers, 1973.
Popham, W.J., and Baker, E.: Establishing Instructional Goals. Englewood Cliffs, NJ, Prentice-Hall, 1970.
————: Systematic Instruction. Englewood Cliffs, NJ, Prentice-Hall, 1970.
————: Planning an Instructional Sequence. Englewood Cliffs, NJ, Prentice-Hall, 1971.
Schurr, E.: Movement Experiences for Children. Englewood Cliffs, NJ, Prentice-Hall, 1980.
Wessel, J.A. (Ed.): Planning Individualized Education Program in Special Education with Examples from I CAN Physical Education. Northbrook, IL, Hubbard, 1977.
Wessel, J.A., and Carmichael, D.L.: The adaptability of the I CAN objective-based instructional system for all handicapped students with specific application to the severely handicapped. J. Spec. Educ. Tech., *3*(3): Spring 1980.
Wickstrom, R.: Fundamental Motor Patterns. Philadelphia, Lea & Febiger, 1977.
Zaichkowsky, L.: Growth and Development: The Child and Physical Activity. St. Louis, MO, C.V. Mosby, 1980.

ACTIVITY 4–1. Identify appropriate program goals.

Objective: To select relevant and defensible program goals.

Materials: List of documented potential contributions of physical activity on growth, development, and general well-being of children and adults.

Worksheet 4–1—Program goal statements with supporting rationale statements based on activity contributions.

WORKSHEET 4–1

Directions:
1. Write goal statements with supporting rationale derived from activity contribution statements. The contribution statements listed may be used and/or additional ones stated and documented.
2. Use the four-step, consensus-forming technique to prioritize the program goals.

Variations:
1. Review the literature, document potential activity contributions, and prepare rationale statements for physical education program in today's schools, and state program goals.
2. Conduct a survey of teachers and other members of the school community, including students, to rate the program goals for the school program.

WORKSHEET 4–1. *Program Goal with Supporting Rationales*

Goal Statement:

_____ TO DEMONSTRATE FUNCTIONAL COMPETENCE _____

Consensus

[   ]

Initial Rating   ( )

Second Rating   ( )

Supporting Rationale Statement

ACTIVITY 4–2. Select program objectives for each goal.

Objective: To select potential program objectives for each program goal.

Materials: Worksheets 4–2A and B
Goals, selection criteria, and program objectives
Goals and prioritized list of program objectives by rank order

WORKSHEET 4–2

Directions:
1. Prepare a list of selection criteria to serve as guidelines for selecting potential program objectives for goals.
   —review and revise as needed selection criteria provided
   —list criteria for selecting objectives for each goal on Worksheet 4–2A
2. Complete Worksheets 4–2A and B.
   —write in goal statements
   —list potential program objectives for each goal
   —for fundamental motor skills, health/physical fitness, and body management objectives, write the name of content area (locomotor skills) and list the specific program objectives for the content area
   —for dance, sport, and leisure skills, write the name of the specific activity; do not list the specific program objectives for each activity at this time
3. Use the four-step consensus-building technique to finalize the rating of each objective by averaging these ratings. Record all findings on Worksheet 4–2A.
4. With the average ratings, rank order objectives for each goal area. Use Worksheet 4–2B, goals and prioritized list of program objectives by rank order, to record these results.

Variations:
1. Conduct a survey of teachers and other members of the school community, including students, to identify potential program objectives for each goal statement based on identifiable selection criteria.
2. Use available program objective resource materials such as I CAN content areas with objectives to identify objectives. These objectives can be used (add/delete) with the consensus-building technique to prioritize objectives for the program plan. A list of I CAN objectives for preprimary, primary, and sport/leisure activities may be found at the end of this chapter.
3. The above procedures may be used by a teacher for a particular program level or grade, as well as for a specific student population group or individual student.

Supplemental Materials:
1. List of I CAN Resource Materials: Preprimary, Primary, and Sport-Leisure Recreational Program Objectives

WORKSHEET 4–2A. *Goals, Selection Criteria, and Program Objectives*

Goal Statement:
_____ TO DEMONSTRATE FUNCTIONAL COMPETENCE _____

Selection Criteria Statements

Potential Program Objectives to be Included

	First	Second	Consensus
_____	( )	( )	( )
_____	( )	( )	( )
_____	( )	( )	( )
_____	( )	( )	( )
_____	( )	( )	( )
_____	( )	( )	( )
_____	( )	( )	( )
_____	( )	( )	( )
_____	( )	( )	( )
_____	( )	( )	( )
_____	( )	( )	( )
_____	( )	( )	( )
_____	( )	( )	( )
_____	( )	( )	( )

WORKSHEET 4–2B. *Goals and Prioritized List of Program Objectives by Rank Order*

Goal Area: _____   Goal Area: _____   Goal Area: _____   Goal Area: _____

ACTIVITY 4–3. Place selected objectives in program levels for each program goal.

Objective: To select program objectives for each program goal by program levels.

Materials: Worksheets 4–3—
Relative Goal Emphasis by Program Levels for Each Program Goal
Identification of Specific Program Objectives to be Included for Each Dance, Sport, and Leisure Activity included in the Program Plan
Place Selected Program Objectives in Program Levels for Each Program Goal K–12
Place Selected Program Objectives in Program Levels for Each Program Goal in the yearly program plan

WORKSHEET 4–3

Directions:

1. Set up guidelines for placing program objectives in program levels:
   —Focus on important program objectives ranked and selected on Worksheets 4–2A and B.
   —Growth development characterizing each level.
   —Fundamental motor skill sequences.
   —Enabling skills related to specific dance, sport, and leisure activities to be included.
2. Use four-step, consensus-building technique to finalize relative program goal emphasis by program level and program objectives for each dance, sport, or leisure activity to be included.
3. On Worksheet 4–3A, assign relative program goal emphasis by program level. This procedure helps to determine total number of program objectives to be selected by program level for each program goal.
4. On Worksheet 4–3B identify specific program objectives to be included for each dance, sport, and leisure activity included in the program. The number of objectives identified for each activity influences the time needed for instruction and the final determination of total number of objectives to be included in the comprehensive program plan. Following is an example worksheet to be used for this purpose.

Activity	First Rating	Second Rating	Consensus Rating
1. Golf			
Swing	_____	_____	_____
Partial swing	_____	_____	_____
Putting	_____	_____	_____
Participation	_____	_____	_____
2. Tennis			
Forehand	_____	_____	_____
Backhand	_____	_____	_____
Serve	_____	_____	_____
Participation	_____	_____	_____

The consensus-building technique can be used to finalize specific objectives. To assist in this task, available program objectives, such as those identified in the I CAN Instructional Resource Materials, can serve as the initial list. Add or delete objectives for activity to be included. These objectives are listed at the end of this chapter.

5. Place program objectives by program levels for each program goal, using Worksheet 4–3C for a comprehensive program plan or Worksheet 4–3D for a yearly program plan.
   • Write in program goal and relative goal emphasis for each program level.
   • List the objectives to be included for each program goal and indicate rank order number. Use the list of program objectives prioritized in Worksheet 4–2B and the specific objectives for each dance, sport, and leisure activity to be included identified on worksheet 4–3B.
   • Use an unmarked Worksheet 4–3C to list final placement of program objectives in program levels for each program goal.
   • Number of program objectives listed on Worksheet 4–3C or D is consistent with relative goal emphasis for each program level.

Variations:

1. Conduct a survey of teachers and other members of the school community to determine relative goal emphasis for each program level and placement of program objectives in program level for each goal.
2. The above procedures may be used by a teacher for a particular program level or grade, as well as for a specific student population or individual student.

119

WORKSHEET 4–3A. *Relative Goal Emphasis by Program Level for Each Program Goal*

1. Assign a percent value (100 points) each each program goal by program level.
2. Finalize percent value assigned each goal by program level by averaging the ratings.
3. Record final ratings which represent the relative goal emphasis by program levels.

Program Level _____ Goal Areas	Ratings		Relative Goal Emphasis
	No. 1	No. 2	Final
1. Health/Physical Fitness	_____	_____	( )
2. Body Management Skills	_____	_____	( )
3. Fundamental Motor Skills	_____	_____	( )
4. Dance, Games, Sports, Leisure Skills	_____	_____	( )
5. Other	_____	_____	( )
Total			100%

WORKSHEET 4–3B. *Identification of Specific Program Objectives to be Included for Each Dance, Sport, and Leisure Activity Included in Program Plan*

Activity	Objectives	First Rating	Second Rating	Consensus
1. _____				
	_____	( )	( )	( )
	_____	( )	( )	( )
	_____	( )	( )	( )
	_____	( )	( )	( )
	_____	( )	( )	( )
2. _____				
	_____	( )	( )	( )
	_____	( )	( )	( )
	_____	( )	( )	( )
	_____	( )	( )	( )
	_____	( )	( )	( )
3. _____				
	_____	( )	( )	( )
	_____	( )	( )	( )
	_____	( )	( )	( )
	_____	( )	( )	( )
	_____	( )	( )	( )

Reproduce this sheet to include all specific activities in the program plan.

WORKSHEET 4–3C. *Place Selected Program Objectives in Program Levels for Each Program Goal K–12*

Write in name of objective, rank order number, and relative percent for each goal and program level.

PROGRAM GOAL AREA	PROGRAM LEVEL/GRADES: ___	PROGRAM LEVEL/GRADES: ___	PROGRAM LEVEL/GRADES: ___

Reproduce this sheet to include all goal areas.

WORKSHEET 4–3D. *Place Selected Program Objectives in Program Levels for Each Program Goal in the Yearly Program Plan*

Write in the name of the objective, a rank order number, and relative percent for each goal.

| PROGRAM GOAL AREA | LIST OF OBJECTIVES IN THE YEARLY PROGRAM PLAN |
	PROGRAM LEVEL: _____ GRADE: _____

Reproduce this sheet to include all goals.

ACTIVITY 4–4. Determine essential program objectives for each program goal by program level.

Objective: To select essential objectives in each program level for each program goal for a comprehensive or yearly program plan.

Materials: Worksheets 4–3C or D

School calendar: Available instructional time

—number of weeks

—number of days

—instructional time per class for each program level

Worksheets 4–4A through D

A. Calculation of Available Instructional Time

B. Time Estimations for Attainment of Meaningful Performance Gain

C. Determine Total Number of Program Objectives for Meaningful Performance Gain by Program Level

D. Comprehensive Program Plan: Selection of Essential Program Objectives by Goal and Program Level

E. Yearly Program Plan: Selection of Essential Program Objectives by Goal and Program Level

WORKSHEET 4–4

Directions: **1.** Complete the calculation on Worksheets 4–4A, B, and C to determine:
- available instructional time in the school calendar year in program level
- time estimation for attainment of meaningful performance gain
- total number of program objectives for meaningful performance gain by program level

2. Complete Worksheet 4–4D or E—Comprehensive or Yearly Program Plan: Selecting Essential Program Objectives by Goal and Program Level. Write in grades/program levels, total number of objectives, and relative goal emphasis (%). Next, select and list essential objectives for each program goal by program level for a comprehensive or yearly program plan.
- If objectives are defined for each activity, they should be listed under each activity.
- If estimations of objectives are made, the number of objectives should be listed in parentheses next to each activity to be included.
- The rank order for each objective on Worksheet 4–3C or D is used to select the essential objectives to be included.

Variations: **1.** Prepare a checklist of the essential objectives to be taught by program level. Conduct a survey in an actual school or school district to determine essential objectives. The sample should include teachers, parents, administrators, and students.

2. Rank order the results. Prepare a report to submit to the school or school district or present at a meeting if this is possible.

WORKSHEET 4–4A. *Calculation of Available Instructional Time*

Complete the calculations below based on school calendar and program level.

_____Level/Grades

1. *Total number* of instructional weeks available: _____Weeks
   —180-day school year = 36 instructional weeks
   —230-day school year = 47 instructional weeks
   (Christmas, spring, summer vacations already excluded.)

2. Subtract _____ weeks of the total time available to allow for *cancelled*   _____Weeks
   physical education classes due to: conference time, psychological testing
   (Brigance), swimming schedule, snow days, field trips, voting days (gym
   in use), holiday assemblies, beginning and ending school,

3. Subtract _____ weeks of the total time available to allow for flex time   _____Weeks
   (unplanned adjustment that needs to be made to allow for additional
   instructional needs).

4. Total weeks available (number) minus 2 and 3 above =   _____Weeks

5. Total days available:
   A. Multiply 4 by the number of gym classes per week: ×_____Days Gym/Week
       =_____Days Gym/Year

   B. Multiply total number of days by the length (minutes) of your PE class   ×_____Min Gym/Day
   (instructional time, not dressing or setup time).   =_____Min Gym/Year

WORKSHEET 4–4B. *Time Estimations for Attainment of Meaningful Performance Gain*

Using the time estimations provided as guidelines, determine the time need for students in your class and/or individual students to achieve meaningful performance gain on selected program objectives for each goal and program level.

PROGRAM GOAL/LEVELS	MINUTES PER OBJECTIVE
Program Level/Grades: _____	
Body Management Skills	_____
Fundamental Motor Skills	_____
Health/Fitness	_____
Play, Sport, and Leisure Skills	_____
Other:	_____
	_____
	_____
Program Level/Grades: _____	
Body Management Skills	_____
Fundamental Motor Skills	_____
Health/Fitness	_____
Play, Sport, and Leisure Skills	_____
Other:	_____
	_____
	_____
Program Level/Grades: _____	
Body Management Skills	_____
Fundamental Motor Skills	_____
Health/Fitness	_____
Play, Sport, and Leisure Skills	_____
Other:	_____
	_____
	_____

Reproduce this sheet to include all program levels. If you selected other goals, adapt this worksheet.

WORKSHEET 4–4C. *Determine Total Number of Program Objectives for Meaningful Performance Gain by Program Level*

1. Class/Level _____

	Number of years/grades			
_____	_____ =	_____ ×	_____ =	_____
Total Time Available	Minutes/ Program objectives needed	Total number of program ob- jectives	Number of year/grades	Total number of objectives

2. Class/Level _____

	Number of years/grades			
_____	_____ =	_____ ×	_____ =	_____
Total Time Available	Minutes/ Program objectives needed	Total number of program objectives	Number of year/grades	Total number of objectives

3. Class/Level _____

	Number of years/grades			
_____	_____ =	_____ ×	_____ =	_____
Total Time Available	Minutes/ Program objectives needed	Total number of program objectives	Number of year/grades	Total number of objectives

4. Class/Level _____

	Number of years/grades			
_____	_____ =	_____ ×	_____ =	_____
Total Time	Minutes/ Program objectives needed	Total number of program objectives	Number of year/grades	Total number of objectives

Grand Total: _____

WORKSHEET 4–4D. *Comprehensive Program Plan: Selection of Essential Objectives by Goal and Program Level—Kindergarten through Upper Elementary*

Write in the number of objectives and relative percent for each goal and program level.

PROGRAM GOAL AREA	PROGRAM LEVEL/GRADES ____ List of Objectives	PROGRAM LEVEL/GRADES ____ List of Objectives	PROGRAM LEVEL/GRADES ____ List of Objectives

Reproduce this sheet to include all goal areas.

WORKSHEET 4–4E. *Yearly Program Plan: Selection of Essential Program Objectives by Goal and Program Level*

Write in the number of objectives and relative percent for each goal.

Program Level/Grade _____

PROGRAM GOAL AREAS	LIST OF OBJECTIVES

Reproduce this sheet to include all goal areas.

ACTIVITY 4–5. Arrange program objectives into instructional units.

Objective:	To design sequential instructional plans for the school year.
Materials:	Worksheets 4–4D or E: Comprehensive Program Plan or Yearly Program Plan
	Worksheet 4–5: Yearly Program Plan: Instructional Units

WORKSHEET 4–5

Directions:

1. With the list of essential program objectives and number to be included for the year, identify clusters of objectives:
   —like content: similarities in equipment and facilities to those highlighted during sport seasons of the year
   —those objectives taught periodically across the entire program plan (across all units, such as fitness objectives) which may be grouped together as a warm-up across one or more units

2. Identify the instructional sequence of the unit groups you identified above. Which unit will be taught first, which second, and so forth. Consider these situations, and assign each unit a number:
   —outdoor units in fall and spring
   —seasonal activities
   —availability of facilities, equipment, and staffing
   —prerequisite objectives, enabling to those objectives taught later

3. Determine time allotments per unit using the time estimates (days and weeks per year) of available instructional time. Assign time in weeks or days to each unit. The days and weeks assigned across all units add up to the total number of days and weeks calculated. Consider these points in making this determination:
   —some units may take more time than others, there may be more program objectives within the unit
   —some units may take more time to achieve student gains owing to difficulty of the program objectives
   —some units may take less time if they are focused on review and retention rather than on skill development
   —the time of some units is predetermined by availability of facilities and equipment

4. Determine time allotments per program objective in each unit. Using the estimate of minutes needed per program objective computed earlier, enter projected minutes for each program objective. To help in this determination, consider these points:
   —some program objectives may require less time if they are repeated across two or more units, or if only review or retention is the focus
   —some program objectives may require more time owing to difficulty of the objectives
   Make sure that the minutes add up to the total amount allocated to each unit. To determine this, multiply the number of weeks or days for each unit by the number of minutes for physical education per week or day.

5. On Worksheet 4–5, list the units in sequence for the year and record the
   • time allotments/minutes
   • number of weeks
   • time in minutes for each objective

WORKSHEET 4–5. *Development of Yearly Instructional Units—Kindergarten, Lower Elementary, Upper Elementary*

Class/Level: _____

Available Instructional Time: _____   Instructional Time: _____
                                                            Meaningful Gain per Objective

Total Number of Objectives: _____

Sequential Instructional Units

	Weeks	*Time*
1.		

ACTIVITY 4–6.   Arrange program objectives into unit lesson plans.

Objective:	To design sequential unit lesson plans.
Materials:	Worksheet 4–5. Yearly Program Plan: Instructional Units
	Worksheet 4–6: Unit Lesson Plans

WORKSHEET 4–6

Directions: **1.** On Worksheet 4–6—
- Enter the information requested on the top of the worksheet.
- Each box is a teaching or class period. The boxes are sequential daily lessons. Enter the number of days in the top right-hand corner of each box. If a unit runs longer than 15 days (one worksheet), continue on to a second worksheet.
- For each new unit, begin a new worksheet. This allows for easier organization later by filling in the unit lesson plans and student/class performance score sheets.
- Write the name of each objective to be assessed/taught/reassessed during that class period. Show the amount of class time to be spent on each objective. Enter the objectives according to the desired sequence. Consider how often the objectives should be taught, every class period, alternating classes, once a week, and so on. Be sure that the amount of time for each objective across all days (boxes) in each unit matches the projected number of minutes for each objective in the yearly program plan. Unit lesson plans can be developed on each unit in the yearly program plan.

2. The data recorded on unit lesson plans are used to plan instruction in subsequent units and/or yearly program plans.
- Upon completion of a lesson, enter the date in each box. If snow days, assemblies, or other cancellations of class occur, begin where you left off. If this happens, adjust future unit(s) accordingly.
- Upon completion of each unit lesson, enter the total actual time worked on for all program objectives. The actual length of the unit is determined by counting the number of boxes with dates in them. Unit lessons may be shortened or lengthened to adjust to the needs of the students in the class.

WORKSHEET 4–6. *Development of Weekly Unit Lesson Plans—Kindergarten, Lower Elementary, Upper Elementary*

Class: #_____Days/Weeks Program Objective(s) MINS. Program Objective(s) MINS.

#_____Mins./Days

Projected Timeline:

_____ to _____

CLASS LEVEL _____ NAME _____ UNIT _____

Reproduce this sheet as needed

I CAN PREPRIMARY SKILLS AREAS WITH PROGRAM OBJECTIVES

LOCOMOTOR SKILLS	Ascend stairs	Jump over
	Crawl	Run
	Descend stairs	Walk
	Jump down	

OBJECT CONTROL SKILLS	Bounce a ball	Kick a ball
	Catch a ball	Roll a ball
	Hit a ball	Throw a ball

BODY CONTROL SKILLS	Climb down a ladder	Log roll
	Climb onto an object	Walk on a balance beam
	Climb up a ladder	

PLAY EQUIPMENT SKILLS	Hang from a bar	Slide down a slide
	Pull an object	Swing on a swing
	Ride a tricycle	Travel on a scooter board

| PLAY PARTICIPATION SKILLS | Free play | |
| | Organized games | |

| HEALTH FITNESS SKILLS | To perform sit-ups | |
| | To walk/run for endurance | |

I CAN PRIMARY SKILLS AREAS WITH PROGRAM OBJECTIVES

FUNDAMENTAL MOTOR

LOCOMOTOR SKILLS AND RHYTHM		OBJECT CONTROL	
Run	Slide	Underhand roll	Underhand strike
Leap	Skip	Underhand throw	Overhand strike
Horizontal jump	Move to even beat	Overhand throw	Forehand strike
Vertical jump	Move to uneven beat	Kick	Backhand strike
Hop	Accent	Continuous bounce	Sidearm strike
Gallop	Communication	Catch	

BODY MANAGEMENT

BODY AWARENESS		BODY CONTROL	
Body parts	Directions in space	Log roll	Static 1-pt balances
Body actions	Personal space	Shoulder roll	Dynamic balances
Body planes	General space	Forward roll	Inverted balances
Shapes and sizes		Backward roll	Bounce on trampoline
		Static 2-pt balances	Airborne on trampoline
			Drops on trampoline

PHYSICAL FITNESS

FITNESS AND GROWTH		POSTURE	
Abdominal strength and endurance	Relaxation	Standing	Pulling
	Trunk/leg flexibility	Sitting	Pushing
Arm/shoulder/chest strength and endurance	Weight training	Walking	Holding/carrying
	Weight maintenance	Ascending/descending stairs	Lifting objects
Cardiorespiratory endurance			Lowering objects

AQUATICS

BASIC SWIMMING SKILLS		SWIMMING AND WATER ENTRY	
Adjustment to water	Back buoyancy	Front crawl	Tread water
Breath control	Front flutter kick	Back crawl	Survival float
Front buoyancy	Back flutter kick	Finning	Jump into water
		Elementary backstroke	Front dive

BACKYARD/NEIGHBORHOOD ACTIVITIES

BADMINTON	CROQUET	HORSESHOES	ROLLERSKATING	TETHERBALL
Ready position	Strike	Pitching	Forward skating	Forehand strike
Underhand stroke			Backward skating	
Serve			Turn right/left	
Forehand drive				
Backhand drive				
Overhead stroke				

TEAM SPORTS

BASKETBALL	KICKBALL	SOFTBALL	VOLLEYBALL
Chest pass	Fielding	Fielding	Forearm pass
One-hand set shot	Running bases	Batting skills	Underhand serve
Dribbling		Running bases	Spike
Lay-up			Block
Rebounding			Overhead pass
Guarding			
Pivot			

OUTDOOR ACTIVITIES

BACKPACKING	CAMPING	HIKING	CROSS-COUNTRY SKIING
Fundamental technique	Fire building and extinguishing	Hiking technique	Preliminary skills
	Preparing meals		Ski on a flat terrain
	Raising and lowering a two-man tent		Ski downhill
			Change directions
			Ski uphill

DANCE AND INDIVIDUAL SPORTS

FOLK DANCE	BOWLING	GYMNASTICS		TRACK & FIELD
Circle formation	Delivery	Forward tumbling	Turns	Sprinting
Circle formation with partner	Accuracy	Backward tumbling	Horizontal ladder	Long jump
Step-hop		Handstand	Rope jumping	Softball throw
Scottische		Body balances	Stunt combinations	440-yard relay
Polka		Bending skills	Partner stunts	High jump
Two-step		Leaps		Distance running

*Participation is generic to each program objective in each activity except gymnastics and track and field.

Assessment

What is Assessment?

Assessment in the ABC Model is a sequential problem-solving process that uses educational measurements (tests) within a decision-making framework. Assessing is a systematic procedure for observing and measuring the learning behavior and then describing that behavior in some form of numerical or categorical system.

How is it Done?	*Decision Aids*
1. Know the role of assessment in the ABC Model.	Purpose Types of instructional decisions 　Programming 　Placement 　Classification
2. Understand how to evaluate assessment tools.	Characteristics of assessment tools 　Validity 　Reliability 　Norm-referenced tests 　Criterion-referenced tests
3. Know how to make programming decisions.	General assessment procedures 　Test selection 　Task analysis 　Data collection
4. Know how to make placement decisions.	Continuum of placements General assessment procedures Identifying content from the ABC program plan to be assessed
5. Know how to make classification decisions.	Physical educator's role and responsibilities General assessment procedures General needs assessment

---

The key to quality and effective Achievement-Based Curriculum (ABC) in physical education is assessment. Valid placement and instructional decisions cannot be made or evaluated without appropriate assessment data, that is, you must know what a student can and cannot do on a task before you can begin to make a decision. Figure 5–1 contains a schematic of the major procedural steps involved in making appropriate decisions in physical education. These same procedures apply to both small (Does a student have the necessary prerequisite skills to successfully play kickball?) and large (Does a student qualify for special education services?) decisions. All the procedural steps outlined in Figure 5–1 are essential to making valid decisions. This chapter focuses on assessment or data collection procedures because they are the key to the remaining steps—any decision can be only as good as the information used to form it. The interpretation, implementation, and evaluation procedures depicted in Figure 5–1 are discussed in the remaining chapters of this book.

As depicted in Figure 5–1, assessment involves the collection of pertinent information from a variety of sources. The three major information categories that should be considered in all decisions are:

> Student's physical and motor skills
> Student's learning and social needs
> Characteristics of the setting

Although the primary focus of assessment in physical education is measuring physical and motor performance, varying degrees of information are needed in the other categories to conduct and interpret assessment tests and ultimately make valid decisions. For example, a physical educator could be asked to assess the object control skills of a new student. The physical educator might administer several catching, throwing, and striking tests to the new student in a corner of the gym while the rest of the class participates in a game directed by an aide. The new student might subsequently fail all the tests and the physical educator

Information Categories

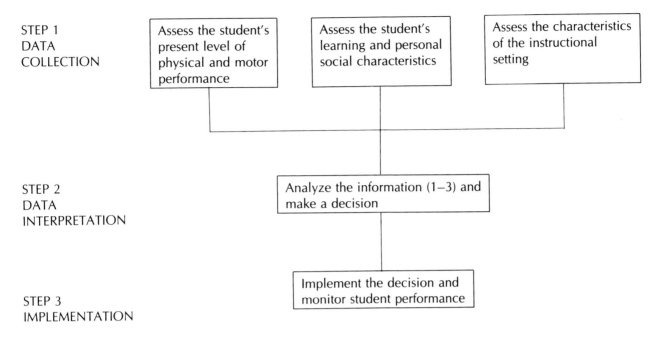

Figure 5–1. *Procedural steps for making appropriate instructional decisions.*

might conclude that the student has very poor object control skills. This conclusion may be invalid, however, because the teacher failed to consider the characteristics of the setting and the unique social and learning characteristics of the new student. The student might in fact have good object control skills, but do poorly on the tests for a variety of reasons such as:

—short attention span;
—inability to understand the test instructions;
—distracted by the game the other students were playing;
—self conscious about being observed by the other students.

The amount of assessment information needed from each of these areas is dependent on the type of decision that must be made. Physical educators in the public schools are faced with a variety of different assessment decisions. These decisions can be liberally categorized into three broad areas:

1. *Programming decisons.* What specifically does a student need to learn on the objectives targeted for instruction?

2. *Placement decisions.* What is the most appropriate and least restrictive physical education setting for a student?

3. *Classification decisions.* Are the student's physical and motor deficits severe enough to qualify for special education services?

Physical educators must play an active role in student assessment and the associated placement and instructional decisions for all students. Failure to play an active role in physical education placement and instructional decisions can have serious detrimental effects on all aspects of the program.

CHARACTERISTICS OF ASSESSMENT TOOLS

The first step in planning an assessment is to select the appropriate data collection instrument. A few basic concepts must be understood to evaluate and select assessment tests. Three important criteria to be considered when selecting assessment instruments are validity, reliability, and the type of data to be collected. Each of these concepts is discussed in the following sections.

VALIDITY

The first criteria for evaluating a test is validity. Does a test measure what it purports to measure? Although this may seem an obvious consideration, many forms of assessment, including commercial assessment instruments, may prove invalid in various physical education applications. Unfortunately, many of the assessment instruments used to measure physical and motor performance depend on "face validity" rather than statistically proven content validity. Face validity implies that it is so obvious that a test measures what it purports to measure that there is no need to statistically substantiate its content validity. Statistical validity of a test is established by measuring the relationship (correlation) between the results obtained with the new test and the results obtained from an already known standard or test with established validity.

The following example is provided to demonstrate the complexity of interpreting validity. Many physical fitness tests, including the AAHPERD Youth Fitness test, use the standing long jump as a test of explosive muscle power of the legs. Both statistical and face validity have been reported in the literature for this item—obviously the more powerful a person's legs are, the farther they will be able to jump. Most of the tests that use this item measure the distance the student jumps and then interpret it in relation to age and sex norms. What the physical educator must ask is under what conditions is this test item valid? Do the standing long jump age and sex standards provide a valid measure of explosive leg power when:

—the student does not know how to perform a proper long jump?
—the student is exceptionally tall or short?
—the student is extremely under- or overweight?
—the student is fearful or otherwise reluctant to perform the task?
—the student has characteristics (i.e., a visual impairment, congenitally deformed arm, hearing impairment) that were not represented in the sample used to create the age and sex norms?

The above example demonstrates that test validity depends on a variety of variables and that interpreting it is not always a simple case of common sense. Regardless of whether a test purports to have face or statistical validity, the responsibility of the physical educator is to be certain that the test is a valid measure for the purpose intended.

RELIABILITY

The second criteria when evaluating potential assessment instruments is reliability, Will the test yield the same information if administered several times by the same or different testers to the same students? Test reliability depends on the clarity of the test instructions and the objectivity of the measurement used to collect the data.

First, let us examine the effect inadequate test instructions can have on reliability. If test instructions are vague or ambiguous, different testers will make different interpretations and consequently will get different results. For example, two physical educators are asked to administer the same test item (bent knee sit-ups for one minute) independently to the same class. Knowing that the students' abdominal strength will not change significantly between the two tests both test results should be the same for each student. Unfortunately, the section of the test instructions pertaining to the degree of knee flexion states only that the student's legs should be bent. The first tester interprets "bent" to mean 90°

flexion of the knees and therefore imposes this standard when administering the test. The second tester interprets "bent" as any degree of flexion and therefore only requires the students to have some degree of flexion in their knees when administering the test. Since sit-ups are more difficult to perform with the knees bent at 90° it is safe to predict that the first tester received lower sit-up scores than the second tester. The important thing to note is that although the abdominal strength of the students remained relatively constant, the measurement of this strength varied markedly because of the ambiguity of the instructions.

The second factor that can affect the reliability of a test is the level of objectivity involved in observing and scoring the behavior being measured. Tests that measure products of a performance are more objective to observe and score than tests that measure the process of the performance. Physical fitness tests are good examples of tests that involve quantitative (product) measures. Most physical fitness tests measure products of performance such as the number of repetitions, distance, or time. Product measures like these are easy to observe and score. Tests of motor performance are good examples of tests that measure the qualitative aspect (process) of the performance. Motor performance tests involve observations of how a skill is performed in comparison with some established standards. Observing and scoring the process of a performance typically requires more training and skill on the part of the tester. Testing diving or gymnastic skills are good examples of tests that require the tester to observe the process of the performance, analyze the performance in relation to established standards, and then score the performance on some scale of measurement (i.e., 1 to 10). Because of the complexity and subjective nature of process measures, these tests usually require more training and experience to administer reliably then do product measures.

NORM-REFERENCED TESTS

The third criteria to consider when selecting and evaluating a test instrument is the interpretative value of the data produced by the test. Tests in physical education can be broadly categorized as either norm-referenced or criterion-referenced tests. Norm-referenced tests primarily focus on qualitative (product) measures of students' performance which then are interpreted by comparing the scores measured to established statistics such as age and sex norms. Table 5–1 gives the AAHPERD Youth Fitness Test normative standards for the 50 yard dash test for girls. Normative data, like that presented in Table 5–1, allow the teacher to interpret an individual student's performance in relation to some established standards. For example, a 13-year-old female student runs the 50 yard dash in 8.0 seconds. Using the values in Table 5–1, this student's score is at the fiftieth percentile, which tells the physical educator that approximately half the students of this age and sex in the normative sample ran the 50 yard dash faster.

Table 5–2 shows another form of a normative table taken from the Bruininks-Oseretsky Test of Motor Proficiency. In this example a student's performance score is looked up in the table and translated into an age equivalence score. The age equivalence score is then compared to the student's chronological age. For example, a male student who is 10 years 2 months old obtains a score of 15 on the Bruininks-Oseretsky strength items. Using the values in Table 5–2, this score can be translated into an age equivalence score of 7 years 11 months. This tells the physical education teacher that this student's strength score is equivalent to that obtained by students 2 years 3 months younger than he.

TABLE 5–1. *AAHPERD Youth Fitness Test Norms for the 50 Yard Dash for Girls** (Percentile Scores Based on Age/Test Scores in Seconds and Tenths)

PERCENTILE	AGE								PERCENTILE
	9–10	11	12	13	14	15	16	17+	
100th	7.0	6.9	6.0	6.0	6.0	6.0	5.6	6.4	100th
95th	7.4	7.3	7.0	6.9	6.8	6.9	7.0	6.8	95th
90th	7.5	7.5	7.2	7.0	7.0	7.0	7.1	7.0	90th
85th	7.8	7.5	7.4	7.2	7.1	7.1	7.3	7.1	85th
80th	8.0	7.8	7.5	7.3	7.2	7.2	7.4	7.3	80th
75th	8.0	7.9	7.6	7.4	7.3	7.4	7.5	7.4	75th
70th	8.1	7.9	7.7	7.5	7.4	7.5	7.5	7.5	70th
65th	8.3	8.0	7.9	7.6	7.5	7.5	7.6	7.5	65th
60th	8.4	8.1	8.0	7.7	7.6	7.6	7.7	7.6	60th
55th	8.5	8.2	8.0	7.9	7.6	7.7	7.8	7.7	55th
50th	8.6	8.3	8.1	8.0	7.8	7.8	7.9	7.9	50th
45th	8.8	8.4	8.2	8.0	7.9	7.9	8.0	8.0	45th
40th	8.9	8.5	8.3	8.1	8.0	8.0	8.0	8.0	40th
35th	9.0	8.6	8.4	8.2	8.0	8.0	8.1	8.1	35th
30th	9.0	8.8	8.5	8.3	8.2	8.1	8.2	8.2	30th
25th	9.1	9.0	8.7	8.5	8.3	8.2	8.3	8.4	25th
20th	9.4	9.1	8.9	8.7	8.5	8.4	8.5	8.5	20th
15th	9.6	9.3	9.1	8.9	8.8	8.6	8.5	8.8	15th
10th	9.9	9.6	9.4	9.2	9.0	8.8	8.8	9.0	10th
5th	10.3	10.0	10.0	10.0	9.6	9.2	9.3	9.5	5th
0	13.5	12.9	14.9	14.2	11.0	15.6	15.6	15.0	0

*Reprinted by permission of the American Alliance for Health, Physical Education, Recreation and Dance, 1900 Association Drive, Reston, VA 22091.

CRITERION-REFERENCED TESTS

The second category of assessment instruments commonly used in school improvement programs is criterion-referenced tests. In contrast to norm-referenced tests, which compare students' performance to various statistical standards for interpretation, criterion-referenced tests compare students' performance to established performance criteria. Good criterion-referenced tests focus on both measuring the process (the quality of how a skill is performed) and the products (time, distance, number of repetitions) produced from the performance.

Figure 5–2 gives an example of a criterion-referenced test item from the Elementary Motor Performance Test designed to assess the fundamental motor skill of catching. In this test the teacher administers the test according to the standardized instructions and then observes and scores the students' performance in relation to the established standards. The teacher then records what standards the students can and cannot perform. Figure 5–3 contains a sample score sheet used for this test to record student assessment data on the catch.

COMPARISON OF NORM- AND CRITERION-REFERENCED TESTS

Both norm-referenced and criterion-referenced tests can provide valuable information needed to make accurate classification, placement, and instructional decisions. Norm-referenced and criterion-referenced tests each have unique strengths and weaknesses that directly affect their suitability in various settings

TABLE 5–2.   *Bruininks-Oseretsky Test of Motor Proficiency Age Equivalency Table**

Age Equivalents Corresponding to Subject Point Scores for the Standardization Sample

Age Equivalent (years-months)	Running Speed and Agility	Balance	Bilateral Coordination	Strength	Upper-Limb Coordination	Response Speed	Visual-Motor Control	Upper-Limb Speed and Dexterity	Age Equivalent (years-months)
15–11 +	12–15	29–32	16–20	29–42	—	13–17	23–24	55–72	15–11 +
15–11	—	—	—	—	—	—	—	—	15–11
15– 8	—	—	—	—	—	12	22	—	15– 8
15– 5	—	—	15	28	21	—	—	54	15– 5
15– 2	—	—	—	—	—	—	—	—	15– 2
14–11	—	—	—	—	—	—	—	—	14–11
14– 8	—	—	—	27	—	—	—	53	14– 8
14– 5	—	—	—	—	20	—	—	—	14– 5
14– 2	11	—	—	—	—	—	—	—	14– 2
13–11	—	—	14	—	—	11	—	52	13–11
13– 8	—	28	—	—	—	—	—	—	13– 8
13– 5	—	—	—	26	—	—	—	51	13– 5
13– 2	—	—	—	—	—	—	—	—	13– 2
12–11	—	—	—	—	—	—	21	50	12–11
12– 8	—	—	—	25	19	—	—	—	12– 8
12– 5	—	—	—	—	—	—	—	49	12– 5
12– 2	—	—	—	—	—	—	—	—	12– 2
11–11	—	—	13	24	—	—	—	48	11–11
11– 8	—	—	—	—	—	10	—	47	11– 8
11– 5	—	27	—	—	—	—	—	—	11– 5
11– 2	—	—	—	23	—	—	—	46	11– 2
10–11	10	—	—	—	—	—	—	45	10–11
10– 8	—	—	—	22	—	—	—	—	10– 8
10– 5	—	—	12	—	18	—	—	44	10– 5
10– 2	—	26	—	21	—	—	20	43	10– 2
9–11	—	—	—	—	—	9	—	42	9–11
9– 8	—	—	—	20	—	—	—	41	9– 8
9– 5	—	—	11	19	—	—	—	40	9– 5
9– 2	—	—	—	—	17	—	19	39	9– 2
8–11	9	25	—	18	—	8	—	38	8–11
8– 8	—	—	10	17	—	—	—	37	8– 8
8– 5	—	—	—	—	16	—	18	36	8– 5
8– 2	—	24	—	16	—	—	—	35	8– 2
7–11	—	—	9	15	—	7	17	34	7–11
7– 8	8	—	—	14	15	—	—	33	7– 8
7– 5	—	23	8	—	14	—	16	31–32	7– 5
7– 2	—	—	—	13	—	—	—	30	7– 2
6–11	—	22	7	12	13	6	15	29	6–11
6– 8	7	—	—	11	12	—	14	27–28	6– 8
6– 5	—	21	6	—	—	—	13	26	6– 5
6– 2	—	20	—	10	11	5	12	24–25	6– 2
5–11	6	—	5	9	10	—	—	23	5–11
5– 8	—	19	—	8	9	4	11	21–22	5– 8
5– 5	5	18	4	7	8	—	9–10	20	5– 5
5– 2	—	16–17	—	6	7	—	8	18–19	5– 2
4–11	4	15	3	5	6	3	7	17	4–11
4– 8	3	14	—	4	4–5	—	6	15–16	4– 8
4– 5	—	13	2	3	3	2	5	13–14	4– 5
4– 2	2	11–12	—	2	1–2	1	3–4	12	4– 2
4– 2 –	0–1	0–10	0–1	0–1	0	0	0–2	0–11	4– 2 –

ADMINISTRATION AND SCORING GUIDE

OBJECT CONTROL

Objective: Catch

Equipment/Materials	Directions	Standards	Position	Distance	Comments
Level I 1. 6 in. playground balls—have 3 balls ready to use 2. Measuring tape—to measure 15 ft distance 3. Marking tape—to mark beginning and end of 15 ft distance. **Level II** 1. 2 to 3 in. balls—tennis balls can be used, have 10 balls ready for use 2. Measuring tape—to measure 60 ft and 10 ft distances 3. Marking tape—to mark beginning and end of 60 ft distance; 10 ft area. 10 ft area X ⊢ 60 ft ⊣ X Student Test Administrator	**Level I** 1. Have the student toss a ball to you to catch to demonstrate a mature catch incorporating all the standards 2. Give the student a practice trial 3. Position student 15 ft from you and give a verbal request to catch the ball you toss to them 4. Observe and score student on 3 consecutive catches of balls tossed in required pattern **Level II** 1. Test the student on Level I standards first. If the student achieves all the Level I standards first then proceed to Level II 2. Give the student a demonstration of a mature catch incorporating all the Level I standards by having the student toss a ball to you 3. Give the student a practice trial 4. Position the student 60 feet from you and give a verbal request to catch the ball you toss to them 5. Observe student on 10 consecutive catches and keep count of number of catches made out of 10	**Level I**—The student will catch a 6 in. playground ball tossed gently to the student between waist and shoulder height from a distance of 15 ft as follows:			
		1. Preparatory position with the hands in front of body, elbows flexed and near the sides	Ⓢide⒮ ide	15 ft 15 ft	
			Ⓢ ide	15 ft	
		2. Extension of arms in preparation for ball contact	Ⓢ ide	15 ft	
		3. Contact ball with hands only	Ⓢ ide	15 ft	
		4. Elbows bend to absorb the force of the ball (hands retract at least 6 in.)	Ⓕ ront	60 ft	
		5. Smooth integration of the above standards			
		Level II—The student will catch a 2 to 3 in. ball thrown at least 10 ft high from a distance of at least 60 ft to a point within 10 ft of the student's initial position using a Level I pattern: 1. Ten consecutive times while moving into position on cue from the ball's flight.			
		2. The student will have caught the ball 10 out of 10 times			

Figure 5–2. *Sample criterion-referenced test item.*

ELEMENTARY MOTOR PERFORMANCE TEST

Class Performance Score Sheet: Catch

Page _____

Teachers Name _____

School: _____
Grade: _____ Class: _____
Physical Education Schedule
Days/Week _____ No. of wk/yr _____
Assessment Dates
Code Day/Month/Year
1 _____
2 _____
3 _____
4 _____

Instructions

Record code for assessment date in Level I to indicate when a standard has been achieved. Record actual criterion achieved for Level II.

Testing Procedures:
• Demonstration
• Verbal Request
• Practice Trial
• Percentile Score
 Pre _____
 Post _____

LEVEL I
CRITERION

1	2	3	4	5
Hands in front, elbows flexed	Extension of arms	Contact ball with hands only	Elbows bend absorb force	Smooth integration

LEVEL II
CRITERION

6	7
No. of catches out of 10	Ten out of ten

RESULTS

A	B	C	D	E			
Number of standards achieved on initial assessment date	Number of standards achieved on final assessment date	Difference = B − A			Sex	DOB	Comments

Name

F = Number of Students in Class _____   G = The Sum of Column D: _____   H = Class % Gain = G ÷ F

Figure 5–3. *Sample criterion-referenced score sheet.*

TABLE 5–3. *Comparison of Norm- and Criterion-Referenced Tests*

SELECTION CONSIDERATIONS	NORM-REFERENCED TESTS	CRITERION-REFERENCED TESTS
Validity	"Face" and statistical validity reported.	Face validity (curriculum).
	Dependent on the nature of the item.	Applies to all content.
	Limited to the normative sample.	Applicable to all students.
Reliability	Instructions are usually standardized and tested.	Instructions standardized but usually not tested.
	Measurements are usually simple and objective.	Measurements are more complex and subjective.
	Overall reliability usually high.	Training required to get reliable data.
Administration	Can be individual or group.	Can be individual or group.
	Administration time is variable.	Administration time is variable.
	Test items cannot be modified.	Test items can be modified easily.
	Limited to students similar to the normative sample.	Applicable to all students.
	Content usually limited in scope.	Applicable to all content.
Interpretation	Normative comparisons possible.	Normative comparisons can be made if normative data is collected.
	Indirect implications for instruction.	Direct implications for instruction.
	Limited in scope of content.	Comprehensive scope of content.
	Limited to normative data.	Applicable to all students.

and types of decisions. Physical educators must be able to evaluate and select the right assessment instruments to meet their unique needs.

Table 5–3 compares the various attributes of norm-referenced and criterion-referenced tests. Each of these factors should be considered and weighed when selecting assessment instruments to address different types of decisions.

Is the test valid for the question being addressed? Obviously if a test is not valid there is no need to even consider the other selection factors. The very nature of criterion-referenced tests ensures that they are reasonably valid. Some variability can exist in criterion-referenced tests in regard to the accuracy of the standards employed. The test documentation should be examined carefully to make sure that a rationale is provided for the standards and that the rationale is appropriate.

Norm-referenced tests must be analyzed carefully to ascertain their validity across several dimensions:

1. Do the test items measure what they purport to measure? Many test items in norm-referenced tests depend on prerequisite skills. The standing broad jump, for example, is frequently used as a test for measuring explosive leg strength. This test is dependent on the student being able to perform a functional standing long jump.

2. Are the interpretation statistics (norms) applicable to the students targeted for testing? If the students being tested are not representative (age, sex, IQ, and so forth) of the sample used to create the test norms, then the normative statistics are not applicable and any interpretations made would be invalid.

3. Are the behaviors measured in the test valid for the conclusions that need to be drawn? If the test items measure only strength then conclusions cannot be made regarding muscular endurance, flexibility, or general fitness.

Can the test be administered reliably? Norm-referenced tests tend to be reliable because of the objectivity of the measurements and the standardization of the test instructions. As long as a norm-referenced test can be administered exactly as described in the test manual it should produce reliable data. Criterion-referenced tests on the other hand can be more variable in terms of reliability. The instructions of many criterion-referenced tests have not been extensively field-tested or standardized. In addition, the more subjective nature of the observations used in these tests requires more training and experience on the part of the tester. Acceptable reliability levels can be achieved with criterion-referenced tests as long as the tester is properly prepared to administer the test.

Can the test be appropriately administered? Administrative factors can limit the use of many norm-referenced and criterion-referenced tests. The amount of time required to administer the test and whether the test must be administered individually or whether it can be administered to groups should be checked. Administration times are usually reported in most norm-referenced tests. These reported times should always be considered minimal times. The time required to administer criterion-referenced tests is more variable since it depends on the complexity of the skill and the tester's expertise in observing the components of the skill. The time investment required to administer the test must be weighed against the value of the data provided by the test.

As already stated under the question of validity, norm-referenced tests must be administered exactly as described in the test manual for the normative data to be applicable. This may limit the use of some norm-referenced tests with students who have special needs that require modifications in the instructions or the actual assessment tasks to perform the test. Criterion-referenced tests are more flexible and can be easily modified to accommodate the unique needs of students without threatening the validity of the tests.

One of the strengths of norm-referenced tests is the statistical data provided for interpretation and comparisons of student performance. To use this data, however, the physical education teacher must be sure that the statistical data provided are applicable to the students they are assessing. The normative data for many norm-referenced tests are limited to specific age and sex groups and usually is not applicable to students with special needs. The flexibility of criterion-referenced tests makes them readily adaptable and applicable to all students.

Finally, the scope of skills assessed in norm-referenced and criterion-referenced tests must be considered. The content assessed in norm-referenced tests is fixed and usually very specific, and in physical education focuses mainly on physical fitness. Criterion-referenced tests, however, cover a broader range of content and can be easily adapted to include additional test items. This quality makes them suitable for use with the ABC model since they can be used for all of the objectives delineated in the program plan.

Can the test be interpreted to address the questions being evaluated? This question has already been indirectly addressed in several of the previous questions. The major strength of norm-referenced tests is that they allow teachers to compare students' performances with established statistical norms and interpret how their students compare to other similar students. This type of information can be particularly useful when administering a general needs assessment associated with a classification or placement decision. The major limitation of norm-referenced tests is that they only identify areas of weakness and do not address why the weakness exists. The results of a norm-referenced test might indicate that an 8-year-old male student who runs the 50 yard dash in 10 seconds is at the fifteenth percentile. Although this information clearly indicates that this student's performance is weak, it fails to provide the teacher with any information on why the student's performance is weak. The reason for this is that the norm-referenced test item only recorded information related to the product of the performance and not to the process.

The strength of criterion-referenced tests is that instructional implications can be drawn directly from the assessment data. A criterion-referenced test of running would indicate what components of the mature running pattern a student could and could not perform. The teacher could then analyze what parts of the skill need to be worked on and then prescribe appropriate instruction to address these needs. The major limitation of many criterion-referenced tests is that they lack normative data to allow for age and sex comparisons. If an 8-year-old male student achieved 5 of 8 standards of the run, would that be above average, below average, or average? Although this is a serious limitation of criterion-referenced tests, it can be corrected. Data can be collected and norms established as to when the average student (age and sex) achieves the various standards within a skill. This information is important for setting student expectations and evaluating student performance. Until such norms are created on a national sample, physical educators will need to create their own local norms on the instructional objectives included in their programs.

CONCLUSION

Norm-referenced tests have traditionally been the most commonly used assessment instruments in physical education. These tests have been the tests of choice largely because they are easy to administer and because of the availability of normative data. Unfortunately, norm-referenced tests are frequently used because of tradition and misconceptions regarding their educational merit. As demonstrated in the above analysis, norm-referenced tests are generally limited in the scope of content they assess, who can be legitimately assessed, and the instructional value of the data collected.

Based on the aforementioned analysis, it is clear that criterion-referenced tests should be used more in physical education. The major obstacle to wide-scale use of criterion-referenced tests is probably due to the training needed to administer these tests accurately and reliably. Criterion-referenced tests are representative of the content actually taught in physical education. They can be modified easily to accommodate the unique needs of all students, and they provide results that are directly applicable to instruction. The major limitation of existing criterion-referenced tests is that they lack normative data.

Based on the previous discussion, it is clear that the ideal assessment instrument should measure both the quantitative (products) and qualitative (process) aspects of a student's performance. Criterion-referenced tests meet these criteria and therefore are the tests of choice to be used in the ABC model. As stated previously, many criterion-referenced tests lack normative standards. This limitation, however, can be overcome. First, teachers can establish their own normative standards for the instructional objectives in their program. Although this is the preferred way, several years of data collecting may be required before enough data are collected to establish sound norms. A second and more expedient approach, which can be used while normative data are being collected, would be to identify normative standards from the motor development literature. If

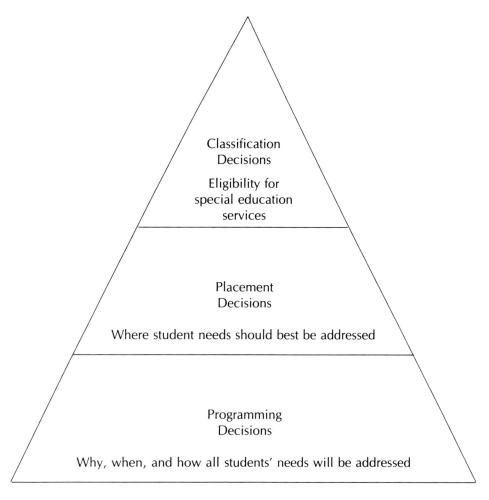

Figure 5–4. *Pyramid of instructional decisions.*

standards cannot be found for all the objectives in the program in the motor development literature, a representative set of standards can be obtained and used until the local standards are developed.

ASSESSMENT DECISIONS IN PHYSICAL EDUCATION

In physical education, there are three major types of decisions that require the use of assessment data. Figure 5–4 illustrates a diagram of these decision categories. The pyramid shape implies the relative frequency with which the different types of decisions are encountered in the public schools. Each of the decision categories is discussed in detail in the sections that follow.

Although the three decision categories discussed later in this chapter are designed to address different questions, they all share some generic assessment procedures. The following general assessment procedures should be considered when conducting any form of assessment.

GENERAL ASSESSMENT PROCEDURES

1. *Know the student:* Physical educators should learn everything they can about their students before making an assessment. Several different sources can provide various types of information. If little information can be obtained about the students from the sources listed below, a screening instrument

like the needs profile, which is discussed in Chapter 3, should be administered before the students are assessed.

(a) Read the students' files and talk to the students' teachers and parents. Specifically find out some of the students' strengths and interests. This information will assist in planning the assessment session and in communicating with the students. Carefully read the students' medical records and identify any potential problem areas or limitations. If the students' medical conditions are a concern, the students' physicians should be contacted and medical clearance obtained prior to conducting the assessment.

(b) Ask the students for their perceptions. Before beginning the assessment ask the students, Do you like physical education? What games and activities do you like to play the most? What games and activities do you like the least? This information can be used to facilitate the testing session by starting with items the students have expressed an interest in and then gradually working into the activities the students have expressed concern over.

(c) Consider the students' unique learning needs. Make sure that there is adequate communication with the students. What if some of the students are nonverbal—how is the teacher going to know the students understand the test items? What if some of the students are visually impaired—how is the teacher going to demonstrate the test items? What are the lengths of the students' attention spans? This will dictate how long the tester can plan to work on any given task. Talking to the students' teachers and parents should provide valuable insights into what preparations need to be made in this area.

(d) Consider the students' unique personal-social needs. The teacher should know how the students react to pressure and failure. Do any of the students act out aggressively or withdraw? What are some of the warning signals that students are under pressure? What are some established procedures that work at home or in the classroom for dealing with these behaviors. As a rule, begin the assessment with tasks the students are likely to be successful with and then gradually increase the difficulty until the students begin to have trouble. This format maximizes the students' success and minimizes their failure, which should facilitate keeping the students focused on the skills targeted for assessment.

2. Prepare the students for the assessment. This applies to both individual and group assessments. For group assessment, students will be more relaxed if they are informed ahead of time what will be happening and why. For individual assessments, the teacher should try to meet the student a few days before the assessment to explain what will be taking place. If such a meeting cannot take place, arrangements should be made to meet the student in the classroom and, while walking to the gym, discuss what is going to take place. The teacher should plan what to say and observe the student to evaluate his or her mood. If the student is extremely nervous or reluctant, some diversions or stops to prolong the introduction and give the student more time to relax could be planned. Finally, it should be determined that the student is not being removed from the classroom during one of his or her favorite activities.

3. Consider how much content can be realistically assessed based on the time available and the students' attributes. Given the limited amount of time that will probably be allotted to conduct many assessments, serious thought should be given to planning the assessment so that the most information is obtained for the time invested. For some students three or four short

assessment periods might be more appropriate and productive than one long period.

4. Make the testing setting as nonthreatening as possible. To young students a large gymnasium filled with equipment can be threatening. The students might immediately react negatively when they enter the gymnasium and see a piece of equipment (high balance beam, trampoline, etc.) they think they are going to be tested on. If possible, reduce the testing space and remove any equipment that will not be used. If equipment cannot be removed, explain to the students as they enter the setting that they will not be using that equipment.

5. Record the students' performance data as quickly and unobtrusively as possible. Use a method of permanently recording the students' performance. Do not depend solely on memory. A variety of recording methods can be used, ranging from a clipboard to tape and video recorders. Explain to the students what is going to be recorded prior to the start of the assessment. If the students are noticeably distracted by the recording process, they should be shown what is being recorded.

PROGRAMMING DECISIONS

The first and most common form of assessment decisions in an ABC model are programming decisions (see Fig. 4–2). Unlike classification and placement decisions, which apply primarily to students with special needs, programming decisions apply to ALL students. Programming decisions address the question of "What specifically do students need to learn on the objectives targeted for instruction?" Instructional decisions are directly related to the assessment component of the ABC model. Although all of the components of the ABC model (plan, assess, prescribe, teach, and evaluate) are necessary and interrelated, assessment at the instructional level is the key to successful implementation of the ABC model. The ABC model will only be successful if accurate assessment data can be obtained. If the assessment data are not collected or are inaccurate, the program implementation phases will all be inaccurate because they are dependent on the assessment phase.

Assessment at the instructional level in the ABC model should be perceived as a continuous process that occurs simultaneously with all instruction in physical education. Too often at the instructional level in physical education, assessment is viewed as a separate time-consuming process that is either rarely administered or administered periodically at the beginning and end of a year or unit of instruction. The purpose of assessment at the instructional level is to provide both the student and teacher with specific information regarding what needs to be learned and how learning is progressing on the targeted objectives.

The reasons commonly offered for not conducting assessments or for employing a pre- or post-instructional assessment in physical education are exemplified by such statements as:

—assessing takes up too much instructional time;

—pre- or post-assessments are the most time efficient to implement; or

—pre- or post-assessments are all that are needed to monitor student performance.

Careful analysis of these arguments reveals that none of them are valid. Although any type of assessment does take time away from instruction, accurate assessment data enables the teacher to use instructional time more efficiently by fine-tuning instruction to meet the unique needs of each student in the class.

The amount of instructional time invested in assessment must also be weighed against the amount and quality of information gained. Pre- or postassessments require only a minimal amount of instructional time to implement and subsequently only provide a minimal amount of useful information. If the post-test data reveal that learning did not occur as planned, something of value has been learned. Unfortunately, the time scheduled for this objective has already been spent, the reasons why learning did not occur are still unknown, and the willingness of the students to continue working on this objective has diminished in the absence of any progress.

The belief that assessment distracts from or wastes valuable instructional time in physical education is a contradiction since appropriate instruction is dependent on continuous assessment. Continuous assessment has the following advantages:

—it relates directly to instruction;

—it provides the teacher with constant feedback regarding student progress and the effectiveness of instruction;

—it allows instruction to be focused on student's specific learning needs (individualized);

—it provides students with specific ongoing feedback regarding their performance;

—it is perceived by students as an integral part of the instructional process and not a punitive or threatening task;

—it maximizes the amount of learning per unit of instructional time;

—it provides the teacher and program with quantitative accountability data; and

—it applies to ALL students' needs.

To reap these advantages, a price must be paid; time spent for preparation. Criterion-referenced tests are the primary assessment instruments used in making programming decisions because they are directly related to the content in physical education, and they can be modified to meet the needs of all students. As discussed earlier in this chapter, however, to use criterion-referenced tests effectively the teacher is required to have more practice and experience. In addition, the teacher must constantly strive to develop innovative ways of combining ongoing assessment with instruction. For example, a teacher might want to focus instruction on three objectives (serve, set, and forearm pass) in a volleyball unit and decide to explain to the students what they should look for in each of the skills targeted for instruction. The students are then divided into small groups and instructed to assess each other. They are then given the responsibility of recording and monitoring their progress on each of the volleyball objectives during the unit. As the teacher works with students throughout the unit, the accuracy of each student's assessment and progress data is verified. At the end of the unit the teacher collects the student progress charts and then may assess each student individually and discuss their progress. This instructional approach to volleyball teaches the students both how to analyze and perform the skills they are being taught. These students are aware of not only what is expected of them, but how it is to be achieved. Instead of having only one set of trained eyes that can provide feedback to 30 students, there are now 31 sets of trained eyes. Although this approach to combine assessment and instruction may take considerably more preparation time to plan and implement, the outcomes far outweigh the investment.

As discussed earlier, instructional assessment is an integral part of the ABC model. To implement assessment at the instructional level in the ABC model involves 4 basic steps: (1) Identification of the content to be assessed; (2) selection and preparation of test items; (3) test administration and data collection; and (4) data organization and interpretation. The procedures associated with each of these steps are discussed in the following sections.

TABLE 5–4. *Sample Achievement-Based Curriculum Unit Plan for Fourth Grade*

Sequential Units	Time (min)	Total Time (min)	Weeks
1. a. Overhand throw	180		
b. Catch	180		
c. Cardiorespiratory	30		
d. Abdominal strength	30	420	7
2. a. Move to uneven beat	180		
b. Accent	180		
c. Cardiorespiratory	30		
d. Abdominal strength	30	420	7
3. a. Accent	180		
b. Cardiorespiratory	60		
c. Abdominal strength	30	270	4.5
4. Basketball			
a. Chest pass	180		
b. Dribbling	180		
c. Cardiorespiratory	45		
d. Abdominal strength	45	450	7.5
5. Softball			
a. Running bases	180		
b. Fielding	180		
c. Cardiorespiratory	15		
d. Abdominal strength	45	420	7
		1,980	33 weeks

STEP 1: IDENTIFICATION OF THE CONTENT TO BE ASSESSED

In an ABC model the content targeted for instruction for any given program level and time of year has been clearly delineated in the program plan. The teacher should review the unit plan and identify which objectives will be worked on first. Table 5–4 shows a sample unit plan for the fourth grade taken from a kindergarten through twelfth grade program plan. From the unit plan in Table 5–4 four objectives have been targeted for instruction in the first unit. These objectives therefore represent the content that needs to be assessed in order to prescribe appropriate instruction.

STEP 2: TEST SELECTION AND PREPARATION

The next task is that of selecting appropriate test items. As discussed earlier, criterion-referenced tests are the preferred tests because they are directly tied to instruction, objectives taught are tested. In addition, through the process of task analysis, criterion-referenced tests can be developed to measure any instructional content and/or modified to assess any degree of ability. Task analysis is a process by which instructional objectives can be broken down into smaller, teachable and measurable units that, when acquired, lead to the attainment of the objective. The following considerations should be addressed when doing a task analysis:

1. The tasks must be simply and clearly stated in observable and measurable terms so that anyone could understand and actually teach the task sequence.
2. The tasks should be sequentially arranged beginning with the lowest ac-

TABLE 5–5. *Task Analysis Checklist*

Instructional Objective: _____

1. What performance level for the objective should be considered as functional competence for the student(s)?

2. Should any of the skill criteria be totally deleted due to specific circumstances (e.g., the weight transfer for overhand throw could appropriately be deleted for a particular student who is in a wheelchair)?

3. Should any skill criteria be added?

4. Should any skill criteria be broken into smaller steps?

5. What subcomponents of the focal points can be identified?

6. Would the performance levels and/or skill criteria be more appropriate if a continuum for degree of assistance was included?
   —Assistance
   —Partial assistance
   —Demonstration
   —Verbal cue
   —No cue

7. Should any of the following performance standards be modified?
   —Distance
   —Number of acceptable repetitions (stability ratio, i.e., 2 out of 3 times)
   —Target size

8. Are the performance levels and skill criteria arranged in an appropriate sequence?

9. Are the size and progression of steps for this objective now appropriate so that measurable gain can be detected?

10. Is the amount of instructional time that must be allotted for the student to achieve functional competence on the objective reasonable?

---

ceptable entry behavior (i.e., with assistance) and ending with the identified exit ability level (i.e., functional competence).

3. The tasks identified should relate only to the important steps.

4. The task sequence should be comprehensive enough to include appropriately sized steps that would facilitate continuous and regular achievement leading to functional competence.

Generally, the processs of task analysis must begin with identifying what will be accepted as functional competence for the particular student(s) on the instructional objective. Once this target performance level has been identified, the skills and/or knowledge the student(s) must have to attain that level must be determined. These skills can be stated in terms of major tasks (skill criteria) to be achieved and then subtasks can be identified. Relationships between tasks should be established, such as the chronological order in which they occur, their interdependence, or whether two or more occur simultaneously.

In the beginning it may seem difficult to develop skill in task analysis. The necessary skills, however, can be learned and mastered with practice. In fact, the teacher may find that the process was intuitively engaged in previously during instruction but never written down. Many unknowns are associated frequently with task analysis. Many times the appropriateness of a given task analysis can be determined for a student only by teaching and evaluating during instruction. Specific guidelines to be used when performing a task analysis on an instructional objective are presented in the checklist in Table 5–5.

Fortunately, many instructional objectives have already been task-analyzed into criterion-referenced test items. Many of these task-analyzed objectives can be found in several of the validated programs listed in the Resources for Teachers section. Teachers are encouraged to select and/or adapt items from these programs rather than engage in the time-consuming work of redeveloping new items for their own program plans.

After the criterion-referenced test items that are going to be used have been identified and modified, appropriate preparations for administering them must be made. In addition to the general assessment procedures discussed earlier in this chapter, the points listed below should be considered when preparing an assessment.

1. Review and study the criterion-referenced test items to be used to measure the objectives. Operationally define all ambiguous terms used to describe movements and/or positions so that they can be consistently interpreted. For example, a term like "almost complete extension of the arm" could be operationally defined as a 30° angle at the elbow or less.

2. Establish how the performance data collected through observation will be recorded. If a score sheet like the I CAN example in Figure 5–5 is used, the teacher must become familiar with it so that data can be recorded quickly and accurately. If it is necessary to read each column heading to recall the standards, a considerable amount of time will be wasted scanning the score sheet and recording the student's performance.

3. Select or design appropriate assessing activities for the class which will allow sufficient opportunity for observation of the students' performance on the objectives being assessed. Table 5–6 shows a sample assessing activity from the I CAN program.

   Regardless of whether an existing assessing activity is selected or one is developed, the following guidelines should be followed:

   a. Select an activity that maximizes student involvement and minimizes the number of students watching the student being assessed. Students waiting to be assessed without any structured activity tend to become restless and frequently disrupt other students in the class. Also, a student's performance on a test may be negatively influenced if the class is observing them.

   b. Organize the class and the assessing activities so that you can move freely to observe all aspects of the skill being assessed and still monitor the class.

   c. Outline the procedures that will be used in observing the students' performances. You should be able to answer the following questions before conducting an assessment:
      —From what distances will you need to observe the various standards of the objective?
      —From what angle or angles do you need to observe the student in order to see all standards of the objective?
      —What standard(s) of the objective will be observed first, second, third . . . ?
      —Approximately how many trials will be needed to completely assess the objective.

Step 3: Test Administration and Data Collection

As discussed, assessment and data collection should be done as efficiently as possible so as not to distract from learning time. Although assessment is directly associated with instruction, the two should be separated during initial and final assessments of student performance on instructional objectives. The purpose of

I CAN

CLASS PERFORMANCE SCORE SHEET
PERFORMANCE OBJECTIVE: Overhand Throw

SCORING

Assessment
X = Achieved
O = Not achieved

Reassessment
A = Achieved
O = Not achieved

FOCAL POINTS
- a Overhand Motion
- b Ball Release
  - a Eyes on Target
  - b Overhand Motion
    - a Arm Exten./Side Orient.
    - b Weight Transfer
    - c Hip and Spine Rotation
    - d Follow Through
    - e Smooth Integration
    - Accuracy
    - Angle of Release 45°

STD.
- 10 ft distance 2/3 times
- 20 ft target at 15 ft 2/3 times
- 2/3 times
- age/sex norm. 2/3 times
- 8 ft. target at 50 ft. 2/3 times

***PRIMARY RESPONSES**
- N • Nonattending
- NR • No response
- UR • Unrelated response
- O • Other (specify in comments)

NAME	1a	1b	2a	2b	3a	3b	3c	3d	3e	4	5	Primary Responses* COMMENTS
1. John J.	O	X	O	O	O	O	O	O	O	O	O	Throws sidearm
2. Katie	X	X	X	X	O	O	O	X	O	O	O	
3. Susan	X	X	X	X	X	X	X	X	X	X	O	Practice accuracy
4. Mark	X	X	O	O	O	X	O	X	O	O	O	Faces target
5. John S.	X	X	X	X	X	X	X	O	O	O	O	Follow through inconsistent
6. Scott	O	O	O	O	O	O	O	O	O	O	O	Throws underhand
7. Judy	X	X	O	X	O	O	O	O	O	O	O	Doesn't look at target
8. Cindy	X	X	X	X	X	O	O	X	O	O	O	Faces target
9. Kirk	X	X	X	X	X	X	X	X	O	O	O	Jerky
10. Joanie	X	X	X	X	O	O	O	O	O	O	O	
11. Larry	X	X	X	X	O	X	X	X	O	O	O	Arm bent
12. Chuck	X	X	O	O	O	O	O	O	O	O	O	Throws underhand or sidearm unless assisted
13. Linda	X	X	X	X	X	X	X	X	O	O	O	Nearly mature
14. Sherry	X	X	O	X	O	X	O	X	O	O	O	Inconsistent beginning position
15. Greg	X	X	X	X	X	X	X	X	O	O	O	Nearly mature

Figure 5–5. *Sample of a completed I CAN class performance score sheet.*

TABLE 5–6. *Sample I CAN Assessing Activity*

I CAN
ASSESSING ACTIVITIES

PERFORMANCE OBJECTIVE: To Demonstrate A Functional Overhand Throw

1. Engage students in overhand throwing activity.
2. While you teach, assess students' entry level status.
3. After sufficient observation, record their status, using the Class Performance Score Sheet.
4. Note which skill level each student has mastered.

5. Observe each student's particular style to determine whether your teaching strategy should involve verbal or nonverbal techniques of communication.
6. Plan lessons according to students' needs and their statuses, based on your physical education goals.
7. Continue to teach and assess students using I CAN Instructional Activities.

Directions	Organization & Materials

Organize the students into stations, with no more than about 4 to 6 per station.
 	
Introduce the overhand throw.
 	
Model the mature overhand throw as defined in the Performance Objective description:
 	
    —extend throwing arm
    —side orientation
    —weight transfer
    —hip and spine rotation
    —follow-through
    —throw smoothly
 	
Tell students: DO THIS. THROW HARD.
 	
Have each student throw at a wall or target.
 	
Physically assist students who do not throw.
 	
At each station the teacher or aide will teach and assess students' performance.
 	
Repeat the activity until all students are assessed, or until students become tired.
	Organization
	
	XXXXX———————————→
	Station 1
	
	XXXXX———————————→
	Station 2
	
	XXXXX———————————→
	Station 3
	
	Materials
	
	Targets
	1 inch masking tape to mark students' position. One 3 to 4 inch ball per station.

initial and final assessment is to determine what the student can and cannot do prior to and/or after instruction. The objective, therefore, should not be taught concurrently while the assessments are being done. This does not mean that a particular activity targeted to be used later as an assessing activity cannot be used prior to assessment. In fact, it may be necessary to do this with many activities to familiarize the students with them. On the days that initial assessment data is collected, however, the teacher should refrain from teaching during that activity. During all other instructional assessments the teacher should assess concurrently during instruction.

General testing procedures should be used to maximize student performance and reduce any factors that might negatively affect performance. Every effort should be made to record the student's performance as quickly and accurately as possible after it is observed. Students should only be given credit for standards they have clearly achieved. If there is any doubt concerning whether a student can perform a standard, the student should NOT be given credit for that standard. In this case the worse that could happen is the student can actually perform the standard and they are successful on the intial instruction. If a student is given credit for a standard he or she cannot perform, future expectations may be unobtainable, which could result in failure. If a student's performance fluctuates considerably, the student's performance should be assessed across several sessions to establish a baseline. The baseline performance profile will provide the teacher with a more accurate picture of what the student's actual performance potential is.

STEP 4:   DATA ORGANIZATION AND INTERPRETATION

The last phase of conducting an assessment is to organize the assessment data into a format that allows for easy interpretation and subsequent prescriptive decisions. Valuable assessment information often is lost or not used because it is poorly organized and cannot be fully interpreted. Although the assessment data could be graphed in a variety of ways to allow for greater interpretation, a well structured data collection form, like the I CAN example in Figure 5–6, is probably the most efficient approach. A well structured score sheet should allow the teacher to observe and analyze the assessment data clearly.

From the assessment data shown in Figure 5–6 the teacher can analyze the individual student's status and set target expectations for both the student and class. The usual method of indicating target expectations is to shade/color in the boxes corresponding to the standards that have been targeted for instruction. After expectations have been established for each student, the teacher can then identify instructional priorities and student groupings based on the patterns of shaded standards depicted on the score sheet. Setting student and class expectations on the objectives targeted for instruction will be discussed in more detail in Chapter 6.

PLACEMENT DECISIONS

The second major type of decision physical education teachers must make are placement decisions. Placement decisions must be considered every time a student's IEP is created or reviewed. PL 94-142 requires that every student with special needs be educated in the most appropriate and least restrictive environment. The intent of the least restrictive environment requirement is to ensure that handicapped children are educated with nonhandicapped students to the maximum extent appropriate. This implies that there should be a continuum of alternative placements available to students with special needs (see Fig. 1–1 and Chapter 1). Placement in an adapted physical education class might be the most appropriate and least restrictive environment for one student, while placement twice a week in a regular physical education class and three times in an adapted physical education class might be the most appropriate for another student.

The concept of a continuum of alternative placements in physical education is commonly misinterpreted in many schools. Instead of a continuum of placements being available in physical education only one (regular) or maybe two (adapted and regular) placements are available. The reasons for these misinterpretations range from simple lack of understanding on the part of teachers and administrators to intentional omissions due to financial factors.

Physical education teachers must become knowledgeable and assume the responsibility for creating optimal alternative placements in their schools. To develop a continuum of alternative placements in many schools, teachers must be:
   —willing to actively participate in IEP meetings;
   —aware of what their responsibilities are in placement decisions;
   —prepared to adequately evaluate students and make appropriate placement decisions;

I CAN

CLASS PERFORMANCE SCORE SHEET
PERFORMANCE OBJECTIVE: Overhand Throw

SCORING

Assessment
X = Achieved
O = Not achieved

Reassessment
A = Achieved
O = Not achieved

FOCAL POINTS

1 a Overhand Motion
   b Ball Release
2 a Eyes on Target
   b Overhand Motion
3 a Arm Exten./Side Orient.
   b Weight Transfer
   c Hip and Spine Rotation
   d Follow Through
   e Smooth Integration
4 Angle of Release 45°
5 Accuracy

STD.

- Overhand Motion — 10 ft distance 2/3 times
- 20 ft target at 15 ft 2/3 times
- 20 ft target at — 2/3 times
- age/sex norm. 2/3 times
- 8 ft. target at 50 ft. 2/3 times

***PRIMARY RESPONSES**

N   • Nonattending
NR • No response
UR • Unrelated response
O   • Other (specify in comments)

NAME	1 a	1 b	2 a	2 b	3 a	3 b	3 c	3 d	3 e	4	5	COMMENTS (Primary Responses*)
1. John J.	O	X	O	O	O	O	O	O	O	O	O	Throws sidearm
2. Katie	X	X	O	X	X	O	O	X	O	O	O	
3. Susan	X	X	X	X	X	X	X	X	X	X	O	Practice accuracy
4. Mark	X	X	O	X	O	X	O	O	X	O	O	Faces target
5. John S.	X	X	X	X	X	X	X	O	O	O	O	Follow through inconsistent
6. Scott	O	X	O	O	O	O	O	O	O	O	O	Throws underhand
7. Judy	X	X	O	X	O	O	O	O	O	O	O	Doesn't look at target
8. Cindy	X	X	O	X	O	X	O	X	X	O	O	Faces target
9. Kirk	X	X	X	X	X	X	X	X	O	O	O	Jerky
10. Joanie	X	X	O	X	X	O	O	X	O	O	O	
11. Larry	X	X	X	X	X	X	X	X	O	O	O	Arm bent
12. Chuck	X	X	O	O	O	O	O	O	O	O	O	Throws underhand or sidearm unless assisted
13. Linda	X	X	X	X	X	X	X	X	O	O	O	Nearly mature
14. Sherry	X	X	O	X	O	X	O	X	O	O	O	Inconsistent beginning position
15. Greg	X	X	X	X	X	X	X	X	O	O	O	Nearly mature

Figure 5–6.   *Completed I CAN class performance score sheet with student expectations shaded.*

—willing to question placement decisions made without their input or without evaluating them.

Positive attitudes and actions like these contribute to the quality of physical education programs for all students. The key to resolving this problem is training teachers to know how to conduct and make appropriate placement decisions. Although this discussion focuses on placement decisions related primarily to students with special needs, the same principles and procedures should be applied to ALL students.

When making a placement decision the teacher's major objective is to determine in what setting the student will have the greatest success in achieving the goals of the physical education program. Although all of a student's strengths and weaknesses should be considered, it is important that the primary reasons for a student's placement in a physical education setting be based on his or her ability to successfully achieve the goals and objectives of that program. Placing a student with special needs in any physical education setting solely for social or other secondary reasons is totally inappropriate. If the IEP committee feels a student should participate in a certain physical education setting for social reasons, then this participation should be in addition to the instructional program provided to address his or her specific physical and motor needs.

A prerequisite for making appropriate placement decisions is an established objective-based program plan that defines the program goals and indicates what content will be taught at the various levels to achieve these goals. With an ABC program plan the necessary foundation for making accurate and justifiable placement decisions exists.

With the general assessment procedures discussed previously, the following points should be considered when making placement decisions. Review the performance objectives scheduled for instruction at the student's targeted placement level. These objectives can be easily identified in an ABC program plan and provide the basis for the content the student should be assessed on. Select a representative sample of objectives to be included in the assessment battery from the pool of identified objectives. It is unlikely that there will be time to assess the student on all the objectives targeted for a given year. The student's performance on a representative sample of objectives should provide sufficient information to predict his or her success in that setting. Both norm-reference and criterion-reference measures should be taken if possible. As discussed in the earlier part of this chapter, criterion-reference measures will probably be the most available and more appropriate.

Conduct the assessment session in a relaxed and nonthreatening manner. Make sure the student understands exactly what is expected of him or her in each test. Allow the student sufficient practice trials to ensure that he or she understands the task. Remember the primary objective is to get a true measurement of performance abilities.

PL 94-142 requires that each student's IEP and the associated placements stated within be evaluated at least once a year. Physical education teachers must play an active role in these evaluations to assure that all students are in the most appropriate and least restrictive physical education placements. To move up the continuum of alternative placements in physical education, each student's ability should be continuously monitored and evaluated. Once a student is placed in an alternative placement, all too often this is seen as a permanent placement for the remaining time the student spends in the program.

CLASSIFICATION DECISIONS

PL 94-142 mandates that students receive 1 of 11 special education classifications prior to receiving special education services. The classification process is initiated by a request or a referral for an evaluation to the school's committee designated to handle this task. The title given to identify this committee varies from state to state. For the purposes of this book the committee will be referred to as the Admission, Review, and Dismissal (ARD) committee since this title implies the committee's purpose. The ARD committee is charged with the responsibility of evaluating students for possible inclusion in special education and for reviewing these decisions at least once every 3 years.

A request for an evaluation can be initiated by any concerned party such as a parent, guardian, teacher, or administrator. Once a request is made, the ARD committee has 30 school days to evaluate the student and make a recommendation. Depending on the student's suspected handicap, the ARD committee appoints an assessment team to evaluate the student and determine what specific special education services are needed. Members of the assessment team will vary in number and areas of expertise depending on what type of need the student has. Committee membership is usually dictated by the criteria needed to qualify for one of the defined conditions. Only rarely will a student qualify for special education services solely because of their needs in physical education. In these cases the student would probably receive the otherwise health-impaired label.

Although physical education teachers are not routinely included on ARD evaluation teams, they should be because physical education is a required content area as delineated in the definition of special education. The input of physical education teachers is particularly relevant when the condition being considered has a significant motor deficit commonly associated with it such as the orthopedic and otherwise health-impaired classifications. In the absence of any formal physical education evaluation, the evaluation committee frequently draws conclusions based on physical and motor data collected from informal observations or from selected motor items in other tests that were administered to the student. The reasons why physical education teachers do not play a more active role in evaluation teams range from lack of understanding on the part of ARD committees to include them to unwillingness and/or inability of physical education teachers to appropriately evaluate, interpret, and report results to these committees. The purpose of this section is to supply the physical education teacher with the necessary knowledge and tools to be a productive member of an ARD evaluation team.

PL 94-142 states that at least two standardized tests administered in the student's native language must be used when making a special education classification. The intent of these requirements is to guarantee that a valid measurement of the student's performance is obtained. Physical education teachers should use both formal and informal observations when assessing students. If norm-reference tests can be appropriately administered, they are recommended because of the interpretative value of the normative data. Unfortunately, norm-reference tests are invalid for many of the students involved in these assessments. In these cases standardized criterion-reference tests should be used and interpretations made based on local standards and developmental landmarks established from the motor development literature.

The major objective in a classification evaluation is to determine if the student's physical and motor needs merit special instructional services in order to learn and make meaningful progress in physical education. The physical education teacher is faced with having to assess the student's performance on a broad range of content in a very short period of time (one or two 45 minute periods). In addition to the general assessment procedures already discussed, the following points should be considered when making a classification decision.

Consider the characteristics of the testing setting and the student's learning and personal-social attributes before beginning an assessment. In most cases a physical education evaluation of this nature is conducted in a one-on-one setting. In many cases the physical education teacher is unable to meet the student prior to the formal assessment. If it can be arranged, however, the teacher should meet the student a day or two before the assessment and explain what will take place the next time they meet. If a meeting cannot be arranged prior to the actual testing, time should be spent at the beginning of the assessment session to explain to the student what is going to take place and generally to relax the student. The teacher should be sensitive to the fact that the student has probably been removed from class several times recently by other strangers and tested intensely. The student might be reluctant and anxious about taking another test.

Consider how much time and content can realistically be assessed in the time available. For example, the teacher might identify performance standards for two key performance objectives within each of the program goal areas (2 physical fitness, 2 body management, 2 locomotor, 2 object control, and 2 body awareness) that are representative of the performance levels of other students of the same age and sex in the program. These 8 performance objectives could then become the basis of the assessment. If the student experienced difficulty on any of these objectives then further testing could be conducted within that given area to determine the student's present achievement level. This format will conserve time and quickly identify the area(s) that need the greatest attention.

In summary, the involvement of physical education teachers in classification decisions is important. It is unfortunate that in order for schools to receive state and federal funds they must label students. Although PL 94-142 does require that each special education student's label be reevaluated at least once every 3 years, there is no way to protect the student from the stereotyping and self-fulfilling prophecies that accompany having a special education label. Physical education teachers must therefore work closely with other educators in the school to make sure that a student's needs and abilities are addressed in making instructional decisions, not the label.

SYNOPSIS

The importance and procedures for conducting student assessments in the ABC model were presented in this chapter. The characteristics of assessment tools were reviewed and analyzed. The merits of norm-referenced and criterion-referenced tests were evaluated and criterion-referenced tests were shown to be the most appropriate form of assessment to be used in the ABC model. Three basic types of assessment decisions commonly faced by physical educators were identified: programming, placement, and classification. General assessment procedures were presented as well as specific guidelines for conducting assessments in the decision areas. Finally, the need for physical education teachers to be adequately prepared and willing to play an active role in student assessment decisions to ensure quality programming for all students was stressed.

RESOURCES FOR TEACHERS

Corbin, C.B.: A Textbook of Motor Development. Dubuque, Iowa, Wm. C. Brown, 1980.
Cratty, B.J.: Perceptual and Motor Development in Infants and Children. Englewood Cliffs, N.J. Prentice-Hall, 1979.
Criterion-Referenced Assessment Kit. (Video and training manual). East Lansing, MI, Instructional Media Center Marketing Division, Michigan State University, 1983.
Dunn, J.M., et al.: A Data-Base Gymnasium. Monmouth, Oregon, Instructional Development Corp., 1980.
Espenschade, A.S., and Eckert, H.M.: Motor Development. Columbus, Ohio, Charles E. Merrill, 1980.
Gallahue, D.L.: Understanding Motor Development in Children. New York, John Wiley and Sons, 1982.

Geddes, D.: Psychomotor Individualized Educational Programs. Boston, Allyn and Bacon, 1981.

McClenaghan, B.A., and Gallahue, D.L.: Fundamental Movement: A Developmental and Remedial Approach. Philadelphia, W.B. Saunders, 1978.

Stein, J.U.: Norm and criterion-referenced tests: A pragmatic approach. American Corrective Therapy Journal, *31*:144–147, 1977.

Thomas, J.R.: Motor Development During Childhood and Adolescence. Minneapolis, Burgess Publishing Co., 1984.

Wessel, J.A. (Ed.): I CAN Instructional Resource Materials: Criterion-Referenced Assessment
   I CAN Preprimary Motor and Play Skills. East Lansing, MI, Instructional Media Center Marketing Division, Michigan State University, 1980.
   I CAN Primary Skills. Northbrook, IL, Hubbard, 1976.
   I CAN Sport, Leisure and Recreation Skills. Northbrook, IL, Hubbard, 1979.

Wickstrom, R.L.: Fundamental Motor Patterns. Philadelphiia, Lea & Febiger, 1983.

Williams, H.G.: Perceptual and Motor Development. Englewood Cliffs, NJ, Prentice-Hall, 1983.

Winnick, J., and Short, F.: The Physical Fitness of Sensory and Orthopedically Impaired Youth. Brockport, N.Y. State University College, 1982.

Zaichkowsky, L.D., Zaichkowsky, L.B., and Martinek, T.J.: Growth and Development. St. Louis: C.V. Mosby, 1980.

ACTIVITY 5–1. Establishing assessment reliability with criterion-referenced tests.

Objective: To practice and develop good assessment reliability using selected criterion-referenced test items.

Materials: Films and/or videotapes of children performing various instructional objectives in the ABC program plan (i.e., locomotor, object control skills, etc.). Films and videotapes are listed in the chapter resources for teachers.

A projector/videoplayer to present the films preferably one with slow motion and stop action capability.

Criterion-reference test items and score sheets that correspond to the skills presented in the films become worksheets for this activity.

WORKSHEET 5–1

Directions:
1. Have the members of the group review the performance standards and score sheets of the objectives they are going to observe on the films.
2. Have the members discuss and define any ambiguous terms used in the standard descriptions.
3. Have the group observe each skill performance three times and assess/record the performance observed on their score sheets. Repeat for each skill on the film.
4. Rewind the film and show the first clip. Summarize the group's composite ratings on the chalk board. Identify the standards that should have been awarded. Have members discuss why they did or did not award certain standards. Repeat the clip in slow motion/stop action to clarify any questions regarding the performance. Repeat this procedure for each clip.
5. Have the group discuss common assessment problems encountered in assessing students on the film and how these problems could be adjusted for in an actual assessing situation.

Variations:
1. Have the group practice independently assessing various film clips and then test them for accuracy and reliability on a novel set of related film clips.
2. Divide the group into subgroups of 3 to 4 members. Have the subgroups simultaneously observe the same child performing a skill and assess the performance independently. Then have the members compare their results, identify any discrepancies, and discuss why they might have occurred.

ACTIVITY 5–2.	Identifying established motor development normative standards that support criterion-referenced test items.
Objective:	To review the motor development literature and identify age and sex performance standards for select instructional objectives that have been task-analyzed into criterion-referenced test items.
Materials:	Existing criterion-referenced test items and/or task-analyzed instructional objectives that correspond to the content in the ABC program plan such as I CAN.
	Access to a library with books and journals in the area of motor development. Worksheet 5–2.

WORKSHEET 5–2

Directions:	1. Have each member of the group select a specific program objective that he or she will be responsible for investigating.
	2. Have members identify criterion-referenced tests and/or task analyze their program objectives into skill levels, sequential instructional objectives, with performance standards. To help with this task I CAN performance objectives can be reviewed and/or revised as needed.
	3. Have the members then decide on which standards they are going to review the literature to identify age and sex standards. For example, if one of the I CAN objectives was being used, an individual might decide to focus on only the standards in skill level 3 since they correspond to the components of the mature pattern.
	4. Have each member investigate and then report his or her findings to the group. Have the group share the problems they encountered and any good sources of information they found.
Variations:	1. The team members evaluate the accuracy of the standards they have found by testing them on a representative sample of students. Members can estimate age and sex standards prior to testing.
	2. Develop standardized criterion-referenced normative standards for a school or school district
	• With the objectives selected for the program plan divided into skill levels, sequential instructional objectives, specify standards of performance for each skill level and the number of learning tasks (criteria). Identify grade level expectancies for students to achieve these learning tasks for each skill level. A sample worksheet is provided to accomplish this task.
	• Conduct a survey. Use one school or school district and the teachers. Have the teachers evaluate the content (skill levels and standards of performance) for each objective. These initial data identify the scope and sequence of the program plan and student expectancies. Using these objectives as criterion-referenced tests, schools or a school district can assess a sample of students and generate standardized criterion-referenced norms.

WORKSHEET 5–2. *Essential Objectives, Content (Learning Tasks) and Expected Grade Level for Achievement*

Program Goal: Demonstrate functional competence on selected fundamental motor skills

Program Objective: Demonstrate a functional overhand throw

	INSTRUCTIONAL OBJECTIVES				
SKILL LEVEL	CONDITIONS		EXPECTED GRADE LEVEL ACHIEVEMENT	OBSERVABLE, MEASURABLE STUDENT BEHAVIORS STANDARD(S): CRITERION USED TO EVALUATE PERFORMANCE	LEARNING TASKS NUMBER
	DIRECTIONS	EQUIPMENT			

Reproduce as needed

ACTIVITY 5–3. Task analysis of instructional objectives.

Objective:	To practice task analyzing instructional objectives into developmentally sequenced steps that can be observed and measured.
Materials:	The task analysis checklist presented in Table 5–5.
	A sample task analysis of an instructional objective to use as a model. Any task analysis can be used for the model. Several sources containing task analyzed objectives, like I CAN, are presented in the Resources for Teachers section in this chapter. Worksheet 5–3.

WORKSHEET 5–3

Directions:	**1.** Have the group review and discuss the sample task analysis. Using an I CAN example, the group might observe that the objective was first divided into skill levels and then standards identified within each skill level.
	2. Divide the group into subgroups of 3 or 4 members and have each subgroup select an instructional objective to task analyze.
	3. Using the checklist in Table 5–5, have the group identify and discuss what criteria must be included in each task analysis.
	4. Have the members in each subgroup develop their task analyses of their objective independently. If time permits, encourage the members to review already existing task analyses of their objective and/or observe children performing their objective to substantiate their standards.
	5. Have the subgroups share their individual task analysis within the subgroups. Encourage the individual members to defend their standards even if they are different from the rest of the group.
	6. Have each subgroup develop a composite task analysis for the subgroups' objective based on the groups' discussion.
	7. Have each subgroup present and share their task analysis with the other subgroups.
Variations:	**1.** Have the group discuss how the task analysis of various objectives could be adjusted to accommodate students with different handicapping conditions.
	2. If the task analyses are developed independent of external sources during the above exercise, have the groups compare their final products with some that already exist.

ACTIVITY 5–4.   Creating a general needs assessment test based on an ABC program plan.

Objective: To develop a functional general needs assessment instrument for various program levels of the ABC program plan that can be employed when making placement and/or classification decisions.

Materials: A completed ABC program plan as described in Chapter 4.
Worksheet 5–4.

WORKSHEET 5–4

Directions:
1. Have the members of the group review their program plans and determine how many different needs assessment instruments might be needed to cover the various levels of their programs. For example, two different instruments may be needed for a kindergarten through 6 program level. The first would be designed to cover the kindergarten through 3 content and the second the 4 to 6 content.
2. Have the group discuss and identify the parameters in which the test will be used: amount of time that will be available for the assessment, type of testing setting, equipment and facilities, and so forth.
3. Divide the group into smaller subgroups of 4 or 5 members and have each subgroup identify what content they will include in their needs assessment instruments.
4. Using one member's program plan, have each subgroup develop a prototype needs assessment instrument for one of the identified program levels. Have the subgroups outline in detail:
   • the sequence in which the test will be administered;
   • how the student's performance will be observed and recorded during the assessment;
   • the organization of the testing setting and the equipment needed;
   • the time required for each test item;
   • how the student will be introduced to the test and handled during the testing; and
   • how the assessment data will be interpreted.
5. Have each subgroup present and explain their needs assessment instrument to the rest of the groups. Have the entire group discuss the relative merits of each instrument.

Variation:
1. Have the group identify several existing needs assessment instruments they feel would be appropriate to use with the ABC model and have them contrast and evaluate these instruments.

ACTIVITY 5–5. Identifying and evaluating student referral procedures used in local schools.

Objective: To explore and understand how different school districts handle student referrals.
Materials: Worksheet 5–5.

WORKSHEET 5–5

Directions:
1. Divide the group into subgroups of 4 or 5 members and assign each group a different school district.
2. Explain to the group the basic protocols that should be followed when setting up a school visitation, conducting an interview, and following up a visit.
3. Have the group identify what questions each subgroup should address when investigating the referral procedures in their school district (especially any specific questions related to how physical education teachers are involved).
4. Have the subgroups actually investigate the referral procedures used in the various school districts they have been assigned.
5. Have each subgroup report to the entire group the procedures they found in their school district. Have the entire group discuss the relative merits of the procedures of each school district.

Variation:
1. Have the group outline the ideal referral system before they complete the above exercise. Then have the group contrast their system with the systems found in the local school districts.

CHAPTER 6

Instructional Planning

What is Instructional Planning?
Instructional planning is teacher decision-making behaviors, before, during, and after instruction to ensure students' success in achieving desired learning outcomes.

How is it Done?	Decision Aids
1. Preassessing students.	Unit lesson objectives: criterion-referenced tests
2. Setting student and class expectancies on objectives to be taught and tested.	Prior available students' data Students' preassessment data Time needed for meaningful gain Time allotted for instruction
3. Prescribing instructional and management strategies for students and class.	Instructional procedures Explicit presentation of lesson Practice Feedback and reinforcement Time-on-task —organizing activities —selecting activities —smooth activity transitions —use of staff including peer tutors and peer teams
4. Teaching and managing time effectively.	Unit lesson plans Preplanning and preparation Structured lesson plans

5. Monitoring and recording student achievement.	Class performance score sheets
	Summary records
	   Unit lesson plans
	    Yearly program plan

6. Reassessing, recording, and modifying the prescription.	Class performance score sheets Lesson plans

---

QUALITY INSTRUCTION: A PERSPECTIVE

No universal prescriptions exist that are appropriate for all students, content, classes, schools, or districts. Rather, our review of research on effective class instruction and experiences points to two indicators of quality instruction focused on student achievement. One indicator highlights two sets of characteristics of quality instruction. These are student and teacher behaviors that are directly linked to improved student achievement. The other indicator is an instructional planning model: teacher decision-making before, during, and after instruction to meet students' needs.

STUDENT AND TEACHER BEHAVIORS: QUALITY INSTRUCTION

What students do in class is directly related to students' achievement. Specifically, three important student behaviors impact on student achievement. These are: (1) *student involvement,* amount of active learning time the student is engaged in learning the objectives of the lesson; (2) *objectives taught and tested,* the content presented by the teacher and tested to determine student achievement; and (3) *student success,* the extent to which the student achieved assigned learning tasks, objectives taught. These three student behaviors are easily observed, readily monitored, and can provide a basis or checklist for teachers to examine their own behaviors in their classes.

What teachers do in their classes impacts on students' achievement, and many teacher behaviors affect student behaviors. The important teacher behaviors fall into three categories: planning, managing, and instruction. Teachers are most effective when they plan, manage, and instruct in ways that keep their students involved in learning the lesson objectives and successfully covering objectives of the lesson. These categories are not new. The challenge now is to plan, teach, and manage time effectively. Examples of teacher behaviors impacting on the three key student behaviors related to student achievement are outlined below:

1. Involvement. Student involvement is the amount of time students spend actively engaged in learning specific lesson objectives. Involvement is a function of allotted instructional time for lesson objectives as determined by the teacher and the time the student is actively engaged in learning—time on task.

Variables	*Examples of Teacher Behaviors*
Amount of time allotted for students to spend on specified lesson objectives.	Instructional time for each objective of the lesson specified.
	Evidence of preparation and preplanning in accord with objectives of the program.
Amount of time students are actively engaged in learning the lesson objectives in the time allotted: time on task.	Maintain purposeful activity in a class climate of mutual respect.
	—Protection of allocated time from necessary disruptions
	—Control of disruptive student behaviors
	—Motivate students to improve performance
	—Feedback and positive reinforcement
	—Explicit presentation of lesson objectives
	—Monitor student performance
	—Keep records and reports information
	—Elicit student participation in planning, conducting, monitoring, and evaluating their performance

2. Objectives Taught and Tested. The appropriateness of the scope and sequence of lesson objectives taught are determined in two ways. First, the objectives covered are appropriate, given student's prior learning. Does the student, prior to beginning instruction, have the prerequisites necessary to learn the new skill? Second, the objectives of the lesson are appropriate, given the achievement test that is used by the teacher to judge student achievement. This is referred to as criterion-related instruction.

Variables	*Examples of Teacher Behaviors*
Prior learning of students	Gathering students' prior data: previous achievement tests and records.
—Prerequisite skills of lesson objectives to be taught	
—Health and safety conditions	
—Students' learning characteristics—record of previous learnings	
Preassessment of students' performance on lesson objectives to be taught.	Preassessing students on each new lesson objective taught; assigning learning tasks; setting class expectancies.
Established sequence of instructional objectives, continuous progress.	Program objectives for each program goal placed in appropriate program level and sequenced yearly in the program plan.
Students' achievements are based on lesson objectives taught.	Criterion-related instructional objectives used to evaluate student and class achievement on objectives, and content taught.

3. Success. Student success refers to the extent to which students achieve assigned learning tasks on objectives and content to be taught.

Variables	*Examples of Teacher Behavior*
Success rate appropriate for students to achieve assigned learning tasks: —daily work —unit —periodic review on a regular basis (weekly, monthly).	Evaluates success levels needed in daily work. Task-analyzing and breaking down difficulty levels of assigned learning tasks or conversely increasing difficulty.
Time needed for high proportion of students to demonstrate meaningful achievement on objectives taught.	Criteria for student performance are established and expectancies set. Evaluates students' achievements in line with objectives of the program. Keeps records of student and class performance scores.

Teachers are most effective when they plan instruction, integrating critical student and teacher behaviors on a day-by-day basis. In the next discussion, attention is focused on such a teaching planning model.

INSTRUCTIONAL PLANNING MODEL: TEACHER DECISION-MAKING

A number of teacher planning models describe planning as a process of selecting lesson objectives, diagnosing learner characteristics, and selecting appropriate instructional and management strategies. Many teachers, however, do not consider these factors during the planning process. Most often they focus their attention on activities or tasks they presented to the class, rather than on instructional objectives of the lesson.

An Achievement-Based Curriculum (ABC) Model is a teaching-planning model that involves teacher decision-making before, during, and after instruction. Teachers' attention is focused on those important student behaviors affecting student achievement. The ABC model helps teachers orchestrate and integrate their behaviors that affect the behaviors of their students. It also provides a process for teachers to continually assess the appropriateness of their instructional and management strategies and modify those strategies when their students' behavior indicates that modification is needed. Figure 6–1 illustrates the sequential, yet cyclic, decision-making process of the model when implemented on a day-by-day basis.

Preassessment, prescription, and teaching decisions are discussed in the next sections.

PREASSESSMENT

Preassessment implies procedures used to assess students' performance on the objectives of the unit before instruction begins. Preassessment procedures are designed to (1) determine whether students have prerequisite skills for instruction to follow; (2) determine whether any student already has the skills and may omit any of the objectives; (3) prescribe appropriate instructional activities; and (4) evaluate the effectiveness of instruction at the end of the unit.

PRIOR STUDENT DATA

Prior student data can help teachers carefully plan, prescribe, and teach. One source of student data is a student progress record, which is a cumulative school record of the student's achievement on previously taught objectives in the program plan. A second source is a checklist such as the needs profile discussed in Chapter 3. Another valuable source of information is a Teacher Tip Sheet that identifies instructional procedures that worked successfully with a student. Table

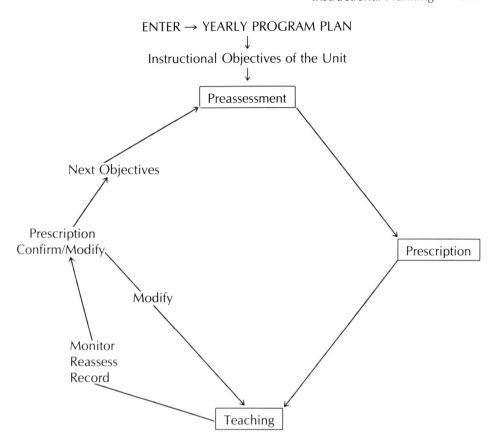

ENTER → YEARLY PROGRAM PLAN
↓
Instructional Objectives of the Unit
↓

Figure 6–1. *Instructional planning model: teacher decision-making before, during, and after instruction.*

6–1 is an example of a Teacher Tip Sheet. A third source of data is health records. The school nurse and other medical personnel may be alerted to any specific health problem, medication, safety conditions, special prosthetic devices or equipment needs. A medical or health record form may be placed in the student's file recommending specific adaptations in activities, environmental conditions, or need for rest and time-out procedures.

ASSESSMENT OF STUDENT'S PERFORMANCE: PRIOR TO INSTRUCTION

This type of assessment evaluates students' mastery of instructional objectives of the unit prior to instruction. It measures students' performance at each skill level and specifies specific skill elements or criteria that the student achieved. For example, in Figure 6–2 assessment data are recorded on an objective-based performance score sheet for the overhand throw. In Figure 6–2, Chuck B's preassessment data show that he has achieved three of the skill mastery criteria for skill level I. Lynn D. has achieved one for skill level I.

Extensive preassessment is most important when beginning a unit of instruction and the instructor is unfamiliar with students' backgrounds and skills. When teachers have the same students for a semester, a year, or longer, extensive preassessment for each unit may be unnecessary. A short or modified preassessment technique can be used to indicate the general level of a student's performance on objectives of the unit. Rather than assessing the learning tasks in each skill level, teachers assess the skill levels of the students. The same performance score sheet as shown in Figure 6–2 is used to record this type of assessment data. Record dates or X's in the shaded skill level column the student

TABLE 6–1. *An Example of a Teacher Tip Sheet*

| Student _____ | Teacher _____ |
| Class _____ | Date _____ |

Student needs

1. _____ frequent change of activity to keep attending.

2. _____ support of one other student or peer group to complete tasks.

3. _____ demonstration, modeling of skill.

4. _____ very specific small steps to achieve success in daily work.

5. _____ encouragement to follow a routine schedule in reporting back for extra help.

6. _____ abundant amount of praise reinforcement in daily work.

7. _____ additional time to achieve certain skills—responds well with parent communication.

Student likes

8. _____ being chosen to make small formal presentations to the class.

9. _____ short, intense activities, such as running.

10. _____ performance contracting to work on learning tasks with partner or in a small peer-group.

is to work on. If a student has none of the criteria for level I, put a O in this column, or leave it blank, indicating the need for prerequisite skills. These students may require teachers to task-analyze the objective for the student to enter skill level I.

Using assessment procedures described in Chapter 5, the teacher selects instructional activities that incorporate the objectives of the lesson. Another example of an instructional assessing activity is provided in Table 6–2.

Peer groups also have been effective in recording the assessment data for students making up the group. Teachers pull the performance score sheets for each objective of the unit. These sheets can be attached to a clipboard, put in a notebook, or enlarged and placed on the wall—any way that enables the teacher or the peer group to have easy access to the skill criteria for the objective and for recording data. Some teachers have the unit lesson plan on the wall, clearly identifying objectives to be taught, as well as class and student expectancies.

THE PRESCRIPTION

Data gathered from preassessments provide teachers with information for prescribing effective instruction. Knowing where the students are on the objectives to be taught, the next decision-making questions are: "Where do I want the students to go?" "How do I get them there?"

Testing Procedures: —Demonstration —Verbal Request —Practice Trial									School: __North__ Grade: __4__ Class: __Brown__ Physical Education Schedule Days/Week __2__ No. of wks/yr __33__ Assessment Dates Day/Month/Year 23/9/'83				
	LEVEL I CRITERION					**LEVEL II** CRITERION		**RESULTS**					
Scoring: Entry Level X = Achieved O = Not Achieved Reassessment X = Achieved O = Not Achieved	Side orientation, weight rear leg	Arm extension behind body to initiate throw	Step in opposition, rotation	Follow-through	Smooth integration	No. of target hits out of 10	10 out of 10 hits	Number of standards achieved on initial assessment date	Number of standards achieved on final assessment date	Difference = B − A Total learning tasks gain			Instructions Record assessment date in Level I to indicate when a standard has been achieved. Record actual criterion achieved for Level II.
Name	1	2	3	4	5	6	7	A	B	C	D	E	Learning Task Assigned / Comments
1. Jay B.	X	X	X	X	X	3/10		6					7
2. Chuck B.	X	X	X	O	O			3					4,5
3. Lynn D.	X	O	O	O	O			1					2,3
4. Steve D.	X	X	X	X	O			4					5,6
5. Ann E.	X	X	O	O	O			2					3,4,5
6. Johnny F.	X	X	X	X	X	2/10		6					7
7. Susan K.	X	X	O	O	O			2					3,4,5
8. Christine L.	X	X	X	O	O			3					4,5
9. Jeff N.	X	X	X	X	O			4					5,6
10. Doug. N.	X	X	O	O	O			2					3,4,5
11. Etc.													

Figure 6–2. *Class Performance Score Sheet: Preassessment data on overhand throw. Students' achievement, average gain of 1 or more learning tasks, class expectancies set at 90% of all students.*

TABLE 6–2. *An Example for Directed Instruction Assessing Activity: Overhand Throw*

	CLASS PERIOD _____
ASSESSING ACTIVITIES	TEACHER _____
	DATE _____

PERFORMANCE OBJECTIVE	INSTRUCTIONAL ACTIVITIES
1. Overhand Throw	Organize the students into stations, with no more than about 4 to 6 per station.
	Introduce the overhand throw.
	Model the overhand throw as defined in the Performance Objective description:
Organization	—extend throwing arm
	—side orientation
XXXXX ⟶	—weight transfer
Station 1	—hip and spine rotation
	—follow-through
XXXXX ⟶	—throw smoothly
Station 2	
	Tell students: DO THIS. THROW HARD.
XXXXX ⟶	Have each student throw at a wall or target.
Station 3	
	Physically assist students who do not throw.
	At each station the teacher or aide will teach and assess students' performance.
Materials	Repeat the activity until all students are assessed, or until students become tired.
Targets	
1 in. masking tape to mark students' positions. One 3 to 4 in. ball per station.	

LEARNING SKILLS TASKS AND STUDENT EXPECTANCIES

By specifying learning tasks for students and setting class expectancies, teachers determine what kind of learning outcomes are expected for a given unit of instruction. Determining these learning outcomes maximizes the efficiency and effectiveness of prescribing, implementing, and evaluating instruction. Teachers will have information to answer two important questions: "How can I tell the difference between successful and unsuccessful students?" and "What instructional procedures worked or did not work in getting this objective across to my students?"

Instructional objectives specify learning tasks in observable, measurable, sequential student behaviors. As illustrated in Figure 6–2, for example, one or more learning tasks for each student with class expectancies set at 90% and individual assignment of tasks and number to be achieved specified on score sheet.

Initially, teachers may use time estimations as determined for the objectives in the program plan. With implementation of the program, teachers gather student performance data along with time required for mastery of the objectives.

With these data, teachers have the prior information to set the criteria for student performance. In some schools, the essential objectives are used to assess all students. With these data, expectancies are set grade by grade or by multigrades, such as end of the third grade, end of the seventh grade, and end of the tenth. On a regular time interval, these expectancies are reexamined using student data collected from the class performance score sheets.

Two important factors should be considered to make these determinations: student success and teacher and student involvement. Student success refers to the extent to which students can complete the learning tasks assigned to them. Student success is one of the most important of all instructional variables. Students differ in amount of success they need during daily work. Success levels vary with student characteristics in learning. For example, students with low motivation and fear of failure may do best when their success rate is 90% or better, and worst when the success rate is below 60%. Conversely, students with high motivation and low fear of failure may perform well at 60% and worst at a 90% success rate. Success in assigned learning tasks is a great morale-building process for both the individual student and for the class as a whole.

Student and teacher involvement in finalizing these determinants is based on the "best fit" between student and teacher objectives in instruction. Procedures to involve students can be done in the large class group, small class group, or by a frank inteview with individual students. These activities also provide a format to elicit the student's own objectives and interests, and to open discussion of their relationships to those in instruction. In using these procedures, the teachers must first decide whether or not students should be involved and the procedures identified and followed. The involvement of individual students, teams, or the class may be carried through in the prescription of activities, monitoring, assessing and recording assessment data, individualizing instruction, and evaluating effectiveness of instruction.

INSTRUCTIONAL PROCEDURES

Extensive coverage of instructional and management strategies are beyond the scope of this book. Five broad areas of teacher behaviors are presented with some examples of effective instructional procedures. The examples are directly related to student achievement variables. Because motivation for learning and class management techniques are critical to increase student involvement, they are treated in more depth in the next chapter. The five broad areas include:

1. Clarity of Presentation: Explicit, Understandable, Task-Related
2. Practice of Skills: Guided and Independent
3. Positive Feedback and Corrective Procedures
4. Maximizing Instructional Time: Time-On-Task
5. Effective Use of Staffing

The appropriateness of the selected instructional and management strategies is continually tested in daily instruction and effectiveness determined by students' mastery of a unit's content and instructional objectives.

Clarity of Presentation: Explicit, Understandable, Task-Related

This area involves teacher behaviors in the introduction and development of the objectives of the lesson taught to the whole class. The importance of a structured lesson, with an introduction and an explanation of what is to be learned, cannot be overemphasized. The first behavior is the teacher's overview of the lesson. This includes a review of previously learned skills with an explanation of the what and why of the lesson. Next is the teacher's explanation of the skills to be learned. This explanation is verbal and nonverbal—a demonstration of the skills to be learned. It is during the explanation that students need to actively respond to the explanation. It is what the student does, not what the teacher does, that will determine the learning outcome. Students need to demonstrate their initial understanding of the skills to be learned. They do this by responding to oral questions and demonstrating their answers. All questions/ answers and demonstrations must be task-relevant to the instructional objective. The teacher continually provides positive feedback and corrective procedures, explaining correct answers or demonstrating correct skill.

The explanations, directions, and demonstrations are instructional cues. These cues focus students' attention on the skills to be learned. An effective and clear cue elicits the intended student response. If teachers speak too rapidly, use vocabulary beyond the grasp of the students, or if students are placed so they cannot see or hear the teacher, the cue is ineffective. Some students learn more easily with verbal cues; others respond more readily to nonverbal cues such as modeling, demonstrating, or physical manipulation. Teachers need to use a variety of cues, which should be used spontaneously in instruction as the need arises, and adapted to individual needs. When students have developed an initial understanding of the lesson, they are ready to practice what they have learned. Drill and practice are other forms of instructional cues.

Practice of Skills: Guided and Independent

Students must know the objectives of each practice session. Practice sessions must be guided and one or two tasks completed under close supervision before they are ready to work independently. Student practice time is most effective when directions are clear and specific and the students know they are accountable for completing their tasks within the required practice time. Students must be provided adequate opportunity to practice and reinforce newly acquired skills. When specific skills are used in a variety of game situations, practice should be provided in each one. For example, after learning the skill of overhand throw, the student should practice throwing different distances, at various targets, and in a variety of game situations. After initial skill acquisition, periodic reviews should be scheduled regularly (weekly, monthly) and structured to be sure students maintain the skills.

Grouping for practice may take many different forms. Alternative grouping formats can help improve practice. One approach that has been used is team-assisted, individualized instruction, teams consisting of students working together on different learning tasks of the objective. These groups are heterogeneous. This approach provides incentives for students to learn by helping one another. It also helps students accept individual differences. The positive effects of teamwork, with the benefits of assigned learning tasks for members of the team, are an effective strategy to individualize instruction and increase active learning time.

Team groups are another aspect of learning center stations. Each team is assigned a space for their learning center. Ideally, the learning center is designed for small team groups or it can be used by individual students doing independent work assignments. The learning center should include the following components: skill criteria for objective to be learned; direction for practice activities; equipment needed for size of group; assessment record of performance: team graph or score sheet; and individual team member's score sheet.

The learning center is used by students incorporating the important processes of making choices and decisions and being responsible for their work. Students can be encouraged to create their own activities at a center in consultation with the teacher.

The team learning center approach provides a structure that allows flexibility of student response. Students work at different speeds on different tasks toward the same objective. The tasks are concrete, discrete, and short. The teams decide when they have successfully completed the tasks assigned each member and if they are ready to move on to the next task. As a team, they can be rewarded for their overall progress. Points can be awarded for each member's achievement. Teams can graph their progress by recording the total number of standards achieved initially and the number achieved each week or at other specified intervals in the unit. A team class performance score sheet can be designed for recording team results on assigned instructional objectives.

The teacher's role is to prepare the learning center stations for the lesson objectives; introduce objectives to the students, explain how equipment is to be used in the space available, where equipment is kept, and where to put equipment; and record results of their work. The teacher continually guides the students in their team work, and assesses or helps them assess and record what they have learned as a team and what each individual member has achieved.

At the same time the teams are working at the learning center stations, teachers may be working with small groups of students of similar abilities. These groups work directly under supervision of the teacher. This provides an opportunity for teachers to help students working on similar tasks, from the highest to the lowest skill abilities. The students are pulled from the team group by teachers according to their abilities. Students stay in a group for one or two objectives. As objectives change, students are reassigned to different team—heterogeneous groups, and teacher-like-ability groups.

This combined approach, guided practice and drills by team and teacher groups, offers several other advantages. It helps build group cohesiveness, establishing learning emphasis and developing positive teacher-student and student-student relationships. In this approach the teachers share responsibility with the students for planning, monitoring, assessing, and recording. It provides an opportunity for teachers to spend time with small groups or individual students. It also provides a class structure for continual peer reinforcement regardless of student ability level and helps establish a system for students' accountability for their behaviors and performances.

Positive Feedback and Corrective Procedures

Task-related feedback and corrective procedures are the most important teacher behaviors. For these procedures to be effective, the predetermined instructional objective, the specific skill criteria to be mastered, is known. Students know when their performances are correct or incorrect. In initial learning of new skills the teacher continually provides feedback as to whether the students' performances are correct. The feedback for correct performance must be for actual achievement of the specific skill criteria for the assigned learning tasks. When students' performances are incorrect, information must be given to correct them. Corrective procedures are always constructive, there are no negative connotations. Teachers need to explain and demonstrate the correct performance, ask students questions, and have them demonstrate their understanding.

Feedback and corrective procedures help students gain self-confidence in their ability to learn. They also generate greater student interest and motivation to learn. Students realize they are capable of learning and teachers and peers expect them to learn. Success in performing daily assigned learning tasks is a positive feedback, a reward. Students making little or no improvement need the objective task analyzed, broken down into smaller units of improvement, for success. For example, in the overhand throw, a smaller unit of improvement in skill level might be a gradual increase in distance thrown to reach the required distance of 40 feet for achievement; or students may need a different reward for successful performance. Students must find their success rewarding if their performances are to be reinforced. For example, the reward may be changed: free choice of activities, demonstration in front of the class, peer tutor status.

Maximizing Instructional Time: Time-on-Task

These teacher behaviors are intended primarily to organize and manage the class to increase students' learning time in instructional time available. What is discussed here includes examples of ways to organize the class and select or adapt activities to maximize instructional time.

Class organization for effective teaching requires preplanning. Some concrete examples are provided below:

- Designate a spot in the room for the activity and bring the students to that spot before beginning the activity. Establish a routine of beginning and ending every lesson in the same spot and formation, such as a circle.
- Choose area(s) for each activity and set up all necessary equipment *before* the students arrive for the lesson. Have enough equipment so that students do not have to wait to use it. Do not clutter the space with equipment that is not to be used in teaching the lesson.
- Clearly define space allocated for each activity area by marking on the floor. Use smaller space areas to eliminate distractions, if needed, for some students. Use mats, screens, or movable partitions to separate teaching areas, which is another way to define the boundaries of an activity or station, as well as for "time-out" areas. Be sure the activity areas are free from extraneous disruptions: balls coming into areas from outside, or persons walking across area to get to another area.
- Orient students to each formation used in teaching the objective: teams, circles, lines, relays, scattered.
- Establish signals for stop and go that are consistent and clearly differentiated from each other. For example, "Go" might always be the signal to start, and a whistle might always be the signal to stop. Be sure signals and class routines are established to move from one activity to another.
- Assume a position that enables continual observation, monitoring, and reinforcing of students' performance. Be certain that all students can see and hear the presentation: whole class presentation or each practice group under guided instruction.
- Maximize equipment and student ratio whenever possible by making homemade equipment; e.g., paper balls; yarn balls; carpet squares; rubber car mats; foam rubber, carpet or contact paper "footprints;" pictures or clown faces for targets; balance beams made by a local high school workshop; or empty drum barrels.
- Increase student involvement by printing on the board or using activity cards listing specific assigned learning tasks before students enter the class. Class performance score sheets can be used as well. Teams can be listed and space assigned in practice and whole class presentation. Activity cards are task cards for team group or independent student learning. They are formatted for instructional objectives and can be compactly packaged. They can be arranged sequentially so that, through essential completion of the specified learning tasks, a particular skill will be achieved. The cards can be stored in a box. Students can pull a card to work on and can either record the results of practice or check with the teacher. The teacher can evaluate the student or suggest that work should be continued on the learning task.
- Use appropriate formations when organizing class activities to match the type of formation with the type of activity required so students can have maximum turns and opportunities to practice, and receive feedback.

Selecting or adapting instructional activities for all students to participate requires teachers to consider:

- Activities that can serve as double "pay-off," such as teaching two objectives or more. For example, teaching the run while students are also running and jogging for a health and fitness-related objective. Using a game or sport activity that requires more than one objective, decrease the time spent on practicing and learning specific objectives.
- Activities that accommodate or can be easily modified to accommodate students at different levels of skill.

Adapting or modifying instructional activities and games for students of varying abilities to participate in helps all students to enjoy and practice their skills. Five strategies have proved effective for modifying activities. These are:

1. *Keep the activity as close to original as possible.* Focus on what students can do, not on what they cannot do.
2. *Keep all students actively involved.* See that losers remain part of the game in elimination-type games: Students in tag games become partners; in dodge ball, students become throwers when hit and score points.
3. *Equalize competition.* Students can use different equipment: larger balls to kick; lighter objects to hit; softer balls to slow down the speed; running to a sound for a target rather than a line; shortening distances or size of playing area; increasing size of target areas for striking or throwing; adjusting height of nets, baskets, or other types of equipment; and decreasing duration of the activity or changing rules.
4. *Be flexible.* If one activity modification does not work well, change the modification.
5. *Involve students in the class.* Students can modify and/or develop new games for all class members to participate and enjoy. Let them have the opportunity to share in the planning and make decisions. Evaluate the effectiveness of the game in terms of stated purposes.

Table 6–3 illustrates ways to modify badminton.

Game equipment may require modification or special equipment may be needed for some students. A multitude of possibilities exist: bowling rails, pushers and special handles on balls, beeper balls, and prosthetic devices for some students to participate in ice hockey, archery, badminton, and other activities, special wheelchairs for students to participate in basketball, track events, field events, and marathons. Modification of existing equipment requires common sense. Examining catalogs of special equipment can be helpful. Often students and/or parents can show how to adjust equipment or to modify or use special equipment.

Effective Use of Staffing

Selection of instructional and management strategies also depends on staffing. Careful planning is required to effectively use peer tutors, aides, or parents. *Parents* are extremely important in meeting the needs of their children who may require more intensive and extensive instructional time to achieve. Home activities program, homework for students, needs to be planned, implemented, and monitored, with periodic reviews and reports. *Peers, aides, and other students* can be trained as tutors. They are all important to individualize instruction and maximize students' learning time. In tutoring, not only is on-task time increased for the student, but in many cases for the tutor as well. Using peers or older students as tutors has other beneficial effects. Not only do peer or older student models provide concrete examples of performance, they also provide positive reinforcement and encouragement for appropriate student behavior in instruction and in free play. They help to establish students' responsibility and ac-

TABLE 6–3.   *Badminton: Activity Modification*

Characteristics	Equipment Regularly Used	Adaptation of Activity	Ability Requirements	Adaptation of Equipment (Special Equipment)
Hit the light shuttle with a racquet over the net and down into the court of opponent(s)	Racquet Shuttle Net	Change size of field Lower or raise net Play in sitting position (on a mat, roller-board, wheelchair, vaulting horse) Allow 2 hits on the shuttle	Run (move quickly in all directions) Balance in standing position Balance in sitting position Balance with or without support (e.g., one crutch) Ability to pick shuttle up from floor	Cane handle (curved handle) racquet Rubber attached on top of the racquet for use as a support for player Glue velcro strips to top of racquet and to shuttle so the shuttle can be recovered from the floor. Adapt racquet handle to fit artificial limbs. Shorten handle of racquet. Make handle of racquet thicker. Use different colors on shuttle Use balloon as "shuttle"

countability for their work and behavior. In addition, there is an increase in understanding and acceptance of individual differences among students in the class. Many teachers provide an opportunity for each student in the class to be a peer tutor. Using the team group approach is one way to achieve this.

In planning effective use of tutors, aides, or parents, teachers need to consider these four general strategies. *First,* orient and train staff as to their roles and responsibilites. Be sure they know students' assigned learning tasks and progressions. Staff needs training in providing positive feedback and constructive procedures. They need to know words and other behaviors that can be used as positive reinforcers. *Second,* assign staff teaching activities comparable to the abilities of the staff. A staff person may need to be assigned specific objectives. This person may be rotated from student to student or group to group all working on the same skill. As the staff person gains mastery, another objective may be assigned. *Third,* set up a system of communication with the staff person. This type of communication is generally nonverbal. It is a concrete record of what happened in instruction with the students. A checklist can be designed such as a tutor tip sheet for recording what worked well with students. A tutor class performance score sheet can be used to record and date successes and also record corrective procedures. *Fourth,* establish a system of monitoring feedback and continuous evaluation of the staff person's performance. This system may take the form of periodic, regularly scheduled observations in instruction. Evaluation can be determined based on a staff person's progress on established objectives. They can write an evaluation of effects on the student. They can list changes they would make in the reinforcement or activity and give rationale. At all times, teachers provide positive feedback and structured corrective procedures to improve the quality of their performances.

Team teaching is another approach to facilitate quality instruction. We have found it helpful for teachers to work in pairs or small groups as they develop specific strategies. This method is particularly helpful with relatively inexperienced teachers and master teachers. It provides a means of promoting personal and professional growth. Team teaching can improve the quality of instruction. Some of the ways include:

—grouping students more efficiently to meet student needs;

—sharing teaching responsibilities to help recognize individual differences and facilitate planning to meet student needs;

—more flexibility in managing blocks of time for the unit;

—more potential to teach those activities that a teacher enjoys most;

—more opportunity to work with different size groups of students;

—learning from one another, sharing ideas and therefore more possibilities for working effectively with students.

Examining the above points clearly indicates what team teaching is not. It is not a procedure

—whereby two teachers and 80 students are divided into classes of 40;

—whereby two teachers, each with a class of 40 students, come together occasionally for a "rainy day," then return to their classes of 40;

—whereby standard-size classes of 40 are rearranged into study groups of 20 without changing what teachers and students do;

—whereby student-teacher ratio is increased;

—whereby time is saved in planning.

The following suggested procedures for effective team teaching are tied directly to the Achievement-Based Curriculum Model. Although the suggestions are at the unit level of the instructional program, they can be applied to program planning as well. The procedures are organized under three categories with examples of questions.

1. The Unit

What are the objectives?

What resources are available?

What assessing activities do we use?

What method do we use to gather prior data?

What criteria do we use to set class expectancies and assign students' learning tasks?

What activities do we use? Do we need to adapt them?

How do we group students for instruction?

What format do we use to structure the lesson?

How can we use this unit to reinforce previously learned skills?

How do we present the unit objectives to catch students' attention?

What method do we use to provide feedback and corrective procedures?

Who will be responsible for each task in implementing the daily lessons?

Who will monitor student behaviors in the class: 60% time-on-task success, covering unit objectives?

2. The Students

Who is having difficulty?

What specific activities do we have to help them?

Is this difficulty showing up in all learning tasks?

What resources within the team can assist the student?

Do we need to modify the difficulty level of the task? Or the activity? Type of feedback or corrective procedures?

Is the student having difficulty in other school areas?

Do we need to communicate with other personnel in the school? With parents? Whose task?

Did students achieve? If not, why not? What needs to be changed? What are our recommendations for improving instruction for students?

TABLE 6–4. *Importance of Structuring the Lesson to Increase Student Involvement, Engaged Time-on-Task: 60% Time-on-Task or Better*

How Instructional Class Time Is Spent: 60 Minute Class

Non-teaching time–14'

Active teaching Whole class

Guided practice 40'

Unengaged student behaviors 6'

QUALITY INSTRUCTION

Non-teaching time 20'

Active teaching time Whole class Guided practice 20'

Unengaged student behavior 20'

OTHER CLASSES

STUDENT NOT INVOLVED IN LEARNING

Management:	Getting ready for instruction, waiting, listening to noninstructional directions or changing activities, getting dressed and undressed for gym class; administrative interruption.
Socializing:	Interacting socially or watching others socialize.
Discipline:	Being reprimanded by an adult, being punished, or watching other students being disciplined.
Unoccupied/ Observing	Wandering about with no evident purpose or goal, watching other people, unassigned activities such as playing with materials.
Out of the room:	Leaving the room temporarily.

3. The Team

How can we improve team functioning? Commitment to team decisions? Organizing so that each member can do more of what each enjoys teaching?

The procedures help to build team cohesiveness and consensus and develop positive team-teacher relationships with emphasis on student learning. They provide direction and content for team-training procedures.

TEACHING

All the planning decisions made earlier culminate in implementing the prescription, teaching. The importance of providing a structured, carefully planned lesson, and explicit instruction of what is to be learned cannot be overemphasized in its relationship to student involvement, engaged time-on-task. For example, Table 6–4 illustrates the importance of carefully planning and sequencing activities for optimal learning time.

STRUCTURING THE LESSON

Structure refers mainly to systematic patterns of instruction and class management. It refers to planned activities relevant to instructional objectives of the lesson. Structure does not connote rigidity. It implies a framework within which much flexibility—spontaneous and creative instruction—is possible and desirable so long as it is relevant to instructional objectives. Following are some points identified by teachers that can serve as the basis of a checklist to help plan and structure the lessons:

1. Identify Activities

Phases	*Activities*
—Introductory Activity	Physical fitness objectives
	Warm-ups
—Body Presentation:	Whole class: what, why of lesson objectives, review previously related skills, explain/demonstrate what is to be learned.
Practice:	Drill, learning center stations for teams, independent work.
	Practice-game activities.
Summary Review	Highlight what was learned.
	Review students' progress and record.
	Relaxation.

2. Choose Activities
    —space and equipment available;
    —ability levels of students to participate in games;
    —health and safety considerations;
    —very active/moderate/inactive;
    —high interest to the students.
3. Identify Organization
    —Formations: circle, line, semicircle, scatter.
    —Consider: visibility and hearing of students; student familiarity with organization and class routine to move from one organization or area to another, characterized by smooth-running transitions.
    —Grouping: team groups—heterogeneous; teacher groups—heterogeneous; other.
4. List time needed for each objective and related activity.
5. List equipment needed opposite each activity.
6. Prepare student/class performance score sheets or activity cards; where to store them, how students pull and use them, and how to collect them.

Each lesson identifies the instructional objectives and time allocations. The lessons are based on unit lessons sequence previously established, unless preassessment prior to instruction changes the sequence or objectives to be taught. With the preassessment data of students' performances and prior data on students' previous achievements and any special needs, the lesson is planned and the students grouped for instruction. Possible instructional groupings for initial lesson planning are based on three considerations: the closeness to the attainment of the objectives, number of learning steps to achieve, and groups of like or different abilities. For example, students may be throwing, but not quite to the required extension: the body rotation is not completed. With a little work on the body rotation, the student can achieve the proper level. Therefore, instruction begins here. As this is achieved, it is recorded and activities planned for the next objective.

In another example, as shown in Table 6–5, students are grouped in heterogeneous groups as teams and in a homogeneous group to work with teachers. Using the assessment data illustrated, 6 students have achieved skill level I, while 18 may need practice on two or three criteria, and the other 12 work on one criterion for skill level I and move to skill level II (learning tasks 6 and 7).

TABLE 6–5. *Students' Assigned Learning Tasks (Overhand Throw and Catch) and Practice Groups: Class = 36 Students*

Number of Students	Throw Learning Tasks							Initial Team Groups	Number of Students	Catch Learning Tasks							Initial Team Groups
	1	2	3	4	5	6	7			1	2	3	4	5	6	7	
6						X		6 teams 6 students Heterogenous ability group	12						X		6 teams 6 students Heterogenous ability group
12			X	X	X				12		X	X	X				
12					X	X			6					X	X		
6		X	X					1 team Similar ability teacher	6	X	X	X					1 team Similar ability teacher

TABLE 6–6. *A Structured Lesson*

Teacher: ___Brown___   Class: _____   Instructional Staff: ___Teacher___

Instructional Time (total): ___30___   Class Size: _____   ___Team Groups___

Total Class Period Time: ___40___

Phase	Instructional Activity	Time (Min)
Introductory Activity Cardiorespiratory Endurance Abdominal Strength	Move to assigned team space for whole class presentation	5'
Lesson—Body Whole Class Presentation Lesson Objectives What, Why Review Team Groups Learning Tasks Practice Overhand Throw Catch	Teacher presents lesson objectives. Explains and demonstrates overhand throw and catch. Students demonstrate, no equipment. Students pin-point learning tasks. Class divided into 6 team groups. Each team assigned practice space.	5'
	Team assigned practice space and equipment. 5 teams—heterogeneous ability groups 1 team—similar ability begin with teacher. On signal, teams change to different objective. Team members monitor each member's progress and record for total team points.	10'
	Play Target Practice game with 4 games going simultaneously. Move to assign team space for whole class presentation.	5'
Summary Review	Teacher reviews lesson objectives, asking students questions. Teams present results of their team and individual members. Results recorded.	5'

In planning a structured lesson, students know their assigned learning tasks on two physical fitness objectives. They have specific spaces for performing the cardiorespiratory and the sit-ups and the time allotted for these activities is recorded. Table 6–6 lists these activities and planned activities and grouping for the other two unit lesson objectives: overhand throw and catch.

MONITORING AND RECORDING STUDENT ACHIEVEMENT

In this section, procedures used to monitor student and class success on objectives covered are discussed. A basic recordkeeping procedure must be implemented. These records must be manageable by the teacher, a student, teams, tutors, or aides, and be designed so they are easily and simply displayed. In addition, such records should provide data for teachers to summarize student and class group achievements. More importantly, such records help teachers determine the appropriateness of the objectives taught and tested, and their time allotments. In the achievement-based curriculum program plan, the basic records are the class performance score sheets, the unit lesson plans, and the yearly program plan.

Monitoring whether content was appropriate for students is done by teachers looking at three student behaviors; objectives covered and tested, success of students, and engaged time (time-on-task). The class performance score sheets and unit lesson plans provide data for teachers to look at these three behaviors. Using the data from these records, teachers are able to summarize the data. A form, such as the one shown below, can be used to summarize the data gathered during instruction and at the end of the unit. These forms are called unit lesson logs.

CLASS	OBJECTIVES TAUGHT	DAYS NEEDED (ALLOTTED)	ACTUAL TIME (TOTAL MINUTES)	DATE/SUCCESS (NUMBER OF STUDENTS ACHIEVING AND NUMBER IN CLASS)	
A	Run	3	180	9/21	21–30
	Jump	4	140	9/21	25–30
	Throw	4	180	9/21	10–30

Using a similar form, all unit lesson logs can be summarized for the yearly program plan. These data provide some indication of the appropriateness of the objectives and time allocations for meaningful class gains. Unit lesson logs also indicate the scope and sequence of the program plan. Teachers can look at these records and determine whether or not they aligned the curriculum with what they taught and tested in class. The yearly program plan, units and lesson plans are modified, based on these data.

Two aspects of student success are monitored, unit lesson plans and the yearly program plan. The class performance score sheets and the lesson plans also provide the data to look at student success and time required for achievement. A basic recordkeeping system needs to be established. The recordkeeping must be manageable by the teacher and students. Records such as the class performance score sheets and unit lesson plans may be enlarged and displayed on the wall. Individual student's record or a team's record can be similarly designed. For example, a large chart with a student's name or a team's name can be developed to record initial standards achieved and progress made, number achieved over specified intervals of time are dated. Students can note their own accomplishments and/or the team's accomplishments. Figure 6–3 gives a graphic illustration of these procedures.

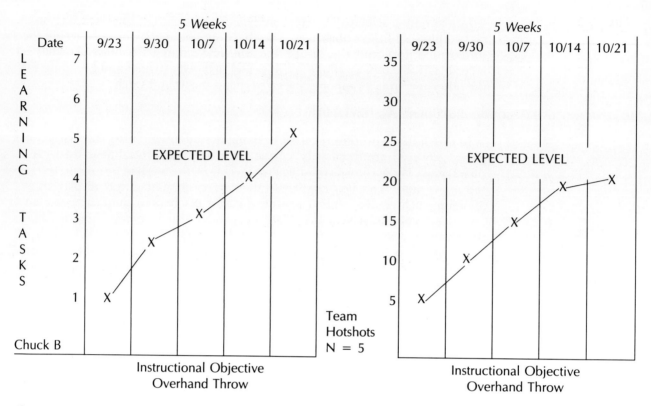

Figure 6–3. *Recordkeeping: Graphing student and team performance data.*

A class progress chart, such as that shown below, can be prepared and displayed on the wall. The data from the class performance score sheet for each objective in the unit lesson plan can be recorded on the chart.

Teacher _____ Class _____ Unit _____ Time Periods _____

STUDENT	NAME OF OBJECTIVE TAUGHT AND MASTERED			
	RUN	JUMP	THROW	OTHERS
Ann	9/20	10/7	10/21	
Jack	—	10/9	10/19	
David	9/19	10/9	—	
Luke	9/20	10/1	10/12	

Teachers and/or students can record dates the objective is mastered in the appropriate column. These class progress charts can be used by teachers to summarize unit or yearly program plan results in terms of student achievement on objectives taught and tested in the program. Hereto, these data provide teachers with concrete data to determine the appropriateness of objectives for each student, as well as the class as a group. Students are not likely to be successful on an objective for which they do not have prerequisite skills, nor are they likely to work on an objective if it is too easy or too difficult.

REASSESSING, RECORDING, AND MODIFYING THE PRESCRIPTION

Reassessment is a continuous process during instruction. The teacher, individual students, and/or teams must have the reasonability to monitor, reassess and record success on the class performance score sheets. Ideally, the reassess-

TABLE 6–7. *Trouble-shooting Checklist: Teacher Behaviors and Example of Possible Instructional Changes*

TEACHER BEHAVIORS: TROUBLE-SHOOTING CHECKLIST	EXAMPLES OF INSTRUCTIONAL CHANGE
1. Are the presentations appropriate and clear; is the vocabulary within the grasp of students, is the rate appropriate, do the cues include verbal, modeling and demonstration?	Decrease the number of directions given at one time. Provide concrete, single-word concepts, using multi-cues. Have student demonstrate understanding of what is presented.
2. Is the practice appropriate? Is enough time spent and are drills provided?	Provide more teacher small-group instruction or peer tutoring. Drill to specific errors only. Change drill to the most simple, straightforward procedure that student practices only until the exact response is achieved; may need physical assistance.
3. Are the reinforcing and corrective procedures appropriate? Amount, kind, and frequency?	Have student correct errors 3 times or 5 times each before beginning next activity with teacher supervising. Have student preview (video-model) skill before beginning instruction in the skill 1:1. Change type of reinforcement most rewarding for the student.
4. Are assigned learning tasks too difficult? Expectations realistic? Objectives appropriate?	Drop back to next lowest skill level or assigned learning tasks of skill level where student achieved success. Task-analyze the learning task criteria, breaking it down into smaller subskill sequential steps. Change expectancies: number of tasks to achieve. Extend instructional time. Delete instructional objective: substitute another one to achieve the same goal.
5. Are there other events occurring in school or home setting that may influence student's work?	Check with other teachers and school personnel. Parent communication.

ment process occurs concurrently. If class size, lack of time, lack of staffing prevent this type of assessment, regular periodic intervals of reassessment and recording during the unit can be planned. The recording of reassessment data can be done at the end of the period or during a planning period. Teachers with video recorders can systematically plan to assess different groups of students periodically and record data. Whatever procedure is developed, teachers should share and discuss the results recorded with students.

Modifying prescriptions during instruction is easily recorded on the lesson. Differences in allotted time and actual time the objective is taught are recorded on the lesson plan. Other changes can be circled, written on the lesson plan itself, or on the back of the lesson plan. Such data provide the teacher with an objective assessment of what worked well with the students and what needs to be changed. These decisions need to be shared and discussed with students. The decision-making process is discussed in evaluation.

Modification of prescriptions takes several forms. If, after several weeks, students are not achieving success in their assigned learning tasks, modification of instruction should be considered. A teacher trouble-shooting checklist can be designed. It helps teachers make decisions on what needs to be changed, and guides selection and implementation of modifications. Table 6–7 illustrates such a checklist.

Whatever the procedures are for monitoring, reassessing, and recording, it

ACTIVITY 6–1. Design and evaluate a structured lesson plan for the four objectives in the yearly program plan, Unit I: overhand throw, catch, abdominal strength, and cardiorespiratory endurance.

Objective: To use established criteria to design a lesson plan and evaluate the design.

Materials: Instructional Objective Standards: criteria to achieve learning tasks of unit lesson objectives. Unit Lesson Objectives: assigned learning tasks for a hypothetical class N = 36. Criteria presented to prepare a structured lesson plan are described in the text.

Worksheets 6–1A   Unit Lesson Objectives: Assigned Learning Tasks N = 36
              B   Structured Lesson Plan
              C   Lesson Plan Evaluation

WORKSHEET 6–1
Case Study: Using Assessment Information

Directions: Examine the unit lesson objective: assigned learning tasks for a hypothetical class N = 36. Using the assessment data recorded, answer the following questions regarding prescription and teaching. Write your answers on Worksheet 6–1.

1. Are most students performing at about the same skill level? If not, how would you plan to group students for guided practice to handle the range of variability?
2. Which criteria of the skill level will you concentrate on to begin initial instruction for each student? Why?
3. How will you group your students in the gym for guided practice based on this initial assessment data?
4. Which instructional activities (dance, games, sports) will you select for students to practice this objective after the initial skill presentation and practice?
5. What materials or equipment will you need to teach these objectives during the lesson?
6. What system will you use to monitor, reassess, and record student achievement, progress on assigned learning tasks?
7. Develop a unit lesson plan incorporating each objective to be taught and indicating time, groupings, and game activities. Write your lesson plan on Worksheet 6–1B.
8. Have a partner evaluate your lesson plan.

Variations:
1. Record hypothetical reassessment data on unit lesson plan objectives: assign learning tasks. Represcribe activities and design a structured lesson plan based on the reassessment data.
2. Observe a class. Assess students on one or two objectives. Assign learning tasks and design a structured lesson plan. Work with a partner and each evaluate the other's lesson plan. (See Worksheet 6–1C.)
3. Three students are having difficulty achieving assigned learning tasks. One is very hyperactive with short attention time. Another one does not seem to comprehend explanations and has difficulty in following directions. What specific strategies would you recommend for these students? Ann C. is the first student, Peter D. is the second student.
4. Design a *teacher tip sheet* that you would like to have to help you plan appropriate instructional and management strategies for students with special learning problems.

INSTRUCTIONAL OBJECTIVE STANDARDS
CRITERIA TO ACHIEVE LEARNING TASKS

CATCH

Skill
Level I
The student will catch a 6 in. playground ball tossed gently to the student between waist and shoulder height from a distance of 15 ft as follows:

1. Preparatory position with the hands in front of body, elbows flexed and near the sides.
2. Extension of arms in preparation for ball contact.
3. Contact ball with hands only.
4. Elbows bend to absorb the force of the ball (hands retract at least 6 in.).
5. Smooth integration of the above standards.

Skill
Level II
The student will catch a 2 or 3 in. ball thrown at least 10 ft high from a distance of at least 60 ft to a point within 10 ft of the student's initial position using a Level I pattern:

6. Ten consecutive times while moving into position on cue from the ball's flight in front of the student with number of catches being recorded.
7. The student will have caught the ball ten out of ten times.

OVERHAND THROW

Skill
Level I
The student will throw a 2 or 3 in. ball a distance of 40 ft three consecutive times toward the target as follows:

1. A preparatory movement—side orientation with weight on the rear leg to initiate throw.
2. Near complete extension of the throwing arm to initiate the throw.
3. Weight transfer to the foot opposite the throwing arm with marked hip and spine rotation during the throwing motion.
4. A follow-through well beyond the ball release and in line with the target.
5. Smooth integration of the above standards.

Skill
Level II
The student will throw a 2 or 3 in. ball using a Level I pattern:

6. Ten consecutive times at a 6 ft square target located 1 ft off the ground 40 ft in front of the student with the number of hits being recorded
7. The student will have hit the target ten out of ten times.

ABDOMINAL STRENGTH

1. Correct sit-up performance 10 times
2. Level I pattern 30 sec, 15 times
3. Level I pattern 45 sec. 30 times
4. Level I pattern 1 min, 40 or more times

CARDIORESPIRATORY

1. Run/jog 600 yards
2. Run/jog ½ mile
3. Run/jog ¾ mile
4. Run/jog 1 mile

WORKSHEET 6–1A. *Unit Lesson Objectives: Assigned Learning Tasks N = 36*

STUDENTS/ DATE	CATCH		OVERHAND THROW		ABDOMINAL STRENGTH		CARDIORESPIRATORY	
	LEARNING TASKS		LEARNING TASKS		LEARNING TASKS		LEARNING TASKS	
	ASSIGNED	ACHIEVED	ASSIGNED	ACHIEVED	ASSIGNED	ACHIEVED	ASSIGNED	ACHIEVED
Jay B	7		7		2		2	
Chuck B.	3,4,5		5,6		2		2	
Lynn B	3,4,5		5,6		3		2	
Steve B	5,6		7		2		2	
Ann C.	3,4,5		4,5		1		1	
Jenny C	7		7		2		3	
Susan C	3,4,5		5,6		3		2	
Christine D	5,6		7		4		3	
Jeff D.	5,6		7		2		3	
Doug D.	3,4,5		4,5		3		1	
Peter D.	3,4,5		2,3		1		2	
Josh E.	3,4,5		4,5		2		1	
Tom F.	1		1		1		1	
Ann G	3,4,5		4,5		4		2	
Judy G	4,5		5,6		1		3	
Luke H.	5,6		4,5		2		3	
John J	4,5		2,3,4		2		3	
Andrew L	5,6		7		2		2	
Allan L	4,5		5,6		3		2	
Barbara L	7		7		4		3	
David M	3,4,5		4,5		1		2	
Bradley M	4,5		4,5		1		1	
James M	5,6		4,5		1		1	
Nick N.	7		5,6		4		4	
Jack N	5,6		7		3		3	
Jill N	3,4,5		4,5		3		3	
Joan O.	4,5		3,4,5		2		3	
Luke O.	5,6		4,5		1		1	
Bernard P.	7		7		3		2	
William R.	4,5		5,6		3		2	
Carol R.	7		7		4		3	
Terry S.	5,6		5,6		2		3	
Cindy S.	4,5		4,5		2		2	
Louis T.	5,6		7		1		1	
Paul V.	3,4,5		4,5		3		2	
Janet W.	4,5		3,5		3		2	
N = 36								

Teacher _____   Level __4th Grade__   PO Time
                                                  Overhand Throw _____   CR _____

Class Size _____   Time __40 Min__   Catch _____   AS _____

Phase	Activity	Time Allotted Actual
INTRODUCTORY ACTIVITY		
LESSON BODY		
SUMMARY		

WORKSHEET 6–1C. *Lesson Plan Evaluation*

Teacher: _____ Lesson Plan #_____ Evaluator: _____

Date _____

Instructions: Use the Scale One to rate each aspect of the lesson plan, unless Scale Two is indicated by an (*). Only circle NA if a question is Not Applicable due to the unique nature of the lesson plan. For example: If the Introductory Activity does not require any equipment, then the question regarding equipment should be rated NA.

SCALE ONE

0	1	3	5
NA	Not stated	Vaguely/	Completely/
Not appropriate		incompletely stated	adequately stated

SCALE TWO

0	1	3	5
NA	Strongly disagree	Neutral	Strongly agree

Introductory Activity

(1) Activity is stated in terms of Performance Objectives   0 1 2 3 4 5

(2) Activity is stated in enough detail so that a substitute could implement.   0 1 2 3 4 5

(3) Type and quantity of equipment required is stated.   0 1 2 3 4 5

(4) Time allocated for the activity is stated.   0 1 2 3 4 5

Lesson Body Activities

(5) Activities are stated in terms of Performance Objectives.   0 1 2 3 4 5

(6) Activities are stated in enough detail so that a substitute could implement.   0 1 2 3 4 5

(7) Instructional groupings are stated.   0 1 2 3 4 5

(8) Organizational strategy is stated.   0 1 2 3 4 5

(9) Type and quantity of equipment required is stated.   0 1 2 3 4 5

(10) Time allocated for each activity is stated.   0 1 2 3 4 5

Summary Activity

(11) Summary activity is related to the Performance Objectives in the lesson.   0 1 2 3 4 5

(12) Activity is described in enough detail so that a substitute could implement.   0 1 2 3 4 5

(13) Organizational strategy is stated.   0 1 2 3 4 5

(14) Type and quantity of equipment required is stated.   0 1 2 3 4 5

(15) Time allocated for the activity is stated.   0 1 2 3 4 5

Overall Plan

(16) The Introductory, Lesson, and Summary activities complement each other.   *0 1 2 3 4 5

(17) The time allocated for each part of the lesson plan appears to be appropriate.   *0 1 2 3 4 5

(18) The lesson plan states who will implement, when the lesson will be conducted, and what class it is designed for.   0 1 2 3 4 5

ACTIVITY 6–2. Design a form to observe and evaluate a teacher's performance in instruction.

Objective:	To use established criteria to design and observe teacher's actions in the lesson.
Materials:	Criteria presented for effective instructional procedures in preparing the lesson.
	Worksheet 6–2A Observation of Teacher's Performance in Instruction

WORKSHEET 6–2

Directions:
1. Worksheet 6–2 provides headings for different phases of the lesson. Examine these phases.
2. For each item in the blank space, write in observable teacher's actions or data that would be available for examination.
3. Work in groups using the consensus-forming technique to determine exact items that you would use to observe the teacher in action.
4. With the final consensus, observe your partner or a teacher in action. If your partner, use the structured lesson previously prepared and teach.

Variations:
1. The form can be used to observe teachers in actual class situations.
2. The most important observable items identified can be used as a questionnaire for teachers in the work place to evaluate and make recommendations.
3. A review of recent literature can be conducted to identify other such forms and synthesize the form or used to develop a form to assess teacher's effectiveness in instruction.

Supplemental Materials
Worksheet 6–2B is a Teacher's Allotted Time Log for a lesson.
This is another aspect of observable teacher's action in instruction. Several of these can be conducted during different units. Such data can help teachers keep time-on-task records.

WORKSHEET 6–2A. *Observation of Teacher's Performance in Instruction*

Teacher _____ Class _____ Unit _____ Time _____

Observer _____ Date _____

ITEM	WRITE IN OBSERVABLE ITEMS
1. Clarity of aims	
2. Appropriateness of aims	

PREPLANNING AND PREPARATION

ITEM	
3. Organization of the lesson	
4. Selection of activities	
5. Selection of equipment	
6. Selection of recordkeeping procedures	

INSTRUCTION

ITEM	
7. Beginning the lesson	
8. Clarity of presentation	
9. Feedback and corrective procedures	
10. Pacing	
11. Pupil participation	
12. Pupil attention	
13. Group instruction	
14. Guided practice	
15. Ending the lesson	
16. Teacher-pupil rapport	

EVALUATION

ITEM	
17. Use of reassessment data to improve teaching and learning	
18. Continuous reassessment and recording data	

Items may be restated or other items added as well as observable items for each item stated.

WORKSHEET 6–2B. *A Teacher's Allocated Time Log*

Teacher _____ Class _____ Unit _____ Time _____

Date _____ Lesson Unit Number _____

Lesson Objectives _____

Activity	Begin	End	Time (min)	Objectives	Total Time
Introductory Activities	9:01	9:31	30	1. _____ _____
Lesson Body Presentation				2. _____ _____
Practice Group	9:35	9:50	15	3. _____ _____
Individual				4. _____ _____
Game				
Summary	9:50	9:55	5	
	Total Time		50	

ACTIVITY 6–3. Observing a class to determine students' time-on-task.

Objective:	To improve students' time-on-task by monitoring their involvement and time-on-task in instruction and learning.
Materials:	Worksheet 6–3 is an instrument to observe student behaviors in instruction and learning focused on time-on-task: objectives of instruction and their assigned learning tasks.

This worksheet was adapted from several sources. (See Supplemental Resources at the end of this activity.) Data collected were based on the following definitions of nontask student behaviors:

Assigned Tasks: Time the students are introduced to and presented the lesson objectives and given assigned learning tasks.

Class Management: Time spent by students changing from one activity to another, waiting for the teacher's help, or listening to unrelated task directions by the teacher or others.

Disciplinary: Time students are being reprimanded or punished, watching other students being disciplined or being punished for inappropriate behaviors, or excluded from the instruction or activity.

Social: Time when students are watching others socialize, not task-related, or interacting socially themselves.

Unoccupied/Observing/Unrelated: Time students are watching other students, not task-related to their assigned tasks; performing unassigned activities; playing with equipment, not task-related; or simply wandering about.

Out of Room: Time students are gone from the room temporarily.

WORKSHEET 6–3

Directions:

1. Examine the completed Worksheet 6–3. These data were collected by an observer of a class using the following procedures:
   - Observe a class. Talk to the teacher before observing the class to learn what the teacher expects to take place. If possible, secure a lesson plan with scheduled time of activities and objectives of the lesson before your observation.
   - Using the definitions provided (adapted from different sources); note nontask time of students in the class, observing in 10 separate intervals of 1-minute observation.
   - Tally your observations in the appropriate columns for the number of students who are not spending time-on-task.
2. At the end of each observation, total the number of students who were not on-task and the number who were on-task.
3. At the end of all ten observations, calculate the total number of students who were observed during all the observations and the total number of students who were on assigned tasks. Since all the students were assigned tasks during the period of observation, the total observed is the total number of students multiplied by 10 observations.
4. Time-on-task is simply calculated by dividing the total number of students on task by the total number of students observed. The time-on-task rate is a percent. To calculate minutes-on-task time, simply multiply the total class time by the percent rate.

Variations: In using the instrument, alternative activities, such as selecting 6 to 10 students to serve as representatives of the entire class, may be used. Another use of the instrument is for a single student. Instead of 10 observations of 1-min intervals, code the total times for the entire class or activity being observed.

Changes in the use of instructional time can be summarized and plotted on a graph. Data can be gathered at regularly scheduled times during the units in the yearly program plan. With improved time-on-task, student achievement should improve. One major benefit in monitoring students' time-on-task during the year is that teachers can take corrective action early.

For example, if the data gathered from two observations during the month average 66% (60% is about average when first using this monitoring instrument), the time might improve to 80% which means that students would spend about 10 more minutes in actual instruction and learning.

Supplemental Resources:

American Association of School Administrators: Time on Task: Using Instructional Time More Effectively. Arlington, VA, n.d.

Huit, W., Caldwell, J., Traver, P., and Graeger, A.: Collecting information on student engaged time. *In* Time Leader's Guide. Edited by D. Helms, A. Graeber, J. Caldwell, and W. Huitte. Philadelphia, Research for Better Schools, Inc., 1980.

McGreal, T.L.: Successful Teacher Evaluation. Association for Supervision and Curriculum Development, 225 N. Washington St., Alexandria, VA 22314, 1983.

Stallings, J.A., and Kaskowitz, D.: Follow Through Classroom Observation Evaluation. Menlo Park, CA, Stanford Research Institute, 1974.

WORKSHEET 6–3. *Observing Students' Time-on-Task Behaviors*

Teacher _____ Class time _____ Lesson Objectives: _____

Observer _____ Number Students ____ _____ _____

Date _____ _____ _____

TIME OBSERVED

| | TIME PERIODS | | | | | | | | | | |
	1 10:01	2 10:02	3 10:03	4 10:04	5 10:05	6 10:06	7 10:07	8 10:08	9 10:09	10 10:10	TOTAL 10 MIN
Assigned Tasks											
Class Management											
Disciplinary											
Social											
Unoccupied/ Observing/ Unrelated											
Out of Room											
Total Students Not on Task											
Total Students on Task											

Time-on-task Rate (%)	Total Time-on-task (min)
$\dfrac{\text{Students observed}}{\text{Total number student observations}}$ = ___ %	Class Time × Time-on-Task (%) = ___ Minutes

Example of Completed **WORKSHEET 6–3.**   *Observing Students' Time-on-Task Behaviors*

Teacher ___E. Pike___   Class time ___60'___   Lesson Objective: ___Basketball___

Observer ___W. Martin___   Number Students _30_   ___Dribbling___   ___Passing___   ___Lay-up shot___

Date ___9/30___

TIME OBSERVED

| | TIME PERIODS | | | | | | | | | | TOTAL 10 MIN |
	1 10:01	2 10:02	3 10:03	4 10:04	5 10:05	6 10:06	7 10:07	8 10:08	9 10:09	10 10:10	
Assigned Tasks	30	30	30	30	30	30	30	30	30	30	300 Students
Class Manage-ment	‖‖‖ ‖‖‖	‖‖‖ ‖‖‖ ‖	‖‖‖ ‖‖‖	‖‖‖ ‖	‖	‖‖	‖	‖	‖		49
Socializing			‖	‖	‖	‖‖‖					8
Disciplinary				‖‖‖		‖‖‖	‖	‖			13
Unoccupied/ Observing/ Unrelated	‖	‖‖‖	‖‖‖	‖‖‖	‖	‖	‖	‖	‖‖	‖‖	30
Out of Room											
Total Students Not on Task	17	16	12	19	3	12	5	5	6	5	100
Total Students on Task	13	14	18	11	27	18	25	25	24	25	200

Time-on task Rate (%)	Time-on-task Minutes
10 separate observations at 1-minute intervals End of observation	Total class time in minutes $\times$ Percent = Minutes
$\dfrac{\text{Total number of students time on task}}{\text{Total number of students observed}}$ $\dfrac{200}{300}$ = 66%	60' Times 66% = 39 Minutes

Teacher behavioral indicators in effective instruction.

Objective:	To identify teacher behaviors promoting the highest possible student engagement rates to increase the probability of student learning.
Materials:	Worksheet 6–4A. Indicators of Teacher Behaviors in Effective Instruction Workksheet 6–4B. Indicators of Teacher Behaviors in Effective Instruction

WORKSHEET 6–4

Directions:

1. Worksheet 6–4A lists statements describing teacher behaviors that have been shown to be highly related to student involvement and success in covering objectives specified for instruction. These statements represent effective instructional and management procedures described in the narrative. The statements have been placed under one of the following headings:

   Clarity of Presentation
   Practice of Skills: Guided and Independent
   Positive Feedback and Corrective Procedures
   Effective Use of Time, Space, and Staff
   Planning in Preparation to Teach

2. Read each statement. Indicate your answer by "Yes" or "No." Indicate how certain you are of your response in the next column: "0"—completely uncertain and "5"—completely certain of the importance of this behavior as an indicator of teacher behaviors reflecting effective instruction. These behaviors become criteria for effective instruction.

3. A consensus-building technique can be used to determine certainty or uncertainty of a particular response. Such data give clues about which behaviors need more data or clues as to what is most important in evaluating teacher behaviors and improving instruction.

Variations:

1. The questionnaire can be used to assess teacher behaviors in an ongoing class.

2. The most important teacher behaviors, identified by consensus, can be used to develop a questionnaire for teachers to use as a self-evaluation checklist at periodic intervals to improve their teaching. (See Worksheet 6–4B.)

3. A review of recent literature can be conducted to identify and synthesize teacher behaviors related to student achievement. The results can be compared to these statements and used to design a questionnaire.

WORKSHEET 6–4A. *Indicators of Teacher Behaviors in Effective Instruction*

Teacher Behavior Categories	Answer Y/N	Certainty 0–5
Clarity of Presentation		
1. An overview of the lesson is provided.		
2. The reason why the lesson is important is presented.		
3. The lesson is presented in a step-by-step sequence from overview to conducting a review at the end of the lesson of previously learned skills.		
4. A demonstration of application of skills contained in the lesson is provided.		
5. Explanations are given in a clear, concise manner—students are not confused.		
6. Students are given an opportunity to demonstrate their understanding of the new skill to be learned.		
7. The presentation is visible and heard by all students in the class.		
8. Directions and instruction are given only when students are ready and listening.		
9. Teacher commands attention of all students and does not talk over student talk.		
10. More class time is allocated to whole group activities rather than individual work.		
11. Teacher assign students' learning tasks and students know what is to be learned.		
12. Teacher sets class expectancies; students know what is to be achieved by class and individual students in instruction.		
13. Teacher uses different cues, verbal and nonverbal to meet students' needs.		
14. Teacher is involved with students on task-related questions and answers or demonstrations.		
15. Teacher is task-oriented and all student interactions are restricted to lesson objectives.		
Practice of Skills: Guided and Independent		
1. Students are provided opportunities to practice skills contained in the lesson during class time.		

2. Students are provided different grouping formats for practicing skills with guided supervision and without supervision.
     Team-assisted individualized approach: all skill levels
     Teacher-directed approach: similar skill levels
     Individual assignments		

3. Teacher provides opportunities for students to practice skills in a variety of game activities.		

TEACHER BEHAVIOR CATEGORIES	ANSWER Y/N	CERTAINTY 0–5
Positive Feedback and Corrective Procedures		
1. Teacher is available to provide assistance to students and spot corrections needed.		
2. Teacher praises, rewards correct response, actual student achievement on assigned learning tasks.		
3. Teacher frequently requests students to demonstrate skill to assess student's understanding of the skill.		
4. Teacher restructures the skill when students are not achieving success after a certain period of time; task-analyzes into smaller units.		
5. Teacher strives to involve all students in class activities (adaptation of game activities) and encourages participation of each student.		
6. Teacher conveys enthusiasm and high interest in objectives and learning activities.		
7. Teacher applies evaluation of students' achievement fairly and consistently.		
Effective Use of Time, Space, and Staff		
1. Use of space is efficient, necessary equipment is readily accessible to both teacher and students.		
2. Teacher handles emergencies with minimal amount of class distraction.		
3. Teacher supervises students' work on assigned tasks, alerting students that they are accountable for their work.		
4. Teacher positions self in class so as to scan the room and pinpoint any student who may require attention.		
5. Teacher does not interrupt students' practice by giving further directions or instruction.		
6. Transition from one activity to another, or one area to another is smooth and does not cause unnecessary disruptions.		
7. Teacher provides activities so that students at varying levels of skills can participate.		
8. Teacher effectively uses different staffing resources; peer tutors, older students as tutors, aides, or provides homework assignments with parents.		
9. Teacher has a system to monitor and record students' work and achievement in assigned learning tasks.		
10. Teacher sets clear expectations and has predetermined standards emphasizing students' responsibility in achieving assigned learning tasks.		
Planning in Preparation to Teach		
1. Teacher has a yearly program plan of objectives (content) to be covered and tested during the year.		
2. Teacher has sequential instructional units and unit lesson plans indicating objectives and time allotments.		
3. Teacher plans lesson activities in advance so that all equipment and activities are closely linked to the objectives taught.		
4. Teacher has the use of student data prior to instruction and preassessment on objectives to be tested and taught.		
5. Teacher has prepared plans to assess students prior to instruction on objectives.		
6. Teacher sets clear expectations on predetermined standards for students to achieve assigned learning tasks.		

WORKSHEET 6–4B. *Indicators of Teacher Behaviors in Effective Instruction*

TEACHER BEHAVIOR CATEGORIES	FIRST RATING	SECOND RATING	CONSENSUS

Motivation and Class Management

What is Class Management?
Class management is teacher behaviors, the skills and techniques primarily intended to develop and maintain appropriate class and individual student's behaviors to increase student's motivation and involvement in learning.

How is it Done?	*Decision Aids*
1. Structuring the learning environment: safe, orderly, task-related and motivated for learning.	Student's motives and needs —attitudes —expectancy for success —class climate —responsibility —roles in instruction
2. Preventing and minimizing disruptive student behaviors; consistently enforcing class routines and rules.	Prior student information Sensible class rules Class routines structured Rewards for appropriate behaviors, positive reinforcement Defined limits, set consequences, consistently enforce Target behaviors
3. Using a variety of strategies to meet student and class management needs to develop and maintain appropriate behaviors.	Strategies to increase student involvement, success in learning, and motivation for learning

---

All students have basic motives and needs for learning. Motivation impels students to learn—to work toward achieving success in learning. Whether or not one takes a position that students' motivation is self-generated, residing totally within each student, teachers do make a difference. They do this by managing and directing instruction to improve students' motivation for learning and to prevent or minimize disruptive student behaviors in their classes.

A safe, orderly, and positive learning climate helps students attend to the work assigned. Need for recognition, approval, acceptance by teacher and peers and the class as a whole are all important needs to consider in planning motivational strategies. Teachers who believe that students' learning is enhanced through their instruction, match their modes of instruction with the abilities of their students.

Teachers' expectations, their belief that what they teach is important, and their belief in their ability to teach and the ability of all their students to learn, influence students' behaviors in learning. Teachers' expectations of success have positive effects on students' motivation to learn and structures the class climate for all students. Each student is expected to achieve. Parents, too, influence their children through their expectations for them. Parents' involvement in the instructional process, their value and attitudes toward program goals and objectives, their supportive efforts for the program and their home instruction all facilitate their children's involvement, their desire to learn and, consequently, their achievements.

FOSTERING STUDENT MOTIVATION FOR LEARNING

A major key to planning appropriate class management strategies is concerted focusing on students' motives and needs for learning. To accomplish this task, a list of pertinent student needs or motives for learning helps to structure the process, to identify class management needs of the students, and to design appropriate strategies. This process helps teachers manage and direct instruction for all students and target their efforts on one or several needs of individual students. Examples of ten pertinent students' motives or needs for learning, identified by different teachers, include the need to:

- trust others;
- feel self-worth;
- act responsibly;
- accept one's own strengths and weaknesses;
- communicate appropriately with others;
- use appropriate behaviors in varied environments;
- interact appropriately with peers and adults;
- cope with stress;
- control anxiety;
- control impulses.

Examples of class management needs, identified by teachers, have included the need for:

- participation in planning, monitoring, and evaluating one's progress in learning;
- clear and detailed statements of rules, procedures, and consequences;
- consistency and predictability in the class routines;
- consistency in enforcing rules and procedures;
- encouragement and support from peers and adults;
- appropriate learning tasks and expectations;
- positive reinforcement, immediate positive feedback in learning new skills or in new situations;
- rewards for success in learning desired by students, positive consequences following learning that motivates the student.

The inclusion of these examples does not preclude the importance of other need areas. These examples focus on students' needs, basic motivations for learning, and consequently, the managing and directing of instruction.

A FRAMEWORK FOR PLANNING

There are many motivational schemes that teachers can consider in planning class management strategies. The chart entitled "Planning Motivation for Learning" on the following pages summarizes the major student motives and needs under three major categories: (1) student attitudes, (2) student expectancies, and (3) class climate.

Each category has example questions that teachers can pose. These questions help teachers identify their perceptions of teacher behaviors that impact on student behaviors. Consequently the questions provide a process whereby teachers can plan motivational techniques to structure the class learning environment.

Using this framework, teachers make value judgments in each category. They can include other categories or revise existing ones. They can pose different questions and activities, personalized to their own perceptions and perceptions of their students' needs and motives. The chart clearly indicates the overlap of many of these activities within each category and the strategies discussed previously. What is highlighted here is the need to consider the students' motivation for learning in planning and delivering effective instruction.

PLANNING MOTIVATION FOR LEARNING

Category	Motivational Plan	Techniques
I. ATTITUDES —toward teacher	**WHAT ARE THE STUDENTS' PERCEPTIONS AND FEELINGS TOWARD ME?**	
	1. Establish a positive relationship with student, sharing something of value. 2. Listen to student with empathetic regard. 3. Treat student with warmth and acceptance.	1. Give student positive attention, task-related. 2. Engage student in conversation demonstrating acceptance and understanding of the meaning and feeling of the student's statements. 3. Provide student equal opportunity to respond and become involved in instruction.
—toward subject and learning: why and what	**WHAT ARE STUDENTS' PERCEPTIONS AND FEELINGS?**	
	1. Make conditions that surround learning positive. 2. Model enthusiasm for the skill(s). 3. Positively confront the possible erroneous expectations and assumptions that may underly the negative student attitudes.	1. Give students questions to work on to demonstrate how skills can be used in positive activities. 2. Relate a story of how you used the skill in different situations. 3. Ask students how many have heard that the skill (activity) is really difficult and discuss their feelings and expectations.
—toward how and what is to be learned, assigned learning tasks and activities	**HOW DOES STUDENT FEEL ABOUT HOW AND WHAT IS TO BE LEARNED?**	
	1. When a student's feelings seem relevant but are unstated or ambiguous, check your impression of them to open communication. 2. When there are strong feelings, misunderstandings or conflicts between you and students, paraphrase the student's message to continue communication and show understanding. 3. Keep communication concrete and task-related on target behaviors disruptive to learning.	1. Investigate feelings and actively listen to the student responses. 2. Keep communication open and ask open-ended questions to facilitate understanding and resolve the issue. 3. Resolve problems with students and avoid continual anger and resentment.
—toward self-esteem: I can learn	**WHAT ARE STUDENTS' SENSE OF WORTH, CAPABILITIES IN ACHIEVING THE ASSIGNED TASKS?**	
	1. Guarantee successful learning at least half of the time working at the levels of skills and less than 5% at a low level of success. 2. Encourage the student. 3. Emphasize student's personal role in learning and responsibility for learning.	1. Task-analyze initial task into achievable increments and give immediate feedback and positive reinforcement. 2. Move among students acknowledging their effort and progress and helping those who need it, restructuring task or redirecting students' efforts if necessary. 3. Have students participate in selecting activities of high interest, monitoring progress, reporting, and evaluating their success.

II. EXPECTANCY FOR SUCCESSES	CAN STUDENTS OBJECTIVELY EVALUATE THEIR SUCCESS?	
	1. Interview students on assigned learning tasks and expectancies. 2. Use predetermined standards on objectives taught. 3. Use sequential learning tasks. 4. Establish reporting and accountability system.	1. Use individual or team-assisted contract system for work assignments. 2. Hold students responsible for monitoring, reporting, and demonstrating performance. 3. Have students evaluate progress in instruction and how to improve.
III. CLASS CLIMATE —atmosphere	WHAT ARE STUDENTS' PERCEPTIONS OF THE CLASS, PERSONAL ACCEPTANCE, OPEN COMMUNICATION WITH TEACHER, ENCOURAGEMENT AND COOPERATION IN ACHIEVING INDIVIDUAL AND GROUP GOALS?	
	1. Use a cooperative structure to maximize student involvement sharing, and establish individual and class expectancies. 2. Involve entire class or teams in open communication and share some of the power typically allocated to teachers. 3. Establish goals and intentions of actions for resolving conflicts and solving problems. 4. Develop an atmosphere of understanding and cooperation rather than control and competition.	1. Have teams of students responsible for drill and practice, monitoring and reporting progress, and evaluating team goals and goals of individual members. 2. Check positiveness of your view of class, team groups, or individual students and directly describe your feelings to resolve problems. Keep it concrete. Take time and interest in listening to task-related or behavioral problems in class situation. 3. Provide positive consequences to follow learning that motivates the class, team, or individual student. Avoid undesirable consequences or negative situations, such as detention, probation, or others specified for nonperformance. 4. Guide group toward examination of the behavior; create an awareness of the problem, and help group clarify problems.
—safety	ARE STUDENTS THREATENED OR FEARFUL IN THE LEARNING ENVIRONMENT?	
	1. Reduce or remove components of the learning environment that lead to failure or fear. 2. Identify intensity of activities and physical environment conditions affecting students' learning.	1. Provide immediate feedback and positive reinforcement for each successive approximation of desired level of skill. Provide tasks that guarantee students' success matched to their performance abilities. 2. Modify activities involving students in adapting or designing new game situations for all to participate.
—responsibility	WHAT ARE STUDENTS' PERCEPTION OF THEIR RESPONSIBILITY AND ACCOUNTABILITY IN LEARNING ASSIGNED TASKS?	
	1. Acknowledge and affirm students' responsibility in completing the learning task. 2. Use a competence checklist or recording system for student to graph his or her progress.	1. Congratulate students for finishing assigned task. Acknowledge their perseverance and cooperation. Discuss with them what part seemed most difficult and see how they conquered the problem. 2. Receive student's monitor report and discuss it and the results with the student as well as steps to be taken.

A Point in Question: Teacher and Student Roles for Achieving Objectives

Teachers who believe that students' learning is enhanced through their participation in managing and directing instruction for achieving objectives, plan class management strategies accordingly. Role expectancies for students to become independent, self-directed learners require planning instruction to match students' level of responsibility at the moment. A continuum of students' role functions is illustrated below:

Dependent			Independent Learner
Listener/ Follower	Mutual Planner/ Performer Peer Team Teacher	Primary/Planner/ and Performer Self Tutor	Self-directed Problem Solver

The shift in students' roles in instruction is sequential. Students' roles are always directed toward task-related activities. Their role in instruction is dependent upon assigned learning tasks and activity options for achieving these objectives (see Fig. 7–1).

Other Considerations: Students with Special Needs

Teachers are often concerned with establishing and maintaining favorable student attitudes, acceptable patterns of behaviors with students who have special needs. Here are some suggestions that have been useful in different classes based on two strategies found in the literature: role playing and source credibility.

Role Playing. Role playing can be an effective technique to introduce students to individual differences in learning. Role-playing techniques are consistent with several instructional activities for learning discussed under motivation. Here are ideas for:

Role Play: A student with special needs.
Objective: Experience a physical condition
Materials: Special equipment to produce a particular condition
Procedure: Create a physical condition in yourself by:
  • fully and partially covering eyes;
  • using earplugs to fully or partially block hearing
  • using a wheelchair;
  • wearing a brace;
  • any combinations.
  GIVE ATTENTION to problems with
  • physical layout of classroom, barriers and obstacles;
  • methods used for giving directions to students;
  • student distractions or outside influence.

Other Activities
Role Play: Puppets
Carnival: Booths (puppet show, adaptive sports equipment, demonstration of adapted game activities, films on special Olympics, wheelchair sports and so forth).

Credibility. At times students need a highly credible source to influence their attitudes. For example, often messages on television are considered a reliable source by students. Here are some things teachers can do to create favorable student attitudes.

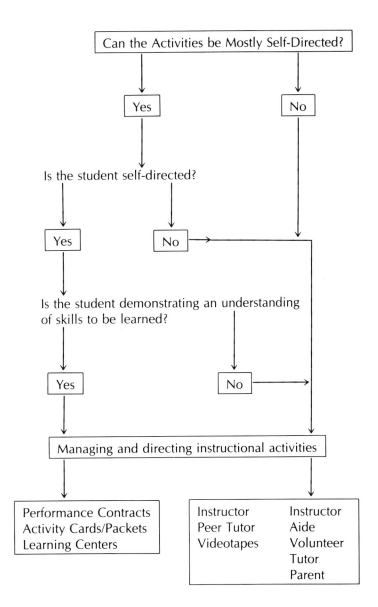

Figure 7–1. *Students' participation in instruction.*

Research Project

Objective: Help students become aware of contributions made by individuals.

Materials: Readings, chalkboard, and chalk.

Procedure: Present a list of persons with handicaps who are living or have died. Ask students to select one person and research his or her life for a report (either written or oral). Each report must include:

- nature of handicap and how it occurred;
- how handicap affected the person—education, home life, friends, job, and recreation/leisure;
- what problems were encountered as a result of handicap;
- what are or were the accomplishments, contributions, goals and future hopes of that person: artists; inventors/scientists; athletes; politicians; others.

Other Activities

Films: Help students become aware of handicaps and their influence on people's lives, reduce stereotypes and myths about individuals with handicaps. Present one or more films pertinent to age group of class. Follow up with discussion.

Other Suggestions.   Although these ideas may increase students' awareness and acceptance of students with special needs, involving students in planning activities is the best procedure. Here are a few more suggestions that have been found effective.

Define: Who has a handicap, a special need?

Objective: Help students examine their perceptions.

Materials: Chalkboard and large charts.

Procedure: Write the word "handicapped" on the chalkboard. Have students give a definition. List words that students suggest. Ask them why they associate each word with the term "handicapped." List reasons on board. List examples of such conditions:

EXAMPLES	AREAS OF POSSIBLE DIFFICULTY			HOW CAN WE HELP?
	SCHOOL	PLAY	HOME	
Seeing Hearing Height Weight Moving				
Other				

Other Activities
Personal Experience
Objective: Gain awareness of the concerns of students with special needs: at home, at school, at play.
   • a buddy or peer in a class or gym class; assist in teaching motor skills in elementary classes.
Visitors: Speakers or sports personalities with special needs.

These strategies focus primarily on preparing classes for students with special needs who are or will be assigned to the teacher's classes. One important strategy is for teachers to get to know the student before entering the class. The student, parents, and related school personnel may be the best sources for helping teachers focus activities for the individual student's needs and motives. Using instructional strategies discussed under motivation for learning applies equally to all students' basic needs and motives for learning.

PLANNING CLASS MANAGEMENT STRATEGIES

Class management strategies include all the skills and techniques that are primarily intended to control student's behaviors. These strategies are most relevant when they are used to increase students' involvement in learning and, consequently, student achievement. Strategies that promote student involvement, engaged time in learning within allotted instructional time, tend to improve students' behaviors in learning, preventing or minimizing disruptive or interfering behaviors.

Student behaviors that are disruptive are not always the result of managing and directing instruction. Students can provide their own sources of interference through forms of withdrawal, disinterested, defensive, or hostile behaviors. These behaviors may represent adjustment mechanisms developed by students in trying to deal with what they feel to be intolerable situations. Reasons are numerous. The ultimate cause lies somewhere between the motivational problem and the learning problem. Numerous, but high on the list, are:
   • repeated failures and frustration in past efforts;
   • lack of motivation, purpose, relevance, interest;
   • rejection at home or by significant others;
   • lack of ability and peer relations.
Class management strategies focused on controlling students' behaviors to increase students' involvement are presented under two areas: selecting principles for designing strategies, and using a variety of strategies.

SELECTED PRINCIPLES FOR DESIGNING STRATEGIES

Effective class management strategies to prevent or minimize students' disruptive behaviors are based on seven general principles. These principles provide teachers with guidelines for planning and managing instruction to help students develop and maintain appropriate behaviors in learning.

Know the Learner

Regardless of how many strategies teachers know, they will be of limited assistance without the knowledge of individual students. Managing and directing instruction appropriate for individual students require teachers to know the learner.

Learning. Teachers need knowledge of students' skill levels, learning styles, and interests in the instructional program.

Personal-Social. Teachers need to be aware of their students' frustration levels, self-esteem, expectancy of success, responsibleness, and attitude toward the teacher, peers, and school.

Health-Physical. Teachers need to know what the students can do—strengths and health and safety factors in the environment.

What teachers do makes a difference. Students who are defensive or fearful, for example, require strategies that are quite different from those needed for students with low self-esteem. Defensive or fearful students may benefit from short, simple tasks, guaranteeing success; students with low self-esteem typically respond to positive reinforcement. Students also respond differently to rewards for success in learning. Some respond to tangible rewards, such as award cards, free choice, praise by the teacher, or being selected to demonstrate for the class. In short, individualizing instruction is the selection of appropriate class management techniques to meet class and individual student's needs.

Select Target Behaviors

Teachers need to focus on specific target behaviors. The target behavior must be manageable. Global statements such as, "The student is disruptive." or "The student does not pay attention." or "The student is lazy." have little meaning. Similarly, teachers who intervene with too many behaviors, important or trivial, are spreading the effects so thin that it is doubtful that any strategy will be successful.

Teachers must select target behaviors that have greatest disrupting or interfering effect for the student or for the class during instruction. Teachers should not attempt to manage each and every inappropriate behavior that occurs within a few seconds. For example, if a student comes late to class, moves noisily about the gym talking loudly to another student, gets equipment clumsily and takes it to assigned space and the teacher uses a series of verbal statements as interventions, such as, "You are late . . . No talking . . . Watch where you are walking . . . Pick up the equipment quietly, please," there is little effectiveness. The teacher's effectiveness is improved if a single target behavior has been selected, such as "being on time." The other behaviors would be unimportant if the class had not started.

Behaviors that are symptomatic of a condition are of critical concern when working with students with special learning needs. Loud vocal noises emitted by hearing-impaired students, the inability of a student with cerebral palsy to remain still in line, the confusion about time and class organization by a learning-disabled student, are examples of symptomatic behaviors. If students have no conscious control of these behaviors, they should be tolerated. Tolerance does not imply a lack of structure for these students. It does imply a "learner's leeway" before the teacher intervenes with direct intervention. The teacher may need to work with related support personnel in identifying manageable target behaviors as well as the most effective intervention strategy.

Focusing on students' target behaviors, teachers are instructional managers. They are not forced into the role of a disciplinarian. By identifying target behaviors, intervention strategies can be planned. The limits of appropriate behaviors can be *defined*. These limits can be clearly communicated to students. Appropriate behaviors can be explained and demonstrated. Students can provide examples of what is desired or not desired. Once behavioral limits are established, these limits need to remain consistent.

Set Routine Structures

A routine structure should be set and followed. Specific student behaviors are defined as appropriate in particular activities. For example, specific assignments to begin and end a class session, moving from one area to another, sharing equipment if necessary, or taking turns in different class formations. Unplanned situations do occur during instruction; for example, interruptions by school announcements, class pictures, school assemblies, or even substitute teachers. Regardless of these interruptions in class routines, structure is important. Students need security of predictability. They need teacher consistency in managing and directing instruction.

Use Sensible Rules

Teachers can make too many rules of conduct. Neither the teacher nor the students can remember all of them. Too many rules provide no consistency in their enforcement and/or reinforcement of appropriate behaviors. Rules established to regulate behaviors that personally annoy the teacher but have no visible impact on learning should be avoided. For example, these might include pulling the hair, picking the nose, or dirty hands and face, which have little impact on learning. These kinds of behaviors need to be handled outside of class time at appropriate times when positive reinforcement of appropriate behavior can be given.

Provide Positive Reinforcement and Feedback

One of the most powerful tools available to teachers is the selective and systematic use of *positive reinforcement*: the continuing use of a stimulus resulting in an increase or maintenance of the target behavior. Positive reinforcement is another name for "what turns the student on."

The reward can take many forms. It is a motivational technique to increase or maintain appropriate student behavior or performance in a skill. A list of example motivational techniques as rewards for performance is provided below. These techniques are easily adapted for use with student behaviors in the learning environment.

1. Decrease the amount of practice time by one minute for each additional correct response/or decrease of one or more error responses.
2. Give points or verbal praise of "beating yesterday's score."
3. Give "free time" for daily, improved performance.
4. Have the student beat "the teacher's best rate."
5. Give days off (from the skill) if the skill is mastered "early" (before the anticipated date).
6. Hand out merit or award cards for aims that were met.
7. Keep a student chart of the skills mastered; follow the mastery of every fifth skill by something specific the student chooses to do (but set the parameters, i.e., help the principal or the folks in the kitchen).
8. Omit practice time altogether if a student demonstrates a better rate of performance today than yesterday (they are probably practicing at home).
9. Have the students select where they would like to practice and continue to let them select the location as long as performance improves.
10. Let students select the person who will monitor the daily check and help chart progress.

Frequently provide reinforcement feedback during the initial learning of appropriate behavior. Reinforcement schedules and timelines for rewarding students vary with each student as well as for the class as a whole. The goal is for students to become self-directing, the reward intrinsic to the act itself: skilled performance and acting appropriately in varied situations.

Teachers can develop, with students or teams, a recordkeeping system of appropriate student behaviors. Charting correct responses, appropriate behavior in a given situation, can serve as a type of reinforcer for student, team, or class. For example, a sample record sheet with a column for desired behavior followed by a column to record reinforcer and dates when given can be drawn on construction paper and covered with a clear, plastic sheet. The sheet can be wiped off and reused.

Team: Hotshots   Student: _____

BEHAVIOR DESIRED	POSITIVE REINFORCER	UNIT: _____								COMMENTS
		DATE USED								
		1	2	3	4	5	6	7	8	
1. Help with equipment	Leader	9/23	9/23							
2.										
3.										
4.										

Reward Appropriate Behavior

Teachers need a systematic plan of rewarding students who are performing appropriately in the learning environment: students who are completing their work, working on target objectives, or working quietly with others. Students who are disruptive can learn from their peers that appropriate behavior is rewarded. Even the most disruptive student performs appropriately sometimes within the class. For every assignment the disruptive student performs correctly, minimal as it may be, should not go unnoticed. Reward the appropriate behavior, "catch the student doing something correctly."

Teachers need to address the current student behavior, i.e., here and now. Reminding the student of past problems in behaviors serves no useful instructional purpose. It may, however, promote feelings of failure or resentment on the part of the student. Teachers must not signal to students that their past behaviors, or behaviors of other students, will continually be used to evaluate current performance. For example, using such statements as, "You did this for the last two weeks." or "How many times must you be told." or "Look how correctly you are performing compared to the number of times I had to tell you."

The current problem should be dealt with and past problems or other students should not be discussed. Teachers must target current behaviors that afford the student the opportunity to change and to achieve success.

Define Limits, Set Consequences, and be Consistent

One of the most important class management strategies is to define limits, set consequences, and consistently enforce them. This strategy helps prevent inappropriate behaviors, thereby reducing the number of discipline problems.

Some students seem to find pleasure, their own reward, or reinforcement, in continuing inappropriate behaviors disruptive to instruction. This is particularly true when there are no defined limits or consequences. Consequences selected need to be practical to carry out, related to the behavior violation, fair and reasonable, and help students learn appropriate behaviors. For example, the students are playing a game of tag and two of them begin pushing and hitting. The teacher approaches the students and asks them to stop. They do not stop. What is the consequence? Send students to the principal's office? Report them for detention? These are too extreme for the violation. Should they be removed from the game until class is over? This consequence may not help them learn to play with appropriate behaviors. The teacher finally decides to have them sit out for two minutes and then rejoin the game. Students finish the game with appropriate behaviors. The teacher praises their performance and the performance of all students in the game.

Whenever possible, teachers should avoid threatening, negative reinforcement of inappropriate behaviors. Negative reinforcement is referred to as aversive control, which motivates students to avoid negative consequences or to escape from undesirable consequences. Examples of this type of motivation include sending students to the principal, threatening detention or loss of privileges, verbal harassment, giving students signals that "they will get it later," or other specified consequences of nonperformance. In some instances, these procedures may be necessary.

Teachers need to communicate clearly the limits and consequences of inappropriate behaviors to all students and explain the appropriate behaviors in instruction for all students. Demonstrating these behaviors and knowing that the students understand them is important. Consistent and predictable enforcement of class rules, procedures, routines, and consequences is required, and periodically reviewing these limits and consequences is important for the whole class. Feedback and positive reinforcement of appropriate behaviors for the whole class, as well as for individual students, are effective class management strategies.

USING A VARIETY OF TECHNIQUES

Teachers must use a variety of techniques to minimize discipline problems. No technique, however, can replace the teacher's knowledge of the students and knowing which situations are likely to create problem behaviors. With this knowledge, teachers can plan and devise instruction to prevent or to minimize the occurrence of the problem behavior. Motivation for learning and instructional and management strategies previously described provide teachers with a variety of techniques. Other techniques that teachers can use in developing and maintaining appropriate student behaviors are presented in the chart entitled "Other Techniques Useful for Teachers" on the following pages.

TABLE 7–1. *Case Study: Positive and Negative Instructional Procedures Used for Socially Withdrawing Behaviors*

CHARACTERISTICS	NEGATIVE STRATEGIES

Withdrawing behaviors
  Inconspicuous in class and ignored by the teacher
  Sitting and playing alone
  Not responding when spoken to
  Failure to talk even though skill is present
  Disturbed peer relations
  Negative self-concept
	Forcing student to become involved
	Embarrassing the student
	Ignoring the behavior
	Asking student why he or she does not want to take part
	Comparing student to other students.

POSITIVE STRATEGIES	
SET BEHAVIORAL GOALS	IMPLEMENT POSITIVE PROCEDURES

1. Direct instruction in social skills to develop competence to interact with peers.
2. Apply these skills with selected peers.
   Watch that student is not traumatized by social contact with peers.
	1. Teach key social skills in one-to-one situation guaranteeing success and establishing guidelines.
	2. Plan activities so student can try skills—socially interacting with selected peers under supervision: parallel activities.
	   These peers may be special helpers in play to facilitate interaction between student and other peers.

3. Motivate student and peers to engage in exchanges with each other.	3. Set up performance contracting for student and classmates to earn daily group activity rewards. Implement program during recess periods or free time when peers are free to concur. Give reinforcement, rewards to student with praise and points for each interaction with peers or for interacting for a certain percent of time available.
4. Exchanges with peers should be positive, of acceptable quality with some verbal interaction.	4. Performance contracting should be initiated by students as well as peers; interaction should be verbal as well as allowing for physical involvement.

TABLE 7–2. *Case Study: Positive and Negative Instructional Procedures for Defensive Behaviors*

CHARACTERISTICS	NEGATIVE STRATEGIES

Defensive behaviors
  Protect themselves from failure, embarrassment, truth, or to take focus from themselves
  Fear of not measuring up
  Avoidance behavior in class
  Unwillingness to accept assignments
  Lack of responsibility and attending to tasks
  Lying
  Continually late or absent
	Telling student that he or she is trying to avoid the task
	Taking away privileges
	Comparing student behavior to another student's actions
	Threatening the student
	Taking student out of activities that student likes or is interested in
	Telling student you are aware of student's gimmicks

POSITIVE STRATEGIES	
SET BEHAVIORAL GOALS	POSITIVE PROCEDURES

1. Realistic success in daily work.	1. Plan activities at success level.
	     Praise student for each small success.
	     Have students evaluate their success and chart each small step.

2. Activities of high-interest	2. Give student choices with teacher selecting parallel activities.
3. Accept responsibility for work and behavior.	3. Set up performance contracting for sharing responsibility with team of selected peers for student to earn daily points.
4. Be truthful	4. Change form of questions when teacher knows student did something wrong. Do not say, "Did you . . .," but, "I saw you, and what shall we do about it?"

TABLE 7–3. *Case Study: Positive and Negative Instructional Procedures Used for Overly Aggressive, Inappropriate, Acting-Out Behaviors*

CHARACTERISTICS	NEGATIVE STRATEGIES
Overly aggressive, inappropriate acting-out behaviors 　Unable to control anger 　Easily distracted 　Disruptive in class 　Refuses to cooperate 　Stubborn, disrespectful 　Fights, abuses other students 　Talks without regard for others, interrupts 　Does not listen 　Does not attend to directions 　Talks back to authority 　Aggressive toward others, always getting his/her way 　Argumentative, swears	Using force Ridiculing behavior Taking away privileges Pushing the student Confrontation over issues Comparing behavior to another student Forcing student to admit lie or error Demanding confession of guilt

POSITIVE STRATEGIES	
SET BEHAVIORAL GOALS	POSITIVE PROCEDURES
1. Student consciously aware of those specific aspects of behavior that are inappropriate. 2. Needs to comply promptly with adult commands and directions or instructions. 3. Needs to decrease argumentative behavior with adults. 4. Needs a more cooperative pattern of interacting with adults.	1. Pinpoint specific inappropriate behaviors and review them with student. 2. Praise student each time they comply on first trial and award them one point. For 80% or more of adult commands followed, exchange special principles. 3. Private role-playing session scheduled and review with student after situations identified when student most argumentative. 　Rewards provided for handling each situation in nonargumentative fashion. 　Planned ignoring in instances of argumentative behavior. 　Brief time-out is another option. 4. Private role-playing sessions scheduled and review with student after situations identified when noncooperative patterns most often occur. 　Other options identified in item 3. In all situations it is helpful to inform parents and, if possible, involve them in supporting student at home.

OTHER TECHNIQUES IN DEVELOPMENT AND MAINTAINING APPROPRIATE BEHAVIORS

Technique	Use	Example
1. Planned ignoring	THE WITHDRAWAL OF A POSITIVE REINFORCER	
	A strategy to decrease disruptive behaviors when you have full control of the consequence and when the behavior must not be stopped immediately.	A student in class is reinforced by the instructor's attention. The student continually complains about everything. Instructor uses planned ignoring of student when student complains and gives student more attention, positive reward, when he or she does not complain.
2. Learning or performance contracting/contingency management	ESTABLISHING A WRITTEN AND/OR VERBAL AGREEMENT WITH STUDENTS TO PERFORM AN EXPLICIT ACTIVITY	
	A strategy for promoting desirable behaviors.	John has trouble working consistently on a task. He could verbalize that this was difficult for him but he had not been able to change his behavior. Teacher and John talked about possible privileges that he might earn if he were able to begin a task and work consistently on it. He mentioned that he would enjoy playing catch. It was agreed that if he were able to begin his task and work 50% of class time for two periods, he would be able to spend 10 minutes playing catch with the teacher.
3. Premack's principle	MAINTAINS THAT FOLLOWING A LESS DESIRABLE ACTIVITY WITH A MORE ENJOYABLE ACTIVITY RESULTS IN MORE PARTICIPATION IN THE LESS ENJOYABLE ACTIVITY	
	A procedure to increase the frequency of appropriate behavior—pleasure principle.	A student likes to play with a ball in the water but does not enjoy participation in floating which is necessary to learn to swim. The instruction allows student to play with ball one minute after two minutes of floating.
4. Reinforcing incompatible behaviors	POSITIVELY REINFORCING BEHAVIORS THAT CANNOT TAKE PLACE AT THE SAME TIME THAT AN UNDESIRABLE BEHAVIOR TAKES PLACE	
	For decreasing the frequency of an undesirable behavior, teacher must identify behaviors that compete with the undesirable behaviors.	Jill occasionally exhibits undesirable behavior of pushing while waiting in relay line. Teacher positively reinforces Jill when she stands with her hands to her sides while in line. Pushing and standing with hands to the sides cannot take place at the same time.

5. Reinforcing schedules	THE RATE AT WHICH POSITIVE REINFORCERS ARE DELIVERED ACCORDING TO TIME INTERVALS	
	To increase frequency of appropriate responses.	There are four basic types of reinforcers: 1. *Fixed ratio.* Reward is given after every response. 2. *Variable ratio.* Requires an average number of responses before reward is given. 3. *Fixed interval.* Reward is given after a specified time interval. 4. *Variable interval.* Reward is provided at variable intervals of time, e.g., after 15 minutes of appropriate behavior, then after 5 minutes, and so forth.

An example of techniques, positive and negative procedures that have been used by teachers to develop appropriate behaviors, is illustrated in the three case studies presented in Tables 7–1, 7–2, and 7–3. Positive approaches foster motivation and management of student behaviors to build teacher and class cohesiveness and consensus. They establish task-related emphasis in learning and develop positive teacher-student and student-student relationships. Techniques that control student behaviors, using pressure and force, appear to be significantly less effective in promoting student achievement, appropriateness of students' behaviors in learning.

The motivation and class management strategies discussed focus on developing and maintaining appropriate student behaviors. They are strategies, teacher behaviors, useful in controlling student behaviors directly relevant to increasing students' involvement in learning—time-on-task. These strategies are designed to prevent or minimize discipline problems and the need for more extreme intervention strategies and consequences for nonperformance. These student behaviors destroy the class climate conducive to learning for all students. Extreme discipline problems—destruction of property, fighting, shouting, profane language, and hostile, argumentative activities—require immediate teacher intervention strategies. These strategies require supportive assistance and a specified set of consequences established by school personnel.

SYNOPSIS

The first part of the chapter discussed fostering students' motivation for learning. Motivational categories for planning and managing instruction focused on students' motives and needs. These included students' attitudes, expectancy for success, and class climate for learning. Concerted focusing on students' motivation for learning provides a framework for identifying effective class management strategies.

The second part of the chapter presented selected principles for designing strategies. These principles focused on topics such as knowing the learner, selecting target behaviors, structuring class routines, using sensible rules, providing positive reinforcement, rewarding present appropriate behaviors and ways to prevent problem behaviors from occurring. Then special considerations were discussed, including some instructional procedures for establishing and/or maintaining favorable learning attitudes toward learners with special needs.

RESOURCES FOR TEACHERS

Brophy, J.: Fostering student learning and motivation. *In* Learning and Motivation in the Classroom. Edited by S. Paris, G. Olson, and H. Stevenson. Hillsdale, NJ, Erlbaum, New IRT, 1983.

Duke, D. (Ed.): Classroom Management. The 78th Yearbook of the National Society for the Study of Education. Chicago, University of Chicago Press, 1979.

Emmer, E., and Evertson, C.: Synthesis of research on classroom management. Educational Leadership, *38*(4), January 1981, 342–347.

Hall, V.H.: Responsive Teaching Services. Rev. ed. Kansas City, H & H Enterprises, Inc., 1979.

Reinert, H.R.: Children in Conflict. 2nd ed. St. Louis, MO, C.V. Mosby, 1980.

Sidentop, D.: Developing Teaching Skills in Physical Education. St. Louis, MO, C.V. Mosby, 1980.

Walker, H.M.: The Acting-Out Child. Coping with Classroom Disruptions. Boston, Allyn & Bacon, 1979.

ACTIVITY 7–1. Design strategies to foster students' motivation and learning.

Objective: To understand students' motives and needs in planning class management strategies.

Materials: Worksheet 7–1 Student and Class Management Needs Resources for reviewing basic student needs.

WORKSHEET 7–1

Directions:

1. List the basic needs of all students on Worksheet 7–1. Use the consensus-forming technique to finalize the list and record on the worksheet. On an unmarked Worksheet 7–1, list the important student needs as determined by the consensus.

2. Match students' class management needs to the student needs determined most important by the consensus and record on Worksheet 7–1 beside each important need. Use the consensus-building technique to finalize the list.

3. On an unmarked Worksheet 7–1, record final student and class management needs determined most important to consider in planning and delivering instruction.

Variations:

1. Examine the planning framework chart for fostering motivation for learning. Match the activities and strategies listed to correlates of the three important student behaviors identified in Chapter 6.

2. An alternative activity would be to accept, add, delete, or revise the activities and strategies listed. Then match them to students and class management needs previously identified.

3. Conduct a survey. Have several teachers rank the needs and the class management needs related to each student need.

4. Have students react to the management procedures finalized in the above procedure. Set up a checklist and have the students assign a point value to each procedure. Rank the procedures in order and discuss these results with the students.

WORKSHEET 7–1. *Student and Class Management Needs*

STUDENTS' BASIC NEEDS	RATINGS			CLASS MANAGEMENT NEEDS	RATINGS		
	FIRST	SECOND	CONSENSUS		FIRST	SECOND	CONSENSUS
1.							
2.							
3.							
4.							
5.							
6.							
6.							
7.							
8.							

ACTIVITY 7–2. Teacher behavioral indicators in effective instruction: motivational and class management strategies for learning.

Objective:	To identify teacher behaviors that foster motivation for learning to increase students' involvement and learning and to prevent frequent discipline problems.
Materials:	Worksheet 7–2 Indicators of Teacher Behaviors in Effective Instruction: Motivation and Management Strategies for Learning

WORKSHEET 7–2

Directions:
1. Worksheet 7–2 lists statements describing teacher behaviors that have been shown to be highly related to student involvement and success in covering objectives specified for instruction. These statements are organized under two major categories: Motivation for Learning and Class Management and Learning.
2. Read each statement. Respond by answering "Yes" or "No." Indicate how certain you are of your response in the next column: 0 = completely uncertain and 5 = completely certain of the importance of this behavior as an indicator of teacher behaviors reflecting effective instruction. These behaviors become criteria for effective instruction.

Variations:
1. Use a team and the consensus-building technique to determine the most important indicators.
2. Survey teachers and have them complete the worksheet.

WORKSHEET 7–2. *Indicators of Teacher Behaviors in Effective Instruction: Motivation and Management Strategies for Learning*

TEACHER BEHAVIOR CATEGORIES	ANSWER YES/NO	CERTAINTY 0 TO 5
MOTIVATION FOR LEARNING		
1. Teachers' expectations affect students' expectations for learning.		
2. Teachers involve students in what they are to learn and how they are to learn.		
3. Teachers provide opportunities for self-directing students to manage and direct their instruction, using no extrinsic rewards.		
4. Teachers structure class climate so that it is pleasant and comfortable from students' perceptions.		
5. Teachers explain importance of learning lesson objectives—the how and why—of value now, and future benefits: play a game, play with others, enjoy TV sports, keep fit.		
6. Teachers provide learning activities that are challenging but that students can succeed in.		
7. Teachers allow students to have as much control over what and how they learn as feasible.		
8. Teachers involve students in selecting learning experiences that interest them.		
9. Teachers use reinforcers that are rewarding for students and produce desirable learning experiences.		
CLASS MANAGEMENT AND LEARNING		
1. Teachers establish class rules and procedures.		
2. Teachers define the limits of students' behaviors and set consequences avoiding negative reinforcers.		
3. Teachers consistently monitor students' behavior and provide positive reinforcement for its appropriateness.		
4. Teachers address specific behaviors that are defined as inappropriate and hold students accountable.		
5. Teachers use a variety of strategies to meet the management needs of students.		
6. Teachers identify or develop effective rewards (reinforcers, things that students want) and systematically deliver rewards for appropriate behavior and withhold rewards for inappropriate behavior.		
7. Teachers use different modes of instruction to provide students with the opportunity to become self-directed problem-solvers.		

WORKSHEET 7–2. *Indicators of Teacher Behaviors in Effective Instruction: Motivation and Management Strategies for Learning*

TEACHER BEHAVIOR CATEGORIES	FIRST RATING	SECOND RATING	CONSENSUS

ACTIVITY 7–3.   Assessing students' perception of learning-related actions in the class.

Objective: To understand effective teaching as described by students relative to the actions of the teacher in the class.

Materials: Teacher behaviors correlated with the student achievement described in Chapters 6 and 7. Activity 6–4:   Teacher Behavioral Indicators in Effective Instruction, and Activity 7–2   Teacher Behavioral Indicators in Effective Instruction: Motivational and Class Management Strategies for Learning.

Worksheet 7–3 Assessing student perception of learning-related actions in class.

WORKSHEET 7–3

Directions:
1. Have a group of teachers select 10 to 15 teacher behaviors. Use the consensus-building technique as needed.
2. Construct a questionnaire for students to evaluate the learning-related teacher behaviors in their class:
   —written statement of each question posed similar to the ones found in Activities 6–4 and 7–2 and understandable for the students;
   —have students answer on a scale from 0 to 5 the importance of the behavior;
   —average all scores and list the most important behaviors as perceived by students to be successful in the class.
3. Report results to the class. Teachers may wish to hold a class discussion and have students present ways that each behavior may be exhibited.
4. The teacher behaviors selected can be used to improve teaching. Productivity circles can be formed with students and the teacher. Each week the group can meet and define successes or problems and identify solutions to be worked on and evaluated the next week. These teaching behaviors can be related to students' role and responsibilities in the learning environment.

WORKSHEET 7–3. *Assessing Student Perception of Learning-Related Actions in Class*

TEACHER BEHAVIOR	RATING SCALE IMPORTANCE OF BEHAVIOR 0 to 5

PART III

Evaluation

The chapters in this section provide information and procedures focused on assessing the effectiveness of the program and principles of the improvement process.

Chapter 8 describes successful procedures for teacher, student, and program evaluation. Report forms and ways to communicate results of instruction in terms of student achievement are presented. A framework for program assessment and instructional effectiveness, based on the indicators discussed, is provided. The elements of effective class instruction, using the achievement-based curriculum (ABC) model, are identified along with specific types of data.

Chapter 9 presents current themes in the numerous reports focused on excellence and quality in education. Procedures that can capitalize on these reports and school improvement efforts are outlined. Specific principles of the improvement process are stated along with potential action plans to develop and/or to improve programs and teaching effectiveness based on school improvement, teaching effectiveness, and the ABC model.

Student and Program Evaluation

What is Evaluation?

Evaluation in the ABC model is a process by which merit is systematically determined. Merit is identified in the evaluation process by comparing program expectancies with actual program products. The program evaluation process can be applied at any level from student achievement on a specific objective to evaluating the overall effectiveness of an entire K through 12 program.

How is it Done?	*Decision Aids*
1. Collect student assessment and reassessment data on instructional objectives.	Data collection procedures Student entry status Student reassessment data
2. Determine the effectiveness of instruction on the targeted objectives.	Changes in student performance related to: —entry —expectancies —skill mastery
3. Report student performance at the unit and program levels.	Report contents Performance profiles Grades
4. Determine if the program plan was appropriate.	Internal review External review Consensus-forming techniques
5. Determine if the program was implemented as intended.	Staff self-monitoring Recording programmatic changes

6. Determine if the program produced the desired results.	Analysis of student change data
	Identification of program
	    Strengths and weaknesses
	Interpretation of why desired
	    changes did not occur

No matter how well an initial ABC program plan is designed, it is never perfect. The initial program plan provides a foundation upon which a dynamic, constantly improving physical education curriculum can be developed. Accepting that all programs can be improved, the question becomes one of how program weaknesses can be identified and remediated. The process of evaluation specifically addresses these issues.

Evaluation in the ABC model is a process by which program merit can be systematically determined. Program merit is the identification of strengths in the program, whereas lack of merit is the identification of weaknesses. The process of evaluation seeks to determine these strengths and weaknesses by comparing program expectations with actual program products. Data related to the identified weaknesses often provide information as to "why" the deficiencies exist and the insight neccessary to design alternatives that will remediate identified weaknesses.

Program, as used in this chapter, can refer to instruction related to a specific objective, a unit, a year, an instructional level, or an entire K through 12 program. It can also refer to a program for an individual or a group. The evaluation process always begins at the instructional objective level and works up. Teachers must evaluate instructional objectives first since they make up the units, and by looking at the effects of several units, they can evaluate the results of a year, multiyear, or the entire program. Therefore, whenever the term "program" is used, simply substitute objective, unit, year, or program.

As indicated, the goal of evaluation is to determine merit. The role of evaluation is multifaceted. Teachers can evaluate a total program, a program component, an individual's program, or the program of a particular population group. Similarly, teachers can evaluate the ends of a program, the means to the ends, or the degree to which the program meets some external standards (i.e., compliance with PL 94-142). The more common purposes of evaluation are to:

1. Document the validity or importance of the expectations (goals, objectives) of the program.
2. Document the way in which the program is being implemented.
3. Determine the effect of the program on its participants.
4. Provide information-based recommendations for revisions necessary to reduce identified weaknesses.
5. Document compliance or noncompliance with legislative mandates.
6. Document the relationship between program costs and effects.

Of particular importance is the information necessary to enhance orderly growth of the program to a stable condition that has benefited from current staff members but is not dependent on them. Such a program is dynamic in that it would improve each year as staff identified and remediated (through applications of evaluation procedures) weaknesses of the program.

The result of the application of evaluation procedures can be as many and varied as the roles that evaluation can serve. The more important for physical education are:

1. To describe the expectations of the program and to communicate the rationale and/or importance of these expectations to everyone involved with the program.
2. To describe how the plans and procedures designed to result in identified expectations (results and compliance processes) are being implemented.
3. To describe the results of implementing the program in terms of student performance gains.
4. To identify strengths and weaknesses of program implementation and effect.
5. To make recommendations for improving the program.
6. To design inservice sessions based on observed weaknesses in the program planning, implementation, and evaluation.

Currently, many models are available to guide educational evaluations; unfortunately, most of them cannot be used readily by physical education teachers. They are too complex, written generically, and designed to be used in a wide variety of educational settings. Consequently, it is often difficult to apply these models to specific physical education evaluation needs. More important, their complexity is overwhelming, not only from the standpoint of evaluation design but also from the standpoint of implementation time. Physical education teachers simply cannot allocate the time necessary to conduct a formal evaluation as described in most models.

A primary value of the evaluation models, however, is that they provide a framework from which a solid evaluation plan can be built. The objective-based structure underlying the ABC model ensures that it has already met certain criteria in its organization and implementation. Teachers, therefore, can cut through much of the content of other formal evaluation models and get right at the evaluative questions that must be answered to continuously refine the program.

The simplified evaluation procedures proposed for use with the ABC model in this chapter are not meant to reduce the quality of the evaluation process. Rather, they are suggested on the premise that a workable evaluation that is completed and results in positive program change is much better than a sophisticated evaluation plan that is not workable and therefore is never implemented. Physical educators must have an evaluation model that:

1. is consistent with the concept of quality;
2. is simple enough to be workable (i.e., completed and resulting in positive change);
3. can be applied to a total program or program elements;

4. can be applied to an individual, group, or groups;
5. can be conducted in a short period of time with little or no data collected beyond that which is already available as a result of implementing the program; and
6. can be conducted as part of the program's regular implementation.

The remaining sections of this chapter are designed to prepare educators in the necessary procedures needed to evaluate an ABC in physical education. Specific procedures will be discussed relative to student evaluation and reporting, and program evaluation and modification.

STUDENT EVALUATION AND REPORTING

Student evaluation is the process of determining and reporting the degree to which targeted goals and corresponding instructional objectives have been achieved by the students in the program. The student evaluation process is based on reassessment and yields information for represcribing and student reporting. The procedures for conducting student evaluations include:

1. assessing student entry status on the instructional objectives selected for inclusion in the program;
2. reassessing student change continuously during the course of instruction to provide:
   —feedback to the student,
   —feedback to the teacher regarding the appropriateness and effectiveness of instruction,
   —information necessary for reporting student status and change at the end of instruction;
3. determining what aspects of instruction were effective and what aspects of instruction were not effective; and
4. determining and reporting to appropriate audiences the amount of change observed subsequent to instruction.

ASSESSING STUDENT ENTRY STATUS

The procedures for assessing student entry status in the ABC model have already been discussed in detail in Chapter 5 (Student Assessment). Student entry assessment data allow the teacher to set student performance expectations, prescribe instruction, and make appropriate placement decisions.

REASSESSMENT AND PRESCRIPTION

Reassessment is designed to measure the performance level of a student subsequent to instruction. Reassessment provides the information necessary to KEEP the student working on the next higher performance level of each instructional objective and thus in the success-breeds-success cycle. For this reason, reassessment should occur continuously during instruction.

Reassessment, in this context, refers to the constant evaluation of student performance included as part of instruction that results in feedback to the student as well as information for the teacher. Each time students attempt a skill and receive feedback regarding some aspect of their performance, reassessment and represcription have occurred. The students have received positive feedback regarding their performance and direction regarding what needs to be worked on next. The teacher has received feedback regarding the quality and effectiveness of the prescribed instruction. Although this form of ongoing evaluation is at the informal end of the assessment-reassessment scale, it nonetheless is associated with good teaching and is a major determinant for improving student on-task-time and thus increases the probability of students making significant gains in performance.

Figure 8–1 shows an I CAN class performance score sheet with assessment and reassessment data. Performance standards that have been achieved are indicated by the date marked in the appropriate column across from the student's name. Each student's expectations have also been established and recorded on the score sheet. Using dates to indicate achievement is preferred over the standard X and O method as it provides a more accurate indication of the amount of time required to achieve the various standards. This procedure requires no more time than the X/O method and provides additional valuable information that can be used in evaluating student progress and program effectiveness.

Not all reassessments are formally recorded. This does not imply, however, that many of these observed changes in performance should not be recorded. It would be desirable if all reassessments were recorded. Such a practice, however, could often demand more instructional time than would be justifiable. Recording methods, as discussed in Chapter 5, that yield timely reassessment information and at the same time do not consume inordinate amounts of instructional time are what are needed. A reasonable amount of time devoted to student evaluation ranges between 10 to 15% of the time available for instruction.

DETERMINING THE EFFECTIVENESS OF INSTRUCTION

Reassessment data, as depicted in Figure 8–1, also provide the teacher with valuable feedback regarding the effectiveness of instruction in regard to both individual students and the class as a whole. Assume, for example, that instruction was specifically prescribed to teach an individual student or group of students a particular standard of a skill. Failure of the student(s) to demonstrate any improvement during reassessment alerts the teacher to a potential instructional problem. The teacher can then evaluate the instruction being prescribed to these student(s) and determine why they are not achieving as expected. A variety of factors exist that separately and/or in combination may contribute to the failure of student(s) to achieve. These contributing factors can be grouped into two broad areas: student characteristics, and characteristics of the prescribed instruction. Table 8–1 highlights some of the common contributing factors in each of these areas. The awareness of the teacher on a lesson-to-lesson basis that the student(s) is having difficulty allows them to examine systematically all the possible contributing factors and determine which one or ones are interfering with instruction. When the competing factors are identified, the teacher can then represcribe appropriate instruction.

Reassessment conducted only at the end of the instructional unit, therefore, yields no prescriptive utility, and much of the benefit of providing feedback and represcriptions is thereby lost. It is most desirable therefore to obtain reassessment data for represcription purposes on a lesson-to-lesson basis. When such data are available, it is possible for teachers to adjust instructional activities to maximize the degree of on-task learning on the objectives targeted for instruction. Assessment provides teachers with information for tailoring initial instruction and reassessment allows constant adjustment of teaching and instruction in accordance with changing student needs. Several techniques for efficiently collecting student assessment data were discussed in Chapter 5.

REPORTS: CONTENT AND GRADING

Meaningful reports to students, parents, and others are extremely important if the program is to maintain credibility. Complete student progress reports should include the following information:

1. The content (instructional objectives) that was taught.

I CAN

CLASS PERFORMANCE SCORE SHEET
PERFORMANCE OBJECTIVE: Skip

SCORING: Record the date, month/day when each focal point is achieved during assessment and reassessment.

*PRIMARY RESPONSES
N —Nonattending
NR—No response
UR—Unrelated response
O —Other (specify in comments)

FOCAL POINT

1. Assisted Skip
2. Unassisted Skip
3. a Step-Hop Alternate feet; b Arm Opposition; c Smooth Integration
4. a Accelerate-Increase Step / Decelerate-Decrease Step; b Incr. or Decr. Arm Action; c Incr. or Decr. Forward Lean
5. Lean on Turns / obstacle course

STD.
- 3 times/50 ft
- 3 times/50 ft
- 10 consecutive cycles, c
- a, b, c

NAME	1	2	3a	3b	3c	4a	4b	4c	5	No. focal points achieved on initial assessment	No. focal points targeted to be achieved	No. focal points actually achieved by final reassessment
1. Peter K.	9/8	9/8	9/8	9/8	10/5					4	2	1
2. Scott H.	9/8	9/15	10/1	10/8						1	3	3
3. Carol J.	9/8	9/8	9/8	9/8	9/8	10/1	10/15			5	1	2
4. Lori K.	9/8	9/8	9/8	9/8	9/8	10/15				5	1	1
5. Deborah M.	9/8	9/8	9/8	9/22	10/5	10/5				3	2	3
6. Denise F.	9/8	9/8	9/8	9/8	9/8	9/28	10/15			5	1	2
7. Larry S.	9/8	10/1	10/15	10/5						1	3	2
8. Billy R.	9/8	9/8	9/15	10/5						2	3	2
9. Donna R.	9/8	9/8	9/8	9/8	9/12	9/28	10/6			4	2	3
10. Joe V.	9/8	9/8	9/8	9/22	10/15	10/15				3	2	2
11. Debbie W.	9/8	9/8	9/8	9/8	9/8	10/15				5	1	1
12. Judy J.	9/8	9/8	9/8	9/15	9/22	10/5				3	2	2
13. Cathy S.	9/8	9/8	9/8	9/12	9/28	10/5				3	2	3
14. Mike M.	9/8	9/28	10/15							1	3	2
15. Eileen D.	9/8	9/8	9/8	9/8	9/8	10/5				5	1	2

Primary Responses* / COMMENTS

Figure 8–1. *Sample I CAN score sheet with assessment and reassessment data.*

TABLE 8–1. *Contributing Factors to Low Student Achievement*

Sample Student Characteristic	Sample Characteristic of Prescribed Instruction
Attention span	Equipment/facilities
Distractibility	Grouping
Attendance	Class climate
Success	Student/teacher ratio
Fear/anxiety	Administrative support
Comprehension	Teacher competence
Communication	Expectancy level/success
Illness/nutrition	Time allocation/objectives taught
Motivation	Instructional approach
Enthusiasm/interest	Type/amount of feedback
Learning rate	Instructional time available
Family/personal problems	Objectives tested/taught
Emotional control	Opportunity to practice
Self-dependence	Clarity of presentation
Prerequisite physical motor skills	Use of staff

2. The student's entry status on the instructional objectives.
3. The student's exit status on the instructional objectives.
4. The amount of change that occurred on each objective.
5. The student's status relative to his or her own continuous progress.
6. The student's status relative to his or her peers.

Not all of the above information needs to be provided on every report. These data should, however, be available on request to the interested student, parent, administrator, teacher, or IEP committee.

Content Information. The reporting of student achievement must be based on the content (instructional objectives) that composes the instructional program. Accordingly, a student progress report should be based on the degree to which the content has been mastered. As simple and logical as this may seem, student performance in physical education has not been evaluated and reported in this manner. Student evaluations (when conducted) are typically based on some standardized test of motor performance, motor development, fitness, and/or selected sport skills. To the extent that these tests measure the objectives included in the program, they may yield some usable information; however, these tests are generally not selected for their match to the instructional content taught in the program, thus making this type of evaluation unacceptable for identifying and reporting student gains.

With an ABC program, student evaluation with respect to test content is clear. Students are tested on the degree to which they have mastered the objectives they were instructed on. The performance standards of the instructional objectives comprise the criterion-referenced test items and the assessment and reassessment process provides the evaluative data. Reporting student progress, therefore, automatically includes the content that was taught by the fact that there are scores reported for each instructional objective.

Student performance data in relation to the instructional content should be reported at two levels. The first is the unit level and the second is the program level. The unit level of reporting is confined to the student's performance on the instructional objectives taught during the specified reporting period. No information is included about objectives covered previously or about those that will be taught in the future. Figure 8–2 shows a sample unit report.

The program reporting level is a cumulative report that indicates the student's

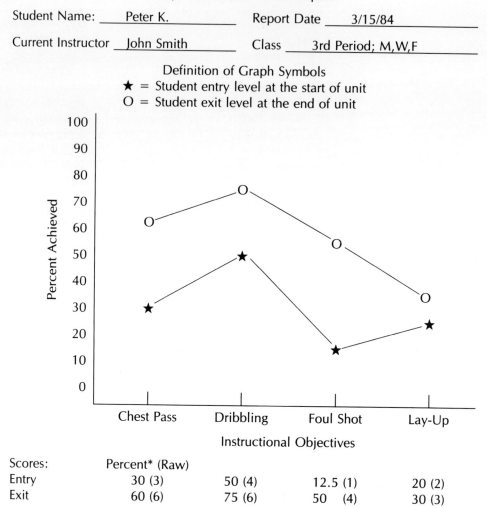

A CITY SCHOOL DISTRICT

Physical Education Unit Report

Student Name: ___Peter K.___   Report Date ___3/15/84___

Current Instructor ___John Smith___   Class ___3rd Period; M,W,F___

Definition of Graph Symbols
★ = Student entry level at the start of unit
O = Student exit level at the end of unit

Scores:	Percent* (Raw)			
Entry	30 (3)	50 (4)	12.5 (1)	20 (2)
Exit	60 (6)	75 (6)	50 (4)	30 (3)

*Percent values are calculated by dividing the number of standards achieved by the total number for that objective.

Figure 8–2. *Sample student unit report.*

performance throughout the program. This report shows the instructional content covered in the entire program and the student's achievement on those objectives to date. Figure 8–3 shows a sample program reporting form. Typically, unit reports would be issued periodically during the year whereas program reports would be issued less frequently, perhaps at the end of each instructional year or level.

Entry and Exit Status.   Entry status on instructional objectives is often omitted from most reporting formats used in physical education. Entry status, however, is necessary for calculating the amount of gain that has occurred on the objectives as a result of instruction. Omitting entry status prohibits the recipient of the report from knowing whether or not any improvement was made. Referring back to Figure 8–2, entry status was depicted by the (★) marks in each column of the graph. Entry status can be reported in raw score form (actual

A CITY SCHOOL DISTRICT

Physical Education Program Report—Elementary Level (K–3)

Student Name: Mike B.   Program Entry Date: 9/8/81

Report Date: 6/15/84   Present Grade/Class: 2nd

Current Instructor: John Smith

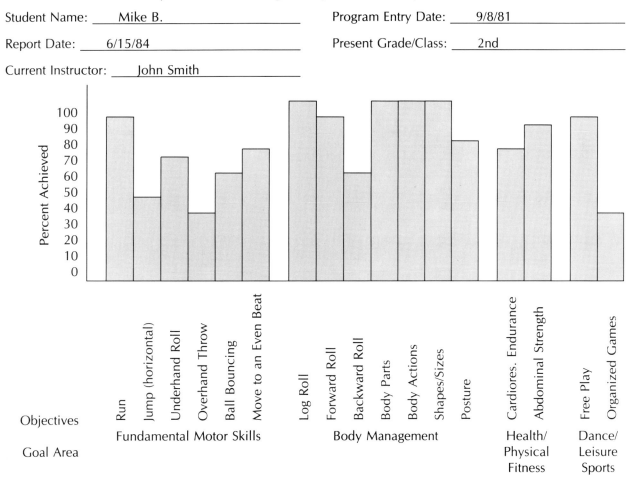

Figure 8–3. *Sample student program report.*

scores) or, more commonly, in the form of a standardized score like the percentiles used in Figure 8–2.

Exit status is more commonly reported in many reporting systems. It may be reported individually for each instructional objective or summarized as a percent or grade representing progress on a cluster of instructional objectives. Exit status is traditional information that most students, parents, and other recipients of the report expect and want to know. Exit status represents the degree of mastery the student has attained on the content covered within a reporting period. More specifically, it indicates the degree to which a student has mastered the components of a skill or skills along an absolute continuum. Exit status alone does not indicate the amount of learning that occurred but instead only the student's present degree of mastery. Although exit status scores allow for comparison between students' degree of mastery, the usefulness of these data is limited in the absence of how much was learned. Student exit status is depicted in Figure 8–2 by the (O) symbols.

Change Status.   Change status is the difference between entry and exit status and indicates the amount of progress (learning) made during the reporting period. Interpreting change status depends on entry and exit status and therefore should not be done independently. The data in Figure 8–4 demonstrate the interdependence between these measures and the need to consider all three when analyzing gain. The graphs show two students' performance on the physical fitness objective, abdominal strength, as measured by a one minute sit-up test. The first student had a low entry status and consequently had much room for potential improvement. At the end of the instructional unit this student had improved 40% as indicated by the difference between the exit and entry status (50% − 10% = 40%) but was only at the 50th percentile of mastery for this objective as indicated by the exit status. The second student had a high entry status (92%) and is probably at a point where increased performance comes very slowly. This student made only a minimal amount of gain during the instructional unit as indicated by the difference between the exit and entry status (96% − 92% = 4%), but had achieved 96% mastery of the objective. As indicated in this example, interpreting change status depends on the student's entry and exit status. To report only gain scores, 40% for the first student and 4% for the second student, would communicate an erroneous lack of progress comparatively for the second student, when in fact the student's performance and progress were excellent.

A second and potentially more meaningful method of calculating and interpreting change status is to compare student's entry status with performance expectations set at the beginning of instruction. Figure 8–5 shows the same abdominal strength example used earlier with the addition of this new dimension (expectations). The (?) in each graph indicates the expectancies set by the teacher for each student at the start of the unit. With this information the teacher can calculate the percent to which the students gained what they were targeted to achieve. The graph in Figure 8–5 reveals that the first student entered with a score of 5 (10th percentile), was expected to achieve a score of 30 (60th percentile) as a result of instruction and practice, and finished the unit with a score of 25 (50th percentile). As indicated earlier, this score indicates a 40% net gain in performance [exit status (50%) − entry status (10%) = gain (40%)], but only represents 80% achievement of the performance expectation set at the beginning of instruction. Expected gain was from 5 to 30 sit-ups or from the 10th to the 60th percentile. Since the student only improved to the 40th percentile, he only achieved 80% (40% divided by 50%) of the expected gain. The second student, on the other hand, was targeted to improve from the 92nd percentile (50 sit-ups) to the 96th percentile (54 sit-ups). Since this student's exit status matched

A CITY SCHOOL

Physical Education

Student Name: ___Peter K.___   Student Name: ___Mike B.___

Current Instructor: ___John Smith___   Current Instructor: ___John Smith___

Definition of Graph Symbols

★ = Student entry level
O = Student actual achievement level

Instructional Objectives

Score: Percent (Raw)			Score: Percent (Raw)		
Entry	10 (5)	40 (8)	Entry:	92 (50)	70 (5)
Actual Exit:	50 (25)	80 (4)	Actual Exit:	96 (54)	80 (4)
Net Change:	40 (20)	40 (4)	Net Change:	4 (4)	10 (1)

Figure 8–4. *Sample student performance profiles reporting change data.*

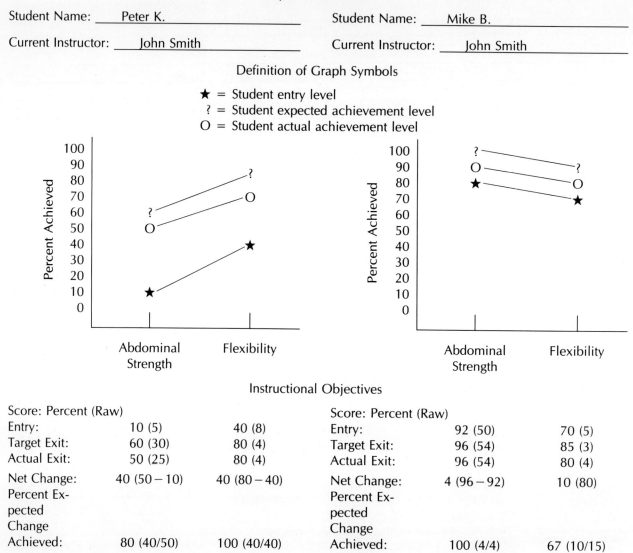

A CITY SCHOOL

Physical Education

Student Name: _____ Peter K. _____   Student Name: _____ Mike B. _____

Current Instructor: _____ John Smith _____   Current Instructor: _____ John Smith _____

Definition of Graph Symbols

★ = Student entry level
? = Student expected achievement level
O = Student actual achievement level

Instructional Objectives

Score: Percent (Raw)				Score: Percent (Raw)		
Entry:	10 (5)	40 (8)		Entry:	92 (50)	70 (5)
Target Exit:	60 (30)	80 (4)		Target Exit:	96 (54)	85 (3)
Actual Exit:	50 (25)	80 (4)		Actual Exit:	96 (54)	80 (4)
Net Change:	40 (50 − 10)	40 (80 − 40)		Net Change:	4 (96 − 92)	10 (80)
Percent Expected Change Achieved:		80 (40/50)	100 (40/40)	Percent Expected Change Achieved:	100 (4/4)	67 (10/15)

Figure 8–5. *Sample student performance profiles reporting both change and expectation data.*

the expectation set at the beginning of instruction, this student achieved 100% of the expected gain. Expected and actual gain both equaled 4% (96% − 92% = 4%). Therefore, the student achieved 100% of the targeted gain set at the beginning of instruction (4% divided by 4%).

As seen from the previous example, the inclusion of change status in comparison to performance expectations adds considerable interpretative power to evaluating student performance. This information can be useful when letter or percent grades must be assigned in physical education. Figure 8–6 shows an example of a profile report that is summarized into a letter grade. Note that the three volleyball objectives are weighted twice as heavily as the physical fitness objectives. These weightings represent the proportional amount of instructional time spent on each objective. Since varying amounts of instructional time are spent on the different objectives in a unit, each can be weighted proportionally in calculating the final grade.

Status Relative To Self and Peers. All of the reports presented thus far have been individual reports. These reports show only the individual student's performance (entry and exit status) in relation to objective mastery and/or targeted expectations. This form of reporting clearly communicates the student's performance on the program objectives. If the student is not achieving as expected, appropriate changes and modifications can be made in the program and/or in instruction.

A second dimension that can be added to these individual reports is peer comparative data. This dimension allows the recipient of the report to also interpret the student's progress and performance on the program objectives in relation to other student populations (class, grade, local, or national norms). This form of evaluative information also aids the teacher in identifying individual student strengths and weaknesses which is helpful in making appropriate programmatic adjustments such as adjusting the amount of content covered, the student's placement, or the level of performance expectations set. Figure 8–7 shows an example of a student report that contains peer comparative data. The (M) symbol indicates the class mean or average degree of mastery the class obtained on each objective. This form of comparative information can be important when evaluating the appropriateness of student placements in physical education.

Profiles represent a comprehensive reporting system that incorporates the content covered, student entry, exit, and change status on the instructional objectives included in the reporting period, information relative to the individual student's own continuous progress, and the student's status in relation to significant others. The pictorial nature of profiles allows them to communicate much information that can be easily interpreted by the report recipients. If percent/letter grades must be assigned, they can by readily derived and justified from the student's profile.

Graphic profiles can be produced by hand or by computers. The greatest obstacle to widespread use of profiles as a reporting format in physical education is the time required to make them. The ever-increasing number of microcomputers in the public schools and the multipurpose data base management programs available to use on them makes the feasibility of using computers to generate profiles a reality in almost all schools. Physical educators must be willing, however, to explore and harness the use of computer technology to best serve their needs. The notion that a teacher must be a computer programmer or a math genius to use a computer is a myth. Many computer programs that could be beneficially used by physical educators only require a few hours of training and practice to use efficiently and effectively.

Student Report Formats. Letter grades (i.e., A, B, C, D, F, S, U) or their

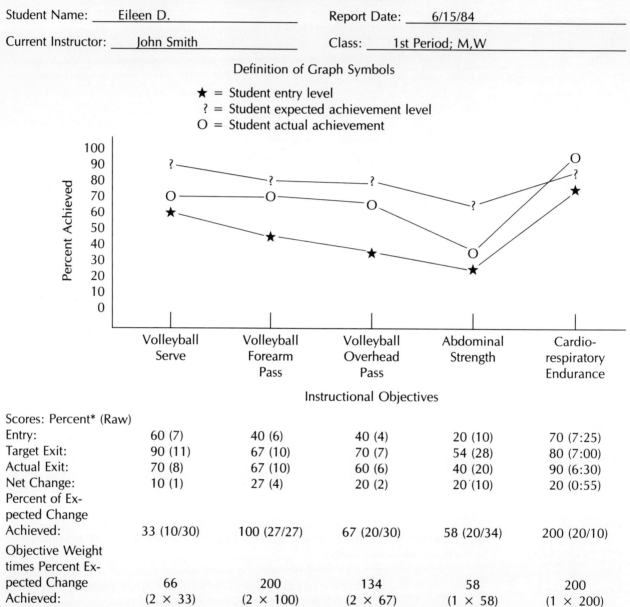

A CITY SCHOOL DISTRICT

Physical Education Unit Report

Student Name: ___Eileen D.___   Report Date: ___6/15/84___

Current Instructor: ___John Smith___   Class: ___1st Period; M,W___

Definition of Graph Symbols

★ = Student entry level
? = Student expected achievement level
O = Student actual achievement

Scores: Percent* (Raw)	Volleyball Serve	Volleyball Forearm Pass	Volleyball Overhead Pass	Abdominal Strength	Cardio-respiratory Endurance
Entry:	60 (7)	40 (6)	40 (4)	20 (10)	70 (7:25)
Target Exit:	90 (11)	67 (10)	70 (7)	54 (28)	80 (7:00)
Actual Exit:	70 (8)	67 (10)	60 (6)	40 (20)	90 (6:30)
Net Change:	10 (1)	27 (4)	20 (2)	20 (10)	20 (0:55)
Percent of Expected Change Achieved:	33 (10/30)	100 (27/27)	67 (20/30)	58 (20/34)	200 (20/10)
Objective Weight times Percent Expected Change Achieved:	66 (2 × 33)	200 (2 × 100)	134 (2 × 67)	58 (1 × 58)	200 (1 × 200)

*Unit grade is calculated by summing the weighted percent expectancies achieved for each objective (66 + 200 + 134 + 58 + 200 = 658) and dividing by the total number of weights (2 + 2 + 2 + 1 + 1 = 8). 658 ÷ 8 = 82.25%. This percent grade can then be converted into a letter grade if needed.

Figure 8–6. *Sample student progress unit report with weighted objectives and letter grade conversion calculation.*

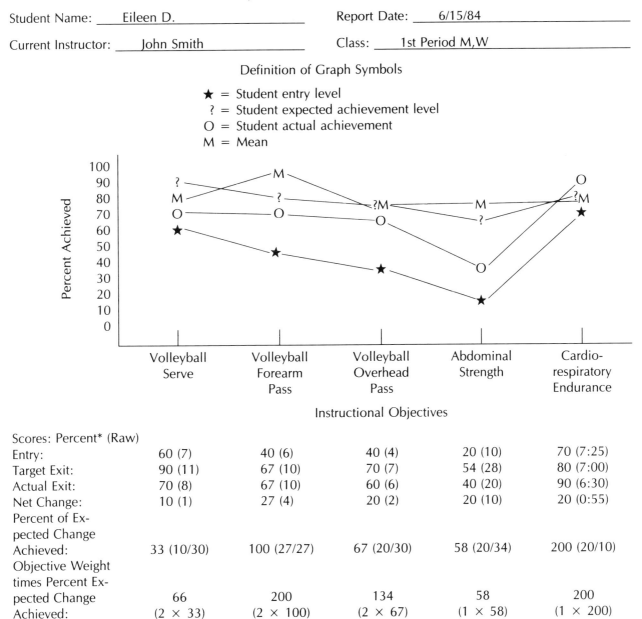

A CITY SCHOOL DISTRICT

Physical Education Unit Report

Student Name: ___Eileen D._____ Report Date: ___6/15/84_____

Current Instructor: ___John Smith_____ Class: ___1st Period M,W_____

Definition of Graph Symbols

★ = Student entry level
? = Student expected achievement level
O = Student actual achievement
M = Mean

Scores: Percent* (Raw)	Volleyball Serve	Volleyball Forearm Pass	Volleyball Overhead Pass	Abdominal Strength	Cardio-respiratory Endurance
Entry:	60 (7)	40 (6)	40 (4)	20 (10)	70 (7:25)
Target Exit:	90 (11)	67 (10)	70 (7)	54 (28)	80 (7:00)
Actual Exit:	70 (8)	67 (10)	60 (6)	40 (20)	90 (6:30)
Net Change:	10 (1)	27 (4)	20 (2)	20 (10)	20 (0:55)
Percent of Expected Change Achieved:	33 (10/30)	100 (27/27)	67 (20/30)	58 (20/34)	200 (20/10)
Objective Weight times Percent Expected Change Achieved:	66 (2 × 33)	200 (2 × 100)	134 (2 × 67)	58 (1 × 58)	200 (1 × 200)

*Unit Grade is calculated by summing the weighted percent expectancies achieved for each objective (66 + 200 + 134 + 58 + 200 = 658) and dividing by the total number of weights (2 + 2 + 2 + 1 + 1 = 8). 658 ÷ 8 = 82.25%. This percent grade can then be converted into a letter grade if needed.

Figure 8–7. *Sample student progress unit report with average class performance indicated.*

percentage equivalents have been used traditionally by many schools to report student progress in physical education. Letter grades by themselves fail to communicate much of the information needed to report student progress effectively, as discussed in this chapter. No information is communicated in a letter grade regarding the content taught, the student's entry or exit status on the instructional objectives, and whether the grade is based on student gain or only student exit status.

If letter grades must be used, they should be accompanied by either a narrative report or a graphic profile to substantiate how they were derived. Although narrative reports can be developed to meet all the report criteria outlined in this chapter, in practice they rarely do in physical education. Most narrative reports used in physical education employ open-ended general descriptions of student performance (i.e., "Mary's performance in physical education continues to show improvement."). Narrative reports of this nature are used quite commonly at the elementary school level; unfortunately, they communicate no more information than the letter grades they were designed to replace.

The graphic profiles as depicted in this chapter are the recommended reporting format to be used in conjunction with an ABC in physical education.

STUDENT EVALUATION SUMMARY

Student evaluation is important for feedback to the student, teacher, and for modification of instructional prescriptions. It is also a prerequisite to accurate reporting of student progress. A complete report of student progress must either incorporate, or have a sound rationale for not incorporating, each of the following elements: the content covered, student entry, exit, and change status on the objectives included in the reporting period, information relative to the individual student's own continuous progress, and the student's status relative to significant others. Though many formats for reporting student progress are available, the student profile, as illustrated in this chapter is the recommended reporting format to be used with an ABC in physical education.

It can be readily seen that the ability to document student progress is a prerequisite to completing any kind of program evaluation and refinement. Physical educators must be able to document the success and failure of students both individually and collectively to systematically alter the instructional program to improve its benefits to all students. The information that students, their parents, and selected other school officials want and need is also essential information needed by physical educators to make appropriate program changes. Data collection and reporting are thereby critical components of instituting a quality ABC physical education program.

PROGRAM EVALUATION AND MODIFICATION

Program evaluation and modifications are an extension of the student evaluation procedures discussed in the first part of this chapter. Program evaluation is necessary to identify program merit and to systematically improve the procedures of planning, implementing, and evaluating instruction to maximize the results or outcomes of the evaluation process. Program evaluation as addressed in this chapter is designed to evaluate three basic questions:

1. Is the program plan appropriate?
2. Was the program implemented as intended?
3. Did the program produce the desired results?

The evaluation and modification procedures associated with each of these questions are discussed in the remaining section of this chapter.

IS THE PROGRAM PLAN APPROPRIATE?

Although the first question reads, "Is the program plan appropriate?", remember the words "program plan" could apply to a K through 12 program, a program level, a unit, an objective, and the question would still be relevant. Similarly, the question could be stated as "Is the program plan appropriate for Johnny, or all children?" The key to the question is the term "appropriate." The program plan must be appropriate for the individual and/or population group for which it was designed. If the program plan is found to be inappropriate, the physical educator should then skip the next evaluation questions, and deal directly with the question "What needs to be changed to improve the program plan?"

Many evaluation questions related to program appropriateness can and should be addressed prior to program implementation. Some of the more prominent questions are presented in Table 8–2.

The checklist in Table 8–2 can be applied to the program plan by a variety of people, either individually or collectively. The outside review of a program by experts, administrators, parents, and students using the consensus technique outlined in Chapter 4 (Table 4–3) provides valuable insights into discrepancies and/or weaknesses in the program plan.

Although the use of internal experts is the most efficient form of evaluation during program development, the use of outside experts to review the final program plan is probably one of the more commonly used evaluation techniques. When this option is considered, it is critical that the experts be selected based on their established experience in program evaluation and demonstrated link with ongoing quality programs and not because they have a fancy title.

The more comprehensive a review undertaken prior to implementation, the greater the likelihood that a number of potential implementation problems will be avoided. When discrepancies or problems are identified, appropriate changes can be made using the procedures outlined in the earlier chapters. When the program is finally judged appropriate, it is ready for the ultimate test—implementation.

WAS THE PROGRAM IMPLEMENTED AS INTENDED?

Before the degree of student gains can be evaluated, it is necessary to identify how the program was implemented. Teachers must know whether they are evaluating the planned program or a modified form. The program can be modified as long as the modifications are known and recorded sufficiently so that the program can be evaluated and replicated.

Self-monitor forms designed to identify program discrepancies can be used by the staff. Table 8–3 depicts a sample checklist that can be used by teachers to monitor their implementation.

The example checklist (Table 8–3) provides several key criteria for determining how an ABC unit was implemented. Completion of the checklist during implementation of each unit provides valuable information necessary to evaluate implementation mastery.

The checklist provides the teacher with a self-check on whether or not the characteristics and procedures built into the program are being followed. Maintaining a record of specific implementation strengths and weaknesses encountered in each unit throughout implementation provides a data base for identifying implementation problems.

Table 8–4 shows the summary of one teacher's unit evaluations across all the units in a given year of the program plan. Summarizing the evaluation data in this way allows for easy identification of implementation of strengths and weak-

TABLE 8–2. *Program Appropriateness Evaluation Checklist*

EVALUATIVE ITEM	YES	NO	COMMENT
1. There is a written statement of program goals that represents physical education content that is directly tied to the evidence that documents the potential contributions of activity to the growth, development, and general quality of life.			
2. The goal statements are written in output terminology (i.e., they represent the *results* of instruction rather than instructional inputs or opportunities).			
3. The goals were derived or updated using both professional and community input to assure their local relevance.			
4. There is a written document that indicates instructional objectives that operationally define each goal statement.			
5. There is a written document that indicates how each instructional objective is subdivided into smaller sequential instructional objectives.			
6. The sequential instructional objectives of each program objective have a sufficient range in difficulty to provide for the assessment of students who range in performance ability from near "zero competence" to at least "functional competence."			
7. The instructional objectives of each program objective are stated in terms that allow for their reliable assessment.			
8. The program objectives are organized into a written structure that identifies a logical progression of content for each grade level in the program.			
9. The program structure (i.e., K through 12) was developed using the expertise of teachers and administrators representative of each level of the program.			
10. Instructional objectives placed into program levels are further arranged into a September to June sequence in some form of logical instructional groupings or units of instruction.			
11. The number of program objectives included in each level of the program were determined based upon creating a match between the amount of instructional time needed to make meaningful gains in student performance and the amount of time available for instruction.			
12. The program content and method were reviewed (and appropriately modified where necessary) for each student placed in the regular education setting.			
13. Individual placements into the program are determined based upon a review of student status in the areas of learning characteristics, personal-social characteristics, and physical and motor performance capabilities.			

TABLE 8–3. *Teacher Unit Implementation Evaluation Checklist*

Evaluative Item	Yes	No	Comments
1. Instructors at each level of the program teach content in accordance with the stated plan.			
2. Lessons are planned in accordance with the skill level of the students as indicated by assessment on the instructional objectives.			
3. Lessons (drills, games, teaching procedures, practice sessions, groupings, time allotments) are selected or developed to facilitate student achievement or instructional objectives included in the program organizational and unit plans.			
4. Lessons are implemented in accordance with program organizational unit and daily plans.			
5. Lessons are implemented in accordance with accepted guidelines for effective instruction.			
6. Efficient use of instructional time available.			
7. Appropriate use of instructional cues, prompts for class and/or individual students.			
8. Positive feedback and corrective procedures for instructional objectives for class group and/or individual students.			
9. Managing student behaviors that interfere with teacher's instruction or on-task-time of other students.			
10. Student achievement or lack of achievement on the instructional objectives is monitored and recorded regularly.			
11. Student achievement information is known and available at the objective, unit, and program levels for review by staff administrators, parents, or significant others.			
12. Evaluation is conducted to determine whether students are making significant gains on a significant number of objectives.			
13. When the evaluation indicates that many students are not making significant gains on many of the objectives, answers to the question "WHY" are systematically sought in areas such as: time alloted, instructional methods, levels of performance expectation, class size, number of aides, and so forth.			
14. Revisions of the instructional program or methods are based on student achievement results in conjunction with answers to the evaluative "WHY" questions.			

nesses. If several different staff members are implementing the same units, the chart in Table 8–4 can be modified to reflect their combined performance. This can be accomplished by replacing the "★" with the percentage of the staff that responded "yes" to each item.

Although the goal of any teacher or staff member would be to achieve 100% mastery on all evaluation items within and across units, each discrepancy must

TABLE 8–4. *Identifying Implementation Strengths and Weaknesses Across Units*

TEACHER IMPLEMENTATION SUMMARY
Teacher Unit Implementation Checklist Items

Instructional Units	1	2	3	4	5	6	7	8	9	10	11	12	13	14	15	16	Sum	% Mastery
1. Physical Fitness	*	*	*	*		*	*	*	*	*	*	*	—	*	*	*	14	93
2. Soccer	*	*	*	*	*	*		*	*	*	*		—				10	67
3. Gymnastics	*	*	*	*	*	*	*	*	*	*	*	*	—	*	*	*	15	100
4. Basketball	*	*	*	*	*	*		*	*	*	*	*	—	*	*	*	14	93
5. Track & Field	*	*	*	*		*	*		*		*		—				8	53
6. Softball	*	*	*	*	*	*			*		*		—				8	53
Sum:	6	6	6	6	4	6	3	4	6	4	6	3	—	3	3	3	69	
Item Percent Mastery: (Sum ÷ by number of units)	100	100	100	100	67	100	50	67	100	67	100	50	—	50	50	50		76

Key: * = Yes response

— = NA not applicable item

blank = a negative response

be interpreted independently. On one item, 80% mastery might be considered acceptable while on another, nothing less than 100% might be acceptable. Acceptance levels therefore should be established in accordance with local values.

When individual or group discrepancies or problems are identified, appropriate modifications can be designed to remediate them. This evaluative data can also be used to determine such things as:

1. inservice priorities for staff training;
2. the need for additional administrative support;
3. rationale for changes in scheduling or class sizes;
4. reallocation of resources; or
5. a variety of other programmatic changes.

In addition, this evaluation process also identifies strengths of both the program and individual staff members. Systematic evaluation of a variety of different approaches to addressing various problems will allow the poor practices to be discarded and the successful practices to be identified and replicated.

If, during the program's implementation, it becomes apparent that changes are needed, they can and should be made. This, however, becomes an evaluation resulting from an attempt to implement the program forcing an immediate refinement to allow implementation to occur. Such a change is the result of a discrepancy between a planned occurrence or expectation and actual implementation and therefore must be resolved. The resolution then becomes the new planned expectation for the next implementation trial. Accumulations of such refinements are what allow the program to grow in its effectiveness and are therefore the desirable products of an evaluation.

When changes are made in the program either as a result of an implementation attempt as suggested, or through the implementation of another evaluation technique like the teacher checklist, they must be recorded in two places. First, the change must be added to the description of the program so that it does not have to be rediscovered during another implementation attempt. Second, the change should be reflected in a modification of the monitoring form, if appropriate, to assure that the form is sensitive to the implementation of the new procedure.

It is critical to the stability of a program (i.e., causing it not to be dependent on a staff that is more transient than the program itself) that such refinements be written into its description or they may be lost and emerge as problems at another time.

When no adequate description of the program exists, this constant refinement and growth is lost. It is not uncommon for refinements that were created over years by an excellent instructor to be lost when he or she leaves the system. This occurs when these changes are not incorporated into the description of the program. A new employee hired to replace the experienced staff person must start all over to build the program without the benefit of information learned and previously integrated into the program. This is a tremendous waste of public resources and a serious disservice to the students.

DID THE PROGRAM PRODUCE THE DESIRED RESULTS?

Evaluation of the program is merely an extension of the evaluation of individual students. Evaluation of individual students within an ABC model is straightforward in that the program's organization, implementation, and evaluation are based on program objectives. As discussed in the previous section, "Student Evaluation and Reporting," teachers evaluate student progress to the degree to which stated instructional objectives are achieved. Student gain is simply the student's status upon entry (assessment) subtracted from their exit performance (final reassessment). Program evaluation concerns itself with the number of students enrolled in the program who are making the desired gains on the objectives taught. If the proportion of gains is large enough, then the program can be said to be effective; if insufficient gains occur, the program is in need of revision.

Program evaluation can be completed by the implementation staff with information primarily available as a result of regular implementation of the program. Professional and legislative mandates require that instruction be delivered based on identified student needs. This requirement can be appropriately met by using an ABC model where instruction is prescribed based on an assessment of student entry status and represcribed as a result of changes monitored during the course of instruction. The student change data necessary to determine program effectiveness therefore are already available in records associated with assessment and reassessment data. Accordingly, program evaluation can be completed by good recordkeeping and simply aggregating the individual student change data already available.

Figure 8–8 shows a completed class performance score sheet for the instructional objective serve from a volleyball unit. The score sheet also indicates the students' initial achievement levels, expected achievement levels, and actual achievement levels. Summing the expected achievement column for all the students in the class and dividing that value by the sum of the actual achievement column for all students indicates the teacher's effectiveness in reaching his or her expectancies. Although the teacher effectiveness value is a good indicator of whether the program is having the desired effect, it must be recognized that this value is dependent on the teacher's ability to set appropriate target expectancy levels for each student. If the teacher consistently underestimates each student and sets a lower expectancy, the effectiveness value achieved would be proportionally too high. Conversely, the opposite would occur if the teacher consistently sets expectations that are too high.

A second indicator, program effectiveness, is the relationship between student actual gain and the standard set for meaningful gain during program planning.

I CAN VOLLEYBALL UNIT
SPORT, LEISURE, and RECREATIONAL SKILLS

CLASS PERFORMANCE SCORE SHEET
PERFORMANCE OBJECTIVE:
Functional Underhand Serve

SCORING
Assessment:
X = Achieved
O = Not achieved
Reassessment:
⊗ = Achieved
∅ = Not achieved
Shaded boxes indicate target expectations

*PRIMARY RESPONSES
NA • Nonattending
NR • No response
UR • Unrelated response
O • Other (specify in comments)

FOCAL POINT / STD.

a Ready position
b Eyes on ball
c Serving arm position and motion
d Serving hand strikes ball
e Stride forward with foot opposite stroking arm
f Follow through
g Foot behind end line
h Smooth integration
   Serve into one of two specified court areas

2/3 times

NAME	a	b	c	d	e	f	g	h	Number of focal points achieved on initial assessment	Number of focal points targeted to be achieved	Number of focal points actually achieved by final reassessment
1. Mary D.	X	X	X	X	∅	⊗	∅	∅	4	2	1
2. Doug D.	X	⊗	⊗	⊗	∅	∅	∅	∅	1	3	3
3. Peter M.	X	X	X	X	X	⊗	⊗	∅	5	1	2
4. Marilyn H.	X	X	X	X	X	⊗	∅	∅	5	1	1
5. Barth T.	X	X	X	⊗	⊗	⊗	∅	∅	3	2	3
6. Joe R.	X	X	∅	X	X	⊗	⊗	∅	5	1	2
7. Jane M.	X	⊗	X	⊗	∅	∅	∅	∅	1	3	2
8. Nancy M.	X	X	⊗	⊗	⊗	∅	∅	∅	2	3	2
9. Dave M.	X	X	X	X	⊗	⊗	∅	⊗	4	2	3
10. Barb G.	X	X	X	⊗	⊗	∅	∅	∅	3	2	2
Sum									33	20	21

Teacher Effectiveness = 20/21 = 95%   Program Effectiveness = 21/30 = 70%
Targeted Meaningful Gain = 3 standards per student per objective

Figure 8–8. *Completed class performance score sheet with teacher and program effectiveness calculations.*

TABLE 8–5. *Yearly Plan Implementation Summary Chart*

Unit/Objectives	Time			Implementation Mastery (%)	Teacher Effectiveness (%)	Program Effectiveness (%)
	Planned	Actual	Difference			
Cardiorespiratory Endurance	70	70		(11/15) 74	75	65
Body Parts	210	120	−90		100	100
Run	150	150			80	72
Low Organized Games	70	160	+90		92	84
Cardiorespiratory Endurance	70	70		(13/15) 87	80	75
Body Actions	150	90	−30		95	100
Run	150	150			90	95
Low Organized Games	150	180	+30		90	90
Cardiorespiratory Endurance	70	70		(12/15) 80	80	85
Hop	150	150			83	72
Underhand Throw	150	180	+30		60	75
Low Organized Games	150	120	−30		67	75
Cardiorespiratory Endurance	70	70		(14/15) 94	85	90
Gallop	150	150			85	95
Kick	150	150			83	85
Low Organized Games	150	150			90	100
Cardiorespiratory Endurance	70	70		(13/15) 87	81	90
Skip	150	180	+30		67	75
Catch	150	210	+70		60	70
Low Organized Games	150	50	−100		45	65
			Average	84.4%	79.4%	82.9%

*Percentages greater than 100% reported as 100%.

Although meaningful gain is also somewhat of a subjective standard, it represents the combined estimate of the staff involved in planning the program. Since the targeted meaningful gain is also directly related to the amount of instructional time scheduled for an objective, failure to consistently achieve meaningful gain on an objective might indicate a need to increase the amount of instructional time allocated. Figure 8–8 also shows the calculation of the program effectiveness value. This value is calculated by dividing the sum of the actual achievement column (21) by the product of the number of students (10) times the standard set for meaningful gain (3). Although actually achieving 100% program effectiveness may be idealistic, it provides the staff with a goal. If 100% effectiveness is achieved or surpassed, it may indicate a need to increase the expected meaningful gain or decrease the amount of instructional time allocated for that objective.

The key to successful program evaluation is the maximum use of available information. Table 8–5 displays a sample chart that summarizes the key indicators of program effectiveness which can be readily derived from the program implementation and monitoring data already collected. The first column (Unit/ Objectives) lists the program units and related objectives scheduled for a given year. The first column under "Time" indicates the (Planned) amount of time scheduled for each unit and objective. The second column under "Time" indicates the (Actual) amount of time spent. Data for this column are obtained from the teacher's comments recorded on either the lesson plans or the class performance score sheets. The third column under "Time" (Difference) gives the difference between the planned and actual time columns. Marked discrepancies in the difference column indicate a need to revise the allocation of instructional time.

The teacher implementation mastery values were taken from the various Teacher Unit Implementation Evaluation Checklists like the one depicted in Table 8–3. Teacher effectiveness and program effectiveness values were calculated from the class performance score sheets as described in Figure 8–8. This composite provides a clear picture of the program's implementation and effect from which strengths and weaknesses can be identified. Where anticipated implementation or effects have been achieved, the teacher can then attempt to refine the program so that the same results can be achieved with less time, effort, and cost. Where expectations were not met, the teacher must determine why and initiate appropriate changes. When the program begins to produce consistent positive results, the physical educator can start a good public relations program advertising the quality of the program. Program evaluation summary data should be reported annually to all relevant audiences (i.e., administrators and the school board).

Although summary implementation and effectiveness evaluation data provide clear indications of where weaknesses exist, they frequently do not explain why. Only by identifying why can revisions be made to remediate the weakness.

It is usually easy to determine why a weakness has surfaced in program implementation. Often it is the result of a lack of knowledge related to planning, implementing, and/or evaluating (suggesting a possible need for inservice), or simply a situation of not following through and doing what was planned.

Determining why a sufficient number of students did not make meaningful gains on one or more of the program's objectives is a more difficult task. There is, however, a simple approach to this problem that is systematic and consistent with procedures recommended in large evaluation projects. The procedure involves systematically identifying the differences between those who made the expected gain and those who did not.

Large evaluation studies investigate this "evaluative why" question by conducting many correlational analyses between student gain data and many other variables. Categories of variables that are typically used include:

1. characteristics of the students;
2. characteristics of the teachers;
3. characteristics of the instructional setting or school-related factors; and
4. implementation characteristics.

In each category there are many variables (anything that might influence learning) measured on many students that are all interrelated in such a way that the strength of the relationships are documented. The stronger the relationship between student gain and some variable or group of variables, the more likely the reasons for insufficient achievement may be attributed to the identified variable or variables.

For example, if the instructional objective RUN were taught to a group of students and only 20% of them achieved the targeted gain, an obvious weakness in the instructional program could be identified. Suppose that an analysis of the relationship between gains in running and other measured variables showed a strong relationship to the variable age. Review of the gain data of the students on running shows that the younger students comprise the majority who made no changes, whereas nearly all the gains were made by the older students. Such an analysis would suggest one or more of the sample reasons listed below regarding why only 20% of the students achieved the expectancy level.

1. The expected amount of gain was too high for younger students.
2. The instructional materials used to direct the lessons were inappropriate for younger students. Games, drills, and/or organization were such that the students did not get a sufficient number of trials and/or appropriate feedback.
3. The teaching method and/or approach was more appropriate for older students or less appropriate for younger students.
4. The instructional context (length and/or spacing of instructional time, facilities, or equipment) was appropriate for older but not younger students.
5. The younger students did not have the necessary prerequisite skills to benefit from the lessons.

This type of analysis can isolate potential causes for an achievement weakness. Such an analysis, however, is fine for large groups of students in large evaluation studies where the resources to do sophisticated computer analyses are available, but what about the single teacher working with one class and only limited data collection on potential relationship variables? Obviously, he or she cannot conduct a large self-investigation into the "evaluative why" question of the same magnitude as a large-scale evaluation project. There is, however, a similar and realistic approach that can yield equally beneficial results.

In essence, teachers can get the same information by informally comparing the characteristics (Table 8–1) surrounding the instruction of the students who were the best achievers with those who achieved the least. Informal implementation of this technique requires no data collection beyond that which is already available.

Assuming there were appropriate recordkeeping, systematic implementation of an ABC model yields the information necessary to identify potential answers to why achievement expectations were not met. For example, a teacher implementing an ABC in physical education would have the following information available:

1. Class performance score sheets that include student entry and exit levels on each of the instructional objectives included in the various units.
2. One page overview of the units showing the amount of time allocated to teaching each instructional objective (including the amount of time actually used for each instructional objective was penciled in).
3. Lesson plans (sufficiently detailed so teachers could repeat good lessons and avoid repeating poor ones).
4. Teacher implementation data for the unit.
5. Information regarding the students' learning, personal-social, and physical and motor characteristics obtained from the student needs profile.

To make a high-low comparison, select 10 to 15% of the highest and lowest achievers on an objective or set of objectives and determine how they differ from one another. Such a comparison can be conducted mentally within a short period of time or by actually comparing the screening profiles of the high and low achievers item by item. Consider every difference for its potential in influencing the lack of learning that occurred for the low group. Where potential influencing factors are detected, they become criteria for making appropriate planning, implementing, or evaluating changes. Often, surprisingly powerful notions emerge regarding achievement. From these notions, changes emerge that must be developed, implemented, and re-evaluated to determine their effect in subsequent implementations of instructional objectives. This process should be continuous. Initially, changes should be identified and remediated to eliminate weaknesses related to student achievement on all possible intructional objectives. When this occurs, the evaluative effort can be shifted away from mere remediation of weak spots toward improvement. Improvement in this context refers to either meeting increased expectation levels or meeting the same levels of expectation while reducing the amount of instructional time. If instructional time can be reduced, additional instructional objectives can be added to the program.

To create a dynamic program, the recommended changes must be included in an updated program description. A program sufficiently described so that its key components can be replicated can be systematically changed to include revision recommendations to be implemented and re-evaluated.

If evaluation is conducted and appropriate changes are not recorded, the students are the losers. If a program is defined, implemented, and evaluated over several years, it will improve. If those changes are not incorporated into revised drafts of the program and the person who implemented these changes leaves the system, the refined program is lost. The new instructor, and more importantly the students, do not have the benefit of the refined program. Although this situation is the norm rather than the exception, it is a tremendous waste of school and district resources. The gains made are lost if the program is totally dependent on the person currently implementing it. By maintaining a dynamic program based on a well-described program plan and evaluation as suggested, the program is truly affiliated with its parent district and is constantly growing in efficiency as new instructors come into the program and contribute their unique expertise through evaluation and description.

A comprehensive program evaluation plan as described is the only acceptable form of evaluation to use in physical education. Some physical educators, however, may feel unable to initially implement this comprehensive form of evaluation in their existing programs due to extremely large classes or a lack of adequate instructional time. The physical educator may elect to *temporarily* monitor only a representative sample of objectives being taught in a unit and/or monitor only a sample of students in the class. This data, although limited, will provide teachers with some useful information with which they can evaluate their programs. These procedures should *not* be interpreted as an acceptable alternative to those procedures discussed in this chapter, but instead only as *temporary* procedures that will be expediently expanded into a comprehensive evaluation program. Teachers should also meet with the chief administrator in their schools and explain the ultimate form of program evaluation they want to achieve and the sequence of steps they are going to follow to achieve this goal. This meeting sensitizes the administrator to both the problems faced by the teacher and the teacher's desire to work on improving the quality of the program.

PROGRAM EVALUATION SUMMARY

Evaluation of a program is necessary to identify program effect and to improve systematically the procedures of planning, implementing, and evaluating instruction to maximize the results or outcomes of the educational process. The program must be described sufficiently so that its key components can be replicated when found effective, or systematically changed when found ineffective or inefficient. Though many comprehensive evaluation models are available for current use in program evaluation, their complexity limits their application in physical education. The evaluation design incorporated into the ABC model encompasses the same criteria used in formal evaluation models and can be used by the instructors within their assigned classes. The yield of conducting the evaluative procedures as outlined in this chapter is a dynamic program systematically changing to the needs of the students and community it serves. Physical education teachers should never settle for anything less.

The ever increasing availability of small powerful microcomputers in the public schools will expand the teacher's ability to efficiently manage and analyze large amounts of evaluation data in the future. The objective-based design of the ABC model allows it to be readily transferred to a computer management system. Schools can develop (or have developed) management programs or use existing database management programs that can be adapted to meet their needs. The Student Performance Management System is an example of a simple database management program that is available commercially and compatible with the ABC model.

Once harnessed, computer technology will allow teachers to manage and analyze evaluation data more efficiently. Computer-managed evaluation will offer many advantages, such as:
  —an increase in the time-efficiency associated with all aspects of student and program evaluation;
  —an increase in the number and complexity of the analyses conducted to investigate "why" evaluation questions; and/or
  —allow for greater frequency and sophistication in student and program reporting.

Computer hardware (microcomputers) and software (programs to manage the data) are already available to meet the basic evaluation needs of most physical education programs. The major obstacle to computer-managed evaluation in physical education today and in the immediate future is the lack of computer literacy (ability to use computers) among teachers. Teachers must learn how to use microcomputers to gain a basic understanding of what computers can and cannot do for them. These competencies could be achieved by taking computer literacy and application courses offered at local colleges, continuing education programs, and computer stores.

RESOURCES FOR TEACHERS

Alkin, M.C., Daillak, R., and White, P.: Using Evaluations. Beverly Hills, CA, Sage Publications, 1979.
Kelly, L.E.: Physical Education Management System. Charlottesville, University of Virginia, 1985.
Kibler, R.J., Cegala, D.J., Watson, K.W., Barker, L.L., and Miles, D.T.: Objectives for Instruction and Evaluation. 2nd ed. Boston, Allyn and Bacon, 1981.
McGreal, T.L.: Successful Teacher Evaluation. Alexandria, VA, Association for Supervision and Curriculum Development, 1983.
Morris, L.L., and Fitz-Gibbon, C.T.: How to Measure Achievement. Beverly Hills, CA, Sage Publications, 1978.
Rutman, L.: Planning Useful Evaluations. Beverly Hills, CA, Sage Publications, 1980.
Safrit, M.J.: Evaluation in Physical Education. Englewood Cliffs, NJ, Prentice-Hall, 1973.
Wessel, J.A., Green, G., and Vogel, P.: An evaluation-based adaptation model for modifying replicable programs for use with alternate population groups. *Journal of Special Education Technology, 11* (4), Summer 1979.

Objective: To develop appropriate unit and program reporting profiles for the ABC program plan.

Materials: A sample program plan developed using the procedures outlined in Chapter 4.
Figures 8–2 through 8–7 from Chapter 8.

WORKSHEET 8–1

Directions: **1.** Using the content delineated in the program plan, identify and develop appropriate reporting profiles for each program level.

    a. Establish program levels, for example, a K through 12 program plan may be divided into three program levels: elementary, middle, and high school.

    b. Identify and sequence objectives that will be taught in each level.

    c. Determine what information will be reported:
- entry status
- exit status
- change status
- expectations
- class average

    d. Determine how progress on each objective will be converted into a percentage score (i.e., if the objective CATCH is composed of 10 standards, each standard achieved would equal a 10% gain. Mastery for another objective like abdominal strength may be defined as 50 sit-ups in 1 minute. In this case each sit-up would equal a 2% gain).

    e. Using the model Program Report Profile provided in Figure 8–3, develop a student program report format for each level of your program.

    f. Complete a program reporting profile for each level of your program using either existing student data or hypothetical student data.

    g. Have your program reporting profiles evaluated for both quality and ease of interpretation by other teachers, parents, and/or administrators.

    h. Revise the program reporting profiles to reflect any feedback received during the evaluation phase.

2. Using the program levels established in the first part of this activity, create appropriate student unit reporting profiles for a given year within each program level.

    a. Select what year will be used for developing the unit reports from each program level. For example, the third grade could be selected as the sample year from the elementary level.

    b. Using the ABC program plan, identify what units and objectives will be taught in each year selected (i.e., what objectives are scheduled to be taught to the third grade in the program plan?).

    c. Determine what information will be reported in the unit reports:
- entry status
- exit status
- change status
- expectations
- class averages
- objective weightings
- letter grade conversions

    d. Determilne how progress on each objective will be converted into a percentage score.

    e. Using the model unit reports presented in Figures 8–4 through 8–7, develop prototype student unit reporting profiles for each of the years selected.

    f. Complete several sample student unit report profiles using either existing student data or hypothetical student data.

    g. Have your unit profiles evaluated for both quality and ease of interpretation by other teachers, parents, and/or administrators.

    h. Revise the student unit reporting profiles based on the feedback received during the evaluation phase.

Variations: **1.** Survey local schools and collect program and unit reporting formats used in their physical education programs. Evaluate these reporting formats using the criteria discussed in this chapter.

ACTIVITY 8–2.	Evaluating the appropriateness of the program plan.

Objective:	To develop and apply appropriate evaluation criteria to an ABC program plan to determine its merit.
Materials:	A sample ABC program plan developed using the procedures outlined in Chapter 4.
	The Program Appropriateness Evaluation Checklist presented in Table 8–2.

WORKSHEET 8–2

Directions:	**1.** Have the group independently review the evaluative items in the Program Appropriateness Evaluation Checklist and add or delete items as they think necessary.
	2. Apply a consensus-forming technique to the list of evaluative items developed in step 1 to identify the final items to be used in the checklist.

      a. Have each person independently rate each item using the following scale:

        0 = totally inappropriate
        1 = not very important
        2 = very important
        3 = extremely important

      b. Summarize the groups ratings and discuss why each item was rated appropriate or inappropriate.

      c. Based on clarification and/or new thoughts resulting from the discussion, have each person rerate each item.

      d. Develop the final version of the checklist using all evaluative items that receive an average rating of 2.0 or better.

    3. Divide the group into small subgroups of 4 or 5 people and have them apply the evaluation checklist to each other's program plans. Identify and discuss why any items were rated "no" and how these deficiencies in the program plan can be remediated. Also identify any items that were consistently rated "no" across all the program plans in the group. These areas should be reviewed and emphasized in the next program planning unit.

Variations:	With access to a school and classes, other columns can be added and answered for each evaluative item. A column headed "What Data Do You Have?" can help answer the question "yes" or "no." Such data can come from the teacher of a particular class, an administrator of a particular school, or from your own experiences. If you have access to the school's record, other sources may be lesson plans, unit lesson plans, yearly or comprehensive program plans, or student performance records.

    Two other columns can be added such as "Who Is Responsible for Task?" and "Who Is Responsible for Checking That the Task was Completed?". These three columns can help to systematize the evaluation data gathering and reporting systems so that a consensus can be generated in making revision recommendations and refining the program.

| ACTIVITY 8–3. | Designing a teacher self-monitoring implementation evaluation checklist. |

Objective:	To develop a teacher self-monitoring implementation evaluation checklist.
Materials:	Teacher Unit Implementation Evaluation Checklist presented in Table 8–3.

WORKSHEET 8–3

Directions:
1. Have the group independently review the evaluative items in the Teacher Unit Implementation Evaluation Checklist and add or delete items as they think necessary.
2. Apply a consensus-forming technique to the list of evaluative items established in step 1 to determine the final items to be used in the checklist.
   a. Have each person independently rate each item using the scale below.
      0 = totally inappropriate
      1 = not very important
      2 = very important
      3 = extremely important
   b. Summarize the group's ratings and discuss why each item was rated appropriate or inappropriate.
   c. Based on clarification and/or new thoughts resulting from the discussion, have each person rerate each item.
   d. Develop the final version of the checklist using all evaluative items that receive a final average rating of 2.0 or better.

Variations:
1. Where appropriate, have the group actually use the revised checklist to evaluate their unit implementation of the program.
2. Have the group examine the activities previously described in Chapters 6 and 7. Many of the indicators of teacher behaviors in effective instruction can be reviewed and added to the implementation checklist. These items, along with the revised checklist, can be compiled and would provide a self-monitoring teacher performance checklist: planning, managing, and teaching effectively. Be sure to check the subjective and objective data identified in Chapter 2 for an ABC model class.

ACTIVITY 8–4.	Creating program effectiveness reporting formats.

Objective: To design a reporting format to demonstrate the effectiveness of the ABC program in meeting its goals and objectives.

Materials: Teacher and student evaluation data on the objectives taught in each unit during the year. The Yearly Plan Implementation Summary Chart presented in Table 8–5.

WORKSHEET 8–4

Directions:

1. Have the group identify what information they feel should be presented to parents, administrators, and/or school boards to demonstrate the effectiveness of their programs. Use the consensus-forming technique described in Activities 8–2 and 8–3 if the group cannot agree on what should be presented.

2. Have the group then delineate how each piece of information to be presented in the report will be obtained. For example, will student achievement be reported in relation to skill mastery, target expectations, or both?

3. Using the Yearly Plan Implementation Summary Chart as an example and the criteria established in steps 1 and 2, divide the group into smaller work groups and have each group design a reporting format.

4. Have each of the smaller groups present and explain their reporting format to the total group. Have the total group discuss the strengths and weaknesses of each reporting format in terms of the target audiences (parents, administrators).

5. Based on the discussion in step 4, design the optimal reporting format for each target audience.

6. Have the final reporting formats evaluated by members of the target audiences for both quality and ease of interpretation.

7. Revise the reporting formats based on the feedback received in step 6.

CHAPTER 9

The Quest for Quality: Shaping Up

KNOW WHAT IS HAPPENING—BE INVOLVED
HAVE DOCUMENTED EVIDENCE
MOBILIZE AND TAKE ACTION
SYNOPSIS
ACTIVITIES

What is the Quest for Quality?

The professional imperative is our continuing quest for quality, shaping up the effectiveness of our program and renewing ourselves as we meet the needs of ALL the children in our nation's schools.

How is it Done?	*Decision Aids*
1. Know what is happening.	Educational reform reports School improvement reports: reports, processes, issues, responses at state, district, and building level
2. Be involved: —issues —responses —body politic	Ways to participate in improvement efforts: school, district, and/or statewide Respond to issues, meeting needs of students in the total education process, not only in physical education. Develop working consensus responses to issues in physical education with supporting rationale for each response. ABC model and procedures.
3. Be accountable or prepare to be accountable: —define quality —develop a school profile —assess program effectiveness —target areas for improvement	Documented evidence of effectiveness: students learn what teachers teach. Indicators of effectiveness, quality criteria discussed in previous chapters to assess program effectiveness. ABC model and procedures
4. Mobilize and take action: —plan a school improvement project —set goals —implement, monitor, and evaluate —institutionalize what is proven effective —inform the public	Eight key assumptions Six-step action plan Commitment: staff, principal, and allocation of resources for the improvement project. Leadership team membership Master schedule Ways to inform the public School profile of excellence
5. Accept change as inevitable: capitalize on educational reform: —renew yourself as well as your program	Know what you teach and what students learn. Examine teaching and student behaviors: self, peers, students, principal. Set target improvement goals that are linked to needs of staff and resources. Plan and implement inservice programs linked to a cluster of schools, making your school a continuous-learning school for staff as well as students. Identify outstanding school programs and share their successes with other educators and persons interested in quality schools.

Education has emerged as an issue of vital importance in the United States in the 1980s. Our nation's schools are currently undergoing the most far-reaching reforms and renewal processes since the turn of the century. Many states already have legislative acts that significantly reform their state systems of schooling.

This resurgence of interest in education is due to the barrage of national and state reports calling for significant reforms in the educational system. Since the early 1980s, over 20 national reports have been issued calling for basic reform of elementary and secondary education in the United States. These reports have been sponsored by the U.S. Secretary of Education, the state governors, national research projects, and noted individuals in the academic field.

All of these reports indicate that the key to solving many of the economic and political problems facing America in the future lies in the improvement in our schools. Although the reports differ in their emphases and audiences, many of the major recommendations are common to all: better curricula, increased and improved use of learning time, improved teaching, more effective leadership in education, and more community involvement in the improvement of our schools.

How do we in physical education respond to recommendations in the national reports and what are the actions required to put these recommendations into practice? To our states' recently enacted bills that reform our state system of schooling? Or to our state's Action for Excellence Commissions for educational reform and curriculum renewal procedures for our school districts and individual schools?

The questions we must ask are: Are we involved, first as educators and second as physical education teachers, in the educational reform and curriculum renewal procedures for our state, our district, and our school? How do we as teachers of physical education gain support for our programs? How do we document what teachers teach and students learn? How do we communicate to other educators, parents, and other persons interested in the quality of schooling, the values of our program in meeting the needs of all students and the community as a whole? Are we knowledgeable about the widely publicized and most important reports that are influential in our state? Are we knowledgeable about the educational reform and curriculum renewal procedures being put into practice to apply these recommendations? Is physical education and health-related physical fitness included in the curriculum for all children and youth?

This chapter presents guidelines of how to respond to the calls for educational reforms and how to put together a general strategy to salute excellence and improve the quality of our physical education programs. It also brings together the concepts and activities discussed in previous chapters relating to building quality programs and highlights the ABC model in the curriculum improvement process. The guidelines are grouped under three broad headings: (1) Know What Is Happening—Be Involved; (2) Have Documented Evidence; and (3) Mobilize and Take Action.

KNOW WHAT IS HAPPENING—BE INVOLVED

We must have knowledge of and invest in learning how to address upcoming educational improvement efforts in our state, district, and school. To do this we must have knowledge of the reports and educational reform issues related to the improvement of our schools—equity and quality in education for all students. We must become involved in the improvement efforts at the state, district, and building level. We, as educators first and physical education teachers second, must play an active role in school improvement efforts and decision-making.

The initiative in response to the national calls for school improvement is coming from the states: from governors, from state departments of education, from state boards of education, and from grassroot coalitions of parents, educators, politicians, and business and industry people. There are more than 240 high-level state commissions studying educational quality and the excellence process. These groups review national reports and studies of school improvement and evaluate implications for their state.

Following is a list of some of the issues being addressed by states. These issues are grouped under five broad headings:

1. *Standards for learning:* student competence and increased testing for all students, increased core requirements in the academics for graduation;
2. *Standards for teaching:* teaching certificate and basic competencies, teacher tenure and evaluation of teacher performance, career ladders/merit pay, and increased teacher salaries;
3. *Increased learning time:* lengthening of the school year/school day, provision of more time for teacher planning in inservice training;

TABLE 9–1.   *Suggested Format for Examining National and State Reports, Studies, and Recommendations*

Targeted Areas	Title of Report or Study	Recommendations	Current District/Building Status	Issues Differences in Program	Response
Time	Commission on Excellence	*Examples:* Six hours available time for learning	Five hours available for schooling	One hour more recommended	Establish a committee to study use of available instructional time and examine need for six-hour program K through 12

4. *Student discipline:* policies on promoting and retaining students and for expulsion or suspension of students;

5. *School organization and structure:* role of principal, students, staff, parents, and community to maximize student achievement and staff effectiveness targeted at the core of instructional policy including what should be taught, who shall teach it, and what resources and financial measures are required.

State, district, and school responses to national reports are important power tools. Information is the number one power tool. We need to know what is happening in our state, district, and school to be able to effectively address the issues for educational improvement. Table 9–1 illustrates a procedure used by states, school districts, and schools for their staff to analyze report recommendations, and the action required to put such recommendations into practice.

Generally, the onward-to-excellence process is organized and managed by a team of leaders in each school district and at the building level. For example, a school district establishes a Committee on School Excellence comprised of administrators, politicians, teachers, parents, students, business and industry personnel, local school board members, and members from institutions of higher education. The goal of the Committee is to develop, communicate, and implement a long-range improvement plan for the district's schools. The tasks of the Committee include:

- examining current national and state reports and recommendations, research findings from studies of effective schools and instruction;
- drawing implications from these reports and studies, making recommendations and providing cost analysis of needed resources to implement, and ways to acquire needed funding;
- establishing continuous communication system with schools and community to inform, listen, receive reactions and recommendations from the staff and community at large; and
- designing a school improvement process by setting up subcommittees (central office and at the building level) that undertake planning, implementation, monitoring, documentation, recommendation, and implementation of activities that proved effective and translate them into standard operating school procedures.

Knowledge of what educational reports are most influential and the states' responses and improvement procedures is essential. Just as important, if not more so, is our active participation in the state, district, and school responses to national educational reform issues.

There are many ways we can become involved in school improvement efforts. We can participate as members of our State, District, or School Committee on

TABLE 9–2. *Example of Rationale and Quality Program Criteria Developed by a Physical Education Staff Based on the ABC Model*

Rationale

No knowledge is more crucial than knowledge about health. Without it no life goal can be successfully achieved, nor can one participate in full measure in society's social and economic benefits. All students should learn about the human body, how it changes over the life cycle, what nourishes it or diminishes its effectiveness. How a healthy life style commensurate with maturation and throughout adulthood contributes to physical and social-emotional well-being. All students need to acquire skills to manage daily living activities efficiently and participate in active sport-leisure activities. Importantly, the purpose of standards or student expectations is not to screen, sort, or select a few students to participate. The aim must be to provide all students, regardless of race, sex, or handicap with those necessary tools, core learnings.

Quality Program Criteria

Quality indicators taken from research and from our experiences with the ABC model provide the following key characteristics that should be stressed to improve the curriculum:

1. Clear-cut physical education program goals that are relevant to the goals of the school K through 12.
2. Program objectives establishing sequence and continuity of core learnings to operationalize these goals.
3. Specific student behavioral objectives to be accomplished for students to progress toward achieving long-range goals.
4. Clear definition of essential learnings, performance criteria, as students progress toward achieving mastery of core learnings.
5. Student expectancies within the instructional time available to make progress toward mastery of the core learnings.
6. Continual and systematic monitoring and evaluation of student performance.
7. Continual feedback and reporting of evaluative data for modifying and purifying the program and instruction.

Excellence. We can react, make recommendations at state and local community educational improvement forums. We can develop a local and state constituency (students, parents, colleagues, business, and industry people) and write responses to the recommendations proposed by the Committee on Excellence.

One of the foremost issues in quality school programming is the definition of excellence. Excellence to what ends? What are the educational goals of the school program? What are the standards of learning for all students? Without a definition of excellence, what is the curriculum? Student expectations? As educators, how do we respond to the recommendations of the specific course requirements for high school graduation? In the establishment of period "promotional gates?" Competency testing and tests through which a student must pass in order to be promoted? As physical education teachers, how do we define excellence, our educational program goals? How do they contribute to the total school goals? What are our standards for learning? Essential learnings? How do we determine student competence? Promotional gates?

By simply providing a definition of excellence, the quality of our physical education program does not improve. Quality program criteria, which are indicators of effectiveness in the program, need to be identified. Without these criteria, efforts to improve the quality of physical education programs will be fragmented. For example, Table 9–2 provides an overview of a physical education staff's rationale for physical education in the school curriculum, along with key quality indicators to improve the program's effectiveness.

With approval by the School Committee on Excellence of these recommendations, the staff outlined a plan to identify core learnings, develop student performance criteria, and conduct an assessment of student performance on the core learnings across grades. The assessment data results were used to set student expectancies across grades, provide physical education opportunities to identify resources needed, and to determine who shall teach what, when, and how data were to be gathered to continually improve the quality of the program in terms of student achievement.

Two other conditions need to be briefly mentioned and considered in planning and implementing procedures to improve the school and/or a program. *First,* no simplistic, short-range approach exists to improve the quality of schooling. The process and the problems of education are far too complex to be amenable to a quick "fix" or solution. No mere tinkering with a curricular area brings about significant improvements. For instance, if the recommendation is to increase time, how is it done? How does one transform the school or a program to make more effective use of time available for learning? Such decisions focus on the goals of education, longer school days, longer school year, deletion of a curricular area such as art, music, physical education, or vocational education, or clocking available instructional time. As mentioned previously, the use of time in learning is a prime area for educational improvement on the basis of its relation to student achievement. Along with instructional time in a specific curricular area, is the importance of the student's engaged time in learning tasks at an appropriate level of difficulty. The issue is how do we increase the amount of time students are engaged in instructional tasks, not just additional time available?

Second, the central focus of the quest for quality programs is the transformation of the individual school by the personnel and the community who run it. The individual school and the school community are the key agents of change. The question is: What can we do to develop the capability of school personnel and the community to run quality programs. For instance, how can we in physical education link our expertise together for staff development and curriculum renewal? Do we develop clusters of schools with resource personnel who are available to help improve the quality of our programs? Do we have available validated programs or models that have proved effective that we might review, adopt, or adapt to our school? Can we, with the help of others, identify and salute excellence in our existing school programs? Provide profiles of quality school programs at the elementary and secondary school levels?

All of these activities and many others provide a beginning in our quest for quality programs in physical education. No one denies that fiscal support and effective management techniques from building principals, superintendents, and state administrators are requirements to successfully carry out the many recommendations to improve schools. But we must initiate activities to shape the quality of our physical education programs in our individual school.

HAVE DOCUMENTED EVIDENCE

Documented evidence of student achievement is our number one power tool. What evidence do we have of our program effectiveness? How will we demonstrate and communicate to others the contributions of our programs and how vital they are to the total education process in meeting students' needs? Not by statements of our program goals and contributions, but by concrete evidence of measurable results of what we taught.

We must be accountable or prepare to be accountable in these times. The future of our programs depends on our ability to have documented evidence of effectiveness and communicate this accountability to all concerned. Past legislation and tradition will no longer support physical education continuance in our schools. The three proposals highlighted in Chapter 1 clearly spell out the need for documented evidence.

In dealing with others we must use the results of our work to show that students

TABLE 9–3. *Suggested Format for Assessing Effectiveness in Physical Education: ABC Model Indicators of Effectiveness, Quality Program Criteria*

Category	Answer Yes/No	What Data Do You Have	Whose Responsibility	Who Checks
STUDENT EVALUATION 1. Are achievement tests (criterion-referenced on content taught) used to evaluate attainment of skills?	Yes	Class Performance Score Sheets Individual Record of Progress	Teacher	Principal
2. Are achievement test results reportable in usuable form for audience intended: students principals teachers school boards community and so on	Yes	Report Cards Student Profiles School Cumulative Records Published Report of Results	Teacher Principal	Principal

do learn what we teach. We need to improve the effectiveness of our programs or develop new programs. We need to improve program effectiveness within the constraints of economic and political reality—doing better with less. We need no great sums of money; the key changes required are staff renewal and a curriculum improvement process that impacts directly on what is taught, such as the ABC model. Programs will not improve much until an entire school staff allows their programs and their teaching to be self-examined and evaluated by peers, parents, and students. Only in this way can we provide for continual shaping of quality teaching skills and the development of effective programs to provide student achievement on core learnings of the physical education program.

Program accountability requires the development and/or selection of practical, valid, and reliable measures for assessing effectiveness. For those teachers who need to develop a curriculum, the ABC model provides systematic procedures for the staff and/or committee to plan, implement, and evaluate a quality program. For others who need documented evidence for accountability now, the indicators of effectiveness described in previous chapters provide questions that can be used to develop a questionnaire for assessing the effectiveness of existing programs and target areas of improvement. The questions are organized according to major categories of indicators: teacher behaviors, student behaviors, program appropriateness (program plan and unit implementation plan), and student achievement. Other categories need to be considered as well; these include supervision, student expectations for success, parent involvement, and the role of the principal.

A sample format for the questionnaire is provided in Table 9–3. The questions represent indicators of effectiveness under the category of student evaluation. Of necessity, the questions are general. A precise answer to a question requires concrete knowledge. The data generated by the questionnaire are used to document and enhance the school's effectiveness. For instance, "yes" answers probably indicate that the program is effective; whereas "no" answers can indicate that this factor is ignored. Inconsistencies indicate that further discussion is needed to build a consensus. After the data are analyzed, priorities for change and target areas for improvement can be identified.

In one sense, the questionnaire becomes a school or district quality program criteria document in that it clearly communicates what the school or district considers a quality program. It presents a school profile of excellence. The questionnaire is a process helper in a program improvement project. By focusing attention on significant questions of what makes a program effective, participants decide what is a quality program, what areas to collect data from, and how the data collected will improve the program's effectiveness. With data collected and analyzed, the team sets priorities for improvement. Selection of an appropriate target area for improvement is important. The staff must perceive the target area as an opportunity to enhance the program. Based on the data collected, staff efforts and willingness to help with what they believe to be needed is markedly increased. In fact, our experience shows that teacher or student behaviors are target areas to implement improvement to build staff support and involvement in a school or program improvement project.

MOBILIZE AND TAKE ACTION

To mobilize and take action now is to plan and implement a program improvement project for the school. This improvement project must be organized and managed by a team of leaders in each school building or district. The team includes the principal, key teachers, a district office representative, and technical assistance personnel as needed. The success of the project depends on several key assumptions and procedures that underline effective action plans. Those presented here are based on school improvement projects, our experiences in training teachers to adopt the ABC model, and/or in curriculum and staff renewal activities. These assumptions are as follows:

1. The school building, principal, and staff are the key units of change.
2. The atmosphere in the school influences the success of the improvement project. A major influence of a healthy climate is the positive attitude of the principal. The single best indicator of success is the principal's estimation, before the project begins, of how successful it is going to be in his or her school.
3. School and community personnel play key roles in the project. Commitment and a sense of partnership comes from shared planning and decision-making at each stage of the improvement process.
4. Improvement goals must be discrete and adopted and supported by all school personnel. Providing an overall picture of what the school program will be when the improvement efforts have been implemented is essential for staff involvement and support.
5. Improvement takes time and hard work and usually costs money. There are no quick solutions. Improvement is not accomplished by a three-hour inservice session, two staff development days, or one-hour staff meetings. The improvement process is a long-range, goal-directed plan with realistic time lines for achieving short-term goals established to progress toward the long-range goals, a 3- to 5-year-improvement project.
6. Each planned activity and its contribution to the improvement goals must be clearly understood by the staff before implementation.
7. The point of departure for improving programs is the ABC model and indicators of quality programs drawn from research. Effectiveness research has a strong face validity that in most cases parallels accepted practice and demonstrates a consistency of findings that seem to cross subject areas, grade levels, and students.
8. Improvement processes in the ABC model that impact directly on teacher

and student behaviors provide the most appropriate entry points for change and by necessity become major improvement goals for inservice.

Action-minded administrators, staff, and/or individuals concerned with the quality of the school's physical education program may decide to embark on a school improvement project. Your superintendent may assign you to lead a school effectiveness project for your school and/or district. You may be part of your school's committee on excellence formed to generate a quality criteria document, a profile for excellence, for the physical education program and instructional practices. You may decide on your own to convince your school to establish a school improvement project in physical education.

In this text, we use the phrase "school improvement project" to include the pursuit of goals that benefit students. These goals, based on our experiences, include the following:

1. Developing and implementing a physical education curriculum for elementary and secondary grades in response to educational reform reports; mandates for essential learnings, student expectancies, teacher competencies, and accountability (documenting and reporting student achievement).
2. Ensuring equitable treatment and increasing the number of opportunities for all students in both regular and special physical education programs, K through 12th grade.
3. Implementing physical education improvement efforts through staff development: a building and/or class level process that involves the staff in planning, trains them to implement changes, and incorporates the new program and practices into the daily operations of the class and the school.

Our efforts have focused primarily on curriculum and instruction. We have observed direct results of successful school improvement efforts—increased student achievement, ongoing use of the ABC model, materials, and correlation of effective instruction, and, the application of computerized physical education management and reporting systems based on the ABC model. At the same time, we have observed the teachers' willingness to support necessary changes and increased capacity to maintain and institutionalize successful practices and new curriculum plans.

In this book, we have transformed our experiences into a series of concrete steps and activities designed to improve the quality of physical education programs and practices in our nation's schools. We have provided tools and strategies that can be used by staff in different situations to meet their needs and experiences. We have outlined a process model, a school improvement action guide for physical education. The six-step action guide, with general guidelines, is briefly discussed in the following paragraphs:

1. *Commitment*—The principal, school staff, and community join to make a commitment to the improvement project following an awareness session. At the awareness session the key characteristics of the ABC model are presented and benefits of implementing the model are discussed along with goals, expectations, and implementation requirements. The School Improvement Project charge is clarified: who, what, why, when, and how. A team is selected at the building level to develop an action guide to systematically organize and manage the improvement efforts of the project. The team includes the principal, key teachers, a district facilitator, and other support personnel as needed.
2. *Assessment and Goal Setting*—The principal and school staff define a quality program. A school profile is developed and improvement goals are set. Developing a school profile is based on the ABC model and indicators of effectiveness. With technical assistance as required, an assessment instrument is designed to evaluate the effectiveness of the existing program. Data

are collected, analyzed, and program strengths and weaknesses identified by the school staff. Improvement goals and expectations are established.

3. *Plan and Prepare to Implement*—The leadership team, with input from the total staff, prepares and implements activities to achieve improvement goals of the project. This plan includes setting short-term goals, target dates for implementing activities to achieve these goals, specific tasks and assignments of persons responsible for each activity, target dates for completion, resources needed and, where available, technical-assistance activities and support procedures. The implementation plan and activities are reviewed by the total staff. Revisions recommended with rationale for inclusion are approved by the staff and incorporated into the plan by the leadership team.

4. *Implement and Monitor*—The implementation activities and tasks are defined, carried out, and continually monitored. The leadership team, or designated persons responsible for each activity, keep track of what is or is not occurring. If the activity was not implemented as planned, or did not occur, there is no way to evaluate whether or not it worked. If it was implemented as planned, then data need to be collected to find out if it worked, or what needs to be changed, or what should be tried. Whatever was started needs to be completed. Postponing an activity that was started decreases future chances of getting staff involved in future improvement efforts. Most importantly, resources to complete the activity are identified and made available before starting any activity. Activities implemented and proved effective need to become part of ongoing operations procedures in the school program and work behavior. For example, preparing and reporting a physical education program plan each year should become as routine as compiling absentee lists. In short, the yearly program plan activity needs to be seen as a standard procedure of an effective program.

5. *Review Progress and Evaluate Results*—The impact of the improvement project activities are recorded and evaluated. The data-gathering suggestions in Chapter 8 can provide information for monitoring and evaluating the program implementation. Documentation and evaluation of the implementation activities provide the information for decision-making. Here the staff decides the next cycle of improvement and how improvement brought about can move quickly from project status to integration into ongoing procedures. The documentation of efforts and evaluation of activities provide a clear signal that plans are being carried out and results are expected. Such documentation and evaluation functions provide the data for reporting to the public the accomplishments made. These data are used to prepare a report for administrators and the Board of Education for project support and incorporation of the new project into district schools' plans.

6. *Institutionalize the Program*—The team presents the case to the board of education and administrators based on the impact on student achievement and the success of the implementation activities as standard operating procedures for continuous staff renewal and Profile of Excellence for the school. Administrative support is ensured when the administrators include the program in the budget and school plans. Plans are prepared; requirements and budget for successful continuation of the program are identified; district personnel are assigned to assist staff in their continued implementation of the program; new teachers receive orientation sessions and training in the program; materials and supplies are available, and community forum activities are planned for continued improvement efforts in the school.

A master implementation schedule is developed by the leadership team and

TABLE 9–4. *A Sample Yearly Schedule Plan to Implement a School Improvement Project*

Training and Assistance	Months	Activities in School	Steps
1/2 Day Awareness Principal Teachers Community Members	1	Awareness ABC Model/Improvement Process Benefits Roles/Responsibilities Commitment	1
1 1/2 Day Training Principal Teachers	2	Develop School Profile Assess Effectiveness Set Long-Term Goals	2
1 Day Training School Leadership Team	3	Select Leadership Team	
	4	Develop School Implementation Plan and Daily Priorities	3
2 Day Training Implementation School Plans	5	Implementing School Plan	4
	6		
Principal Team Teachers	7	Evaluating Outcomes and	5
	8		
Technical Assistance on call for		Reviewing Progress	
	9		
Trouble Shooting Problem-Solving	10		
1 Day Training Evaluating and Reporting Progress Principal Teachers Community	11 12	Report Results Set Goals for Next Year Incorporate Effective Activities into Standard Operating Procedures Renew Efforts Public Informed	6

Next Year's Schedule

approved by the staff. The master schedule provides necessary information so that in any one year everyone concerned knows what is happening in the three-year improvement project. Table 9–4 is an overview of a master yearly schedule for a three-year improvement project.

Having a master schedule has many advantages. Highlighted here are six of the key advantages:

1. Curriculum renewal is scheduled in physical education each year: set goals, identifying target areas, schedule implementation, specify goals and responsibilities of staff, and report results.
2. Inservice education is a practice based on an identified process: specify teaching competencies to implement target areas, plan and implement evaluation, report results, provide inservice assistance as needed on an individual basis.

3. In advance, systematically project allocation of resources, periodic meetings, inservice, and equipment requirements.

4. Continuous communication and feedback between planners, implementors, local school boards, administrators, the school staff, parents, students, and the public at large. Accountability is built-in improvement goal.

5. The long-range plans can be matched to the requirements of ongoing school improvement committees and the local school board plans for district and state.

6. The elements of the program that proved effective can be quickly moved from project status into standard operating procedures and made part of work behaviors. For example, compiling yearly program plans, or individual and class performance results can be as routine as compiling absentee lists. This work is easily computerized to assist teachers in managing and teaching effectively as well as reporting class and student results for the school reports and student report cards.

A school improvement project is a difficult task, but is not an impossible task for anyone who is committed or in a position to be involved. Change in our school programs is inevitable. We choose to accept change and make it work for us—our program in our school as we want it to be. We share strategies and tools that can be useful for students and for school personnel involved in prompting change—developing, adapting, or adopting curriculum and instructional practices—to improve the quality of our physical education programs for all students.

SYNOPSIS

We are in the process of shaping our future and our challenge is to demonstrate that our programs are effective, individualized, and accountable. No simplistic approach exists to meet this challenge. No quick "fix" or solution. No one-hour or three-hour inservice session will improve the quality of our programs. With the current revolution in education reform, we must know what is happening, be knowledgeable about key issues and recommendations to improve our schools, and be able to address these issues both as educators and as physical educators. The focus is on excellence, higher levels of attainment for ALL students. The concern is for equity and quality of education for ALL students in our nation's schools.

Setting goals is clearly emerging as the first task of schools. Excellence is meaningless without goals—instructional intent for what purpose or ends. Excellence is superficial unless we acknowledge that what happens at the building level in each class is the heart of the improvement process. The individual school, the school staff, and the community that run it are the key agents in the improvement efforts. To have accountable programs we need to provide documented evidence of our effectiveness. We need to meet this challenge of accountability within the constraints of economic and political reality. We must look to ourselves to mobilize and take action. Eight key assumptions and guidelines of how to put together a general strategy for an improvement project at the building level were offered. The ABC model with indicators of effectiveness discussed in previous chapters can serve for a staff to plan, implement, and evaluate a quality program. For those who need to provide evidence of effectiveness of their existing program, the ABC model and indicators of effectiveness serve to assist in the development of a questionnaire for assessing existing program effectiveness. Improvement in the quality of our physical education programs will not be easy or quick. But it can be done.

RESOURCES FOR TEACHERS

Adler, M.J.: The Paideia Proposal. New York, Macmillan, 1982.

American Alliance for Health, Physical Education, Recreation and Dance: Shaping the Body Politic. Legislative Training for Physical Educators, 1900 Association Drive, Reston, VA 22091, 1983.

Boyer, E.: High School: A Report on Secondary Education in America. New York, Harper and Row, 1983.

Education Week, P.O. Box 1939, Marion, Ohio 43305.

Goodlad, J.I.: A Place Called School: Prospects for the Future. New York, McGraw-Hill, 1983.

Leadership Up Close: Educational Leadership. Journal of the Association for Supervision and Curriculum Development, *41*(5), February 1984.

Lobbying guidelines. *The American School Board Journal,* April 1983.

A Nation at Risk: The Excellence Report. Using it to Improve Your Schools. Arlington, VA, American Association of School Administrators: 1983.

A Nation at Risk: The Imperative for Educational Reform. National Commission on Excellence in Education, U.S. Government Printing Office, Washington, DC, 1983.

Peters, T.J., and Waterman, R.H., Jr.: In Search of Excellence. New York, Harper and Row, 1982.

School Management Handbook. Reston, VA, National Association of Elementary School Principals, 1983.

Sizer, T.: Horace's Compromise. The Dilemma of the American High School. Boston, Houghton Mifflin, 1984.

Squires, D.C., Huitt, W.G., and Segars, J.K.: Effective Schools and Classrooms: A Research-Based Perspective. Alexandria, VA, Association for Supervision and Curriculum Development, 1983.

State Commission on Excellence: Reports and recommendtions. Each state department of education will have this available upon request. The principal of the school has a copy.

State Programs of School Improvement: A 50-State Survey. Education Commission of the States, Suite 300, 1860 Lincoln St., Denver, CO 80295, 1982.

A summary of selected major reports on education. Education Commission of the States, Suite 300, 1860 Lincoln St., Denver, CO 80295, 1982.

Wessel, J.A.: Advancing school physical education for all handicapped children: Project I CAN via the National Diffusion Network. *Counterpoint,* May/June 1982.

Woodbury, M.: A Guide to Sources of Educational Information. 2nd Ed. Information Resources Press, 1983.

ACTIVITY 9–1. Familiarization with major reports on education: local, school district and building level response.

Objective: To develop awareness of what is happening in educational reform in the search for quality education in our nation's schools.

Materials: The report used at the building level by the School Committee on Excellence or Improvement, or develop a report using the suggested format presented in Chapter 9.
Tables 9–1 and 9–2.

WORKSHEET 9–1

Directions:
1. With a complete form provided for the building level committee, examine the issues and responses.
2. Involve the total physical education staff in the school program in examining the issues and recommendations. Summarize the group's concerns.
3. When physical education staff agrees on concerns, each staff member talks with other teachers in the school, building principal, and members of the school committee at the building level. Build a working consensus of what is happening or might happen to the school's programs and impact on physical education program.
4. Summarize the physical education staff concerns and address the issues and recommendations for the physical education program: Table 9–2.
5. Present your rationale and recommendations—a position paper for physical education to the school committee, principal, and other teachers. Based on reactions and clarification of issues and recommendations or new throughts, revise your report as necessary.
6. With the position paper in hand, discuss plans to implement a school improvement project matched to the school's plans.

ACTIVITY 9–2.   Assessing program effectiveness and target areas for improvement.

Objective: To design a questionnaire using indicators of effectiveness, quality program criteria, and the ABC model to assess effectiveness of existing school programs and target areas for improvement.

Materials: The ABC model and the indicators of effectiveness, quality program criteria, described in the previous chapters.

The questions (written statements) in the tables in the chapter text and accompanying worksheets for chapter activities: see supplemental materials for this activity.

WORKSHEET 9–2

Directions: **1.** Have a group of students design a questionnaire to assess existing program effectiveness using the suggested format in Table 9–3.
  • Using a consensus-forming technique, develop/select:
    —major headings or categories for the questionnaire under which indicators of effectiveness subheadings and questions can be organized.
    —questions, written statements, from the resources presented (supplemental material)
    —the method for analyzing the responses to the questions: Yes, No, Yes/No to evaluate what is effective, not effective, or ignored, and inconsistent data that require that needs be checked, such as
      —Yes to question indicates that the data found demonstrate that the program is effective
      —Yes/No column indicates that there are inconsistent data and suggests the need for further discussion to build a consensus
      —No to the question indicates that the program is ignoring a factor that may lead to an effective program
  2. Have a group of students evaluate existing program using the questionnaire, collect data, analyze data according to responses and method to determine effectiveness of each evaluative item and major heading.
    —With data generated, have students develop a priorities list of target areas that need improvement based on those items that are most likely to improve student achievement.
  3. Have a group of students present an awareness session based on the questionnaire, data generated, data analyzed, and target areas identified for program improvement
    —to the total class;
    —at a conference/professional meeting;
    —to principal and staff of school program evaluated.

Variation: Divide the total class group into subgroups and set up case studies of school programs and instruction for them to assess effectiveness using the questionnaire.

Have the total class or subgroup of students use the data generated—target areas for improvement—and develop a plan to mobilize the school to take action by implementing a three-year improvement project. See Activity 9–3 supplemental materials.

ACTIVITY 9–2. SUPPLEMENTAL MATERIALS

Resources in the Text: Developing/selecting written statements to pose as questions in a questionnaire for assessing program effectiveness using the ABC Model and indicators of effectiveness: quality program criteria.

Evaluative Items for Questionnaire: Indicators of Effectiveness Statements—MAJOR CATEGORIES	ABC MODEL COMPONENTS	TEXT		
		CHAPTERS	CHAPTER WORKSHEETS	CHAPTER TABLES
1. *PROGRAM* Appropriateness of the Plan Unit Implementation Plan Placement Options	Planning Evaluating	3, 4, and 8	3–4 8–3 8–4	8–2 8–3
2. *TEACHER BEHAVIORS* Planning Instruction Management Motivation Class Climate	Prescribing Teaching	6 and 7	6–4 7–2	6–7
3. *STUDENT BEHAVIORS* Success Involvement: Time-on-Task Objectives Covered/Tested Expectations for Success Student Needs	Prescribing Teaching	3, 6 and 7	3–3 4–5 6–4 7–2	6–7
4. *STUDENT ACHIEVEMENT* Assessment Procedures Results Used in Modifying the Program and Instruction Student Profiles/Reports	Assessing Evaluating	5 and 8	5–1 5–2 5–4 8–1	5–4 8–5
Additional Categories for Evaluative Items Consideration Indicators of Effectiveness Identified by Others				
PARENT INVOLVEMENT SUPERVISION SCHOOL ENVIRONMENT ROLE OF THE PRINCIPAL	Check Resources at the end of the following chapters for these evaluative items: Chapters 6, 7, 8, and 9.			

Special Note: The text and worksheets in Chapter 2 present general statements pertaining to the major categories/components of the ABC Model and indicators of effectiveness.

ACTIVITY 9–3.   Organizing and managing a school improvement project in physical education.

Objective: To develop an action guide to organize and systematically manage your school improvement efforts for a program as you want it to be.

Materials: The six-step action guide, assumptions underlying successful improvement programs, and the outline of a master schedule presented in Chapter 9.

The tools and procedures presented in the previous chapters to plan, implement, and evaluate the ABC model for curriculum renewal and staff development and growth; entirely new program and/or to improve existing programs.

The completion of Activity 9–2:
- the questionnaire developed to assess program and instructional practices: the statements under the major headings depict a school and/or district's quality program criteria document— A Profile of Excellence for Physical Education Programs and Instructional Practices;
- the results of administering the questionnaire—identification of the strengths of existing program and practices and identification of target areas for improvement;
- Worksheet 9–3: School Improvement Project Action Guide;
- Worksheet 9–3: Supplemental Materials and Resources.

WORKSHEET 9–3

Directions: 1. Have a group independently review the criteria delineated in the questionnaire developed in Activity 9–2 and the results of administering the questionnaire.
  a. Add or delete items as necessary:
  - selection criteria for the program and instructional practices representing the school or district's statements of quality;
  - strengths of existing program and instructional practices based on these selection criteria;
  - target areas for improvement prioritized.
  b. Apply a consensus-forming technique to the criteria, its strengths, and areas targeted for improvement using an average rating of 2.0 or better for the final version of the quality document for the school and/or district.
2. Divide the group into small subgroups of 4 or 5 people. Each group serves as a school leadership team for the improvement project. The team in a school may be selected by the principal, or the principal and staff, after a commitment is made at the awareness session to embark on a school improvement project.
3. Each team develops a practical action guide and a model framework to plan, implement, and evaluate a school improvement project.
  a. Determine sequential steps to organize and manage the change process in terms of major tasks undertaken at each step.
  b. Identify the major tasks and activities involved at each step that are necessary to complete the task.
  c. Select tools, procedures, and personnel to be involved in the major tasks at each step.
  d. Identify evidence of achievement, indicating completion of each task. (Include the role and responsibility of personnel involved in the improvement process for each task).
4. Have the team present its model to the group and use a consensus-forming technique to develop/select the final version of the model.
  a. The sequential steps and major tasks.
  b. The major activities for each task.
  c. The primary tools, procedures, and roles and responsibilities of personnel involved in the improvement process.
  d. The evidence of achievement and the individual responsible for checking to see that implementation activities are completed.

Variation: With access to a school, have the principal or principal and staff review and evaluate the model framework. Evaluate their opinions and revise your model as needed by developing a rationale for change, if this is decided.

With access to a staff development day for a district, or a regional or state conference, or a parent group, and/or a board of education, present the model framework. Develop a short evaluation checklist for the audience to react to the model (select on criteria model for a quality school program; sequential steps, major task and activities, roles and responsibilities of personnel involved in the improvement process, evidence of achievement and personnel responsible and recommendations):

- divide your audience into small groups, if time permits;
- present each group with your written document (selection criteria for quality program model for your school improvement project);
- prepare a short evaluation checklist for each group to react to the document, including their recommendations;
- use the summary data for all groups (or have each group present material individually to the total group) to open discussion and finalize group reaction and recommendations;
- prepare a report and submit to each member of your audience and welcome any further imput.

WORKSHEET 9–3. *A School Improvement Project Action Guide*

SCHOOL: _____ GRADES: _____ TEACHERS (NUMBER AND GRADES) _____

STEPS	MAJOR TASKS AND ACTIVITIES	PERSONNEL RESPONSIBLE	TOOLS	EVIDENCE OF ACHIEVEMENT

SUPPLEMENTAL RESOURCES

Loucks, S.F., and Hall, G.E.: Implementing innovations in schools: A concerns-based approach. Austin: Research and Development Center for Teacher Education, The University of Texas, 1979.

Horsley, S. and Hergert, L.F.: An Action Guide to School Improvement. Alexandria VA, American Associatin for Supervision and Curriculum Development: 1985.

Wessel, J.A.: I CAN Consultant Manual: Leadership Training Guide for Implementation of the ABC Model. East Lansing, MI, Michigan State Instructional Media Center, 1985.

Wessel, J.A.: I CAN Evaluation Handbook: Tools and Procedures for Implementation of the ABC Model. East Lansing, MI, Michigan State Instructional Media Center, 1985.

ACTIVITY 9–3. SUPPLEMENTAL MATERIALS

A six-step action guide outlined by a school improvement team is presented below. The outline represents the first draft by the team members to develop a structure to systematically plan, implement, and evaluate their school project. The specifics will be given by the team members and reviewed by all personnel involved before implementation of project activities. The guide will be developed in detail for Year One implementation of the project. Evidence of achievement and designated personnel responsible for each activity will be included in the Year One guide. The consensus-forming technique will be employed in all activities requiring a group decision. The action guide was developed by the team after the decision was made by the school staff, principal, and district superintendent to adopt the ABC model, curriculum plan, and instructional practices.

STEPS	MAJOR TASKS AND ACTIVITIES	PERSONNEL AND TOOLS
1. Commitment	1. Establish the school improvement project as a legitimate school activity, K–6th.	Superintendent, principal, school staff and selected team members
	a. Select a school improvement team of 5 to 10 members: principal, district physical education director, building level physical educator, 2 teachers from grades K through 3 and 2 from 4 through 6, 2 parents, and a district facilitator:	
	• identify roles and responsibilities of team members, including channels of support; • identify consultant to serve as trainer; • identify team leader to serve primarily as director of the implementation process.	Team members
	b. Build a base of support for the project with the administrators (school and district), school staff, parent groups, student groups, and community at large: • identify vehicles to provide information to the public throughout the project such as slide tape shows, open house for parents, periodic newsletters, announcements in newspapers, briefings for staff and community members; • provide preliminary awareness sessions (formal and informal) and complete these within a short time span (about a month) once the project is underway.	Team members Any school staff member or community members
	c. Clarify your change: • goals and expectations for all people involved in the project, the relationship of the new curriculum and instructional practices to the school's plan, and yearly outcomes when the project is successfully implemented;	Team members ABC model and benefits Documentation of yearly outcome, student expectations/achievement, program effectiveness, teacher effectiveness, and recommendations.

STEPS	MAJOR TASKS AND ACTIVITIES	PERSONNEL AND TOOLS
	• personnel to be directly involved in the project and their selection; • grades and pilot school(s) and how they are selected for the first year of the project: one school and grades K through 6; • identify and negotiate for resources to support planning, implementing, and evaluating the project.	Money: substitute teachers, consultant(s), supplies, and materials. Services: secretarial help, district facilitator, volunteers, meeting rooms, release time for teachers involved to plan and take part in the inservice staff development program, for team leader and/or school members, for committee work, or to assume other responsibilities during the implementation of the project.
2. Assessment and Goal Setting	**2.** Develop a shared mission for the future: curriculum and instruction as it is now and as you want it to be on completion of the implementation. **a.** Define long term goals and expectations for the project: • define excellence and quality selection criteria for the curriculum and instructional practices; • develop a profile of excellence for the school's physical education program; • define the essential learnings for students to achieve (program objectives). **b.** Conduct an assessment of existing curriculum and instructional practices of the school's program: • develop a questionnaire based on the ABC model and correlate effective instruction identified in the text chapters as indicators of effectiveness; • implement the assessment activity including student achievement on essential program objectives (criterion-referenced test items). **c.** Review and evaluate findings, pinpointing strengths in the existing program and targeting areas for improvement.	Team members and school staff Definitions in Chapters 1 and 2, Table 9–2. Written statements (criteria) in the questionnaire developed in Activity 9–2. School Program Plan K through 6 Grade Mandates: state, district, school team members and staff. Questionnaire (Activity 9–2) Student Achievement: Use and/or adapt I CAN Performance Objectives or other sources related to essential program objectives identified in the program plan. Questionnaire results

Steps	Major Tasks and Activities	Personnel and Tools
	d. Set short-term (year) and long-term goals for the project improvement efforts: • consider local resources and constraints; • consider goals and expectations for parents, students, teachers, administrators, community at large.	
3. Plan and Prepare to Implement	**3.** Make shared decisions and prepare to implement the project activities as a dynamic process involving all concerned. **a.** Define implementation requirements for short-term and long-term goals and expectations: • training, facilities, equipment, materials, implementors, volunteers, and outside consultant help are considered; • roles and responsibilities designated for all personnel for first year implementation; • identify mastery expectations levels and for whom: teachers, students.	Team members and staff ABC model teaching competency requirements Student Achievement Levels (locally determined for success).
	b. Prepare for implementation of the project for year one: • set the time lines for all implementation activities and events—three years and detail for the first year; • set up awareness sessions and schedule for school, district, and the community—what and how for the first year; • make arrangements for training school staff, for continuous monitoring and support procedures for teachers, and for ordering the materials needed for training and the curriculum; • select implementors, four teachers for pilot project for the first year, and spread the program to other teachers within the school and schools in the district for second and third years;	 Consultant Manual: Leadership guide for implementation of the ABC model. (see Activity 9–3 supplemental resources).

Steps	Major Tasks and Activities	Personnel and Tools
	• establish procedures and develop report forms to document and evaluate results for teachers and students: teachers master the curriculum and instructional practices the first year; the second and third year collect data on students when the teachers have achieved mastery.	Evaluation Handbook: Implementation of the ABC Model. (See Activity 9–3 supplemental resources).
	c. Set up a staff development training plan in steps for teachers to master the curriculum and instructional components of the ABC model: assess, prescribe, teach, evaluate, and plan: • initial training focused on "what it is" and "how do I do it?"; • subsequent training focused on implementation skills using the components in the class setting with follow-up support and monitoring; • end of the year training focused on planning the program, reviewing and evaluating the training plan, making refinements as needed for successful implementation.	Consultant manual: leadership guide for implementation of the ABC model (see Activity 9–3, supplemental resources).
4. Implement and Monitor Project Activities	**4.** Develop a systematic management and monitoring plan focused on organizing the logistics of the implementation activities and addressing the concerns of all individuals involved in the project. a. Continuously review roles and responsibilities of team members, volunteers, and outside consultant help. Assign different roles as needed for successful implementation at different points in the process.	Team members and staff
	b. Continuously monitor, document, and review implementation activities being carried out as planned for intended effects and/or problems encountered.	Evaluation Handbook: Implementation of the ABC model. (See supplemental resources for Activity 9–3).
	c. Identify problems encountered, determine why, and document the solution found to that problem and produce desired outcome.	

STEPS	MAJOR TASKS AND ACTIVITIES	PERSONNEL AND TOOLS
	d. Address individual concerns as they emerge: sharing in decision making, training goals and expectations, follow-up help, use of volunteers, designated support personnel, time lines for activities and project events, and recognition and reinforcement needs.	Concerns-Based Adoption Model (CBAM). (See Activity 9–3 supplemental resources).
5. Review Progress and Evaluate Outcomes	**5.** Analyze progress, evaluate outcomes, and make reports to the public and all individuals involved in the project.	Team members, staff, and principal
	a. Data gathered the first year that will indicate progress includes: teacher mastery levels in the implementation of the ABC model, curriculum and instruction; implementation activities and events, concerns of individuals involved in the project, and continuing support of the project.	Evaluation Handbook: Implementation of the ABC Model (see Activity 9–3 supplemental resources).
	b. Second and third year data includes the previous section, and when teacher has mastered the components of the ABC model, student achievement data.	Criterion-Referenced Test Items: representing essential objectives, target and tested.
	c. Make changes in the implementation activities and events, program benefits, goals and expectations for second year, resources needed, implementation requirements, team members, support personnel, and the six-step action guide based on implementation data gathered: • make refinements in the ABC model components only after the teacher has mastered the components and knows their effect on student achievement assessment; • educate audiences (teachers, parents, students, community at large) on the specific goals and expectations and the reason why the data gathered at the end of year is important; • provide opportunities for teachers to get together to review the results and recommend changes with rationale stated at the end of each year.	

STEPS	MAJOR TASKS AND ACTIVITIES	PERSONNEL AND TOOLS
	d. Make reports on the first year implementation data gathered, analyze changes made, and overview of activities for the second year of the project: • determine audiences for briefings (parents, teachers, administrators, students, and community at large); • ensure administrative support for project's continuation: plan and budget for Year Two, present a strong case to the administrators and the board of education, based on data gathered and long term goals and expectations; • present action guide for second year.	
6. Institutionalize the Program	**6.** Establish the new program (curriculum and instructional practices) as part of the school's ongoing operation, moving from project status to standard operation activities as soon as possible: **a.** Decision for the incorporation of the program into the school's plan made by superintendent, board of education, principals, and staff of schools involved: • prepare a report for the program's continuation based on its impact on student achievement and the success of the implementation activities; • plan how the program will be maintained, identify resources needed for operation. **b.** Decide where the program will operate: pilot schools, certain designated schools, district-wide schools, or as an alternative approach, in special centers. **c.** Ensure administrative support to include the programs resources and requirements in the school's budget and district school plans.	Team members, staff, principal, board of education, and superintendent Documented Report. (See Evaluation Handbook: Implementatin of the ABC Model).

Steps	Major Tasks and Activities	Personnel and Tools
	d. Prepare plans for staff commitment and continuous renewal of skills to effectively implement the program: • assign a person responsible for checking with teachers and principals, providing support services as needed, and monitoring the continuous implementation by a staff trained in the pilot project and by new teachers. • orient new teachers and train them in implementing the program; • prepare written guidelines for use of the program's materials; ordering supplies, receiving ongoing support, making concerns known, and reviewing effective school and teaching research for incorporation into the program; • provide staff development activities for the continuous improvement efforts in your school.	Team members, staff and principals

A Case Study

A COMPLETED SCHOOL PROGRAM PLAN IN PHYSICAL EDUCATION (KINDERGARTEN THROUGH ELEMENTARY)*

The definition of the school setting and the completed Chapter 4 Activity Worksheets illustrating each step in the planning process are presented. There may be several steps in the process within a single Chapter 4 Activity. For each step, a completed Activity Worksheet is presented.

Activity	*Steps*	*Worksheets Completed*
4–1	1	Program Goals with Supporting Rationale
4–2 and 4–3	2	Relative Goal Emphasis by Program Level for Each Program Goal
	3	Place Selected Program Objectives in Program Levels for Each Program Goal
4–4	4	Calculation of Available Instructional Time
	5	Time Estimations for Attainment of Meaningful Performance Gain
	6	Determine Total Number of Program Objectives for Meaningful Performance Gain by Program Level
	7	Comprehensive Program Plan: Selection of Essential Objectives by Goal and Program Level—Kindergarten through Upper Elementary
	8	Development of Yearly Instructional Units: A. Kindergarten B. Lower Elementary C. Upper Elementary
4–6	9	Development of Weekly Unit Lesson Plans A. Kindergarten B. Lower Elementary C. Upper Elementary

A SCHOOL PROGRAM PLAN
DEFINITION OF THE SETTING

School   Elementary School
City School District

*This completed school program plan was developed by Jeff Walkley, a graduate student at the University of Virginia.

Population	Kindergarten Age Children
	Elementary Age Children
	Lower: Grades 1–3
	Upper: Grades 4–6
	Coeducational
	2 to 3 children with handicapping conditions (school classification of Learning Disabled and Emotionally Impaired) in each grade

Day and Time	Tuesday	9:00– 9:30 a.m.	Kindergarten
		9:30–10:00	Grade 1
		10:00–10:30	Grade 2
		10:30–11:00	Grade 3
		12:30– 1:00 p.m.	Kindergarten
		1:00– 1:30	Grade 4
		1:30– 2:00	Grades 4 and 5
		2:00– 2:30	Grade 6

Teacher	Physical Educator, Jeff Walkley
Facilities↔	Playground, elementary gym

Step 1. Program Goals with Supporting Rationale

1. *Goal Statement:*

   Develop competence in selected *Fundamental Motor Skills* (FMS). Supporting rationale:

   a. Fundamental motor skills are prerequisites to successful participation in most other games, sports, and dances common to leisure or competition.

   b. Competence in fundamental motor skills provides the skill base for future learning and participation in leisure and competitive sports which may not be available in the current program.

   c. Acquisition of qualitative fundamental motor skill patterns do not automatically occur for large numbers of students without instructional assistance.

   d. Competence in FMS enhances the chance of success in various activities, which in turn enhances a person's self-worth.

2. *Goal Statement:*

   Develop and maintain a functional level of selected *Physical Fitness Skills.* Supporting rationale:

   a. Physical fitness capabilities are necessary to meet biological needs for activity (normal growth and development).

   b. Physiological adaptions to stressors promote the ability to adapt to stress through increasing the body's physiological efficiency.

   c. Physical fitness capabilities are necessary to provide sufficient strength, endurance, and flexibility to meet the demands of daily living plus maintaining a residual for extra needs.

   d. Fitness capabilities provide the base (necessary prerequisites) for the efficient acquisition of skill and leisure objectives.

   e. Incremented levels of fitness provide motivation for developing and maintaining fitness levels in a "snowballing" fashion.

   f. Physical fitness capabilities contribute to effective weight control.

   g. Incidence of injury can be reduced and in some cases prevented due to maintaining physical fitness capabilities.

   h. Maintenance of desirable levels of fitness contributes to preventing ill health and delays aging process.

i. Recovery from injury (time) is enhanced by a desirable level of fitness.

3. *Goal Statement:*

Develop competency in selected *Body Management Skills.* Supporting rationale:

   a. Body management skills promote functional body structure (posture-alignment) which in turn positively affects body function.
   b. Control of the body in assorted postures promotes kinesthetic awareness.
   c. Selected body control activities provide a deterrent to injury from mishaps such as falling.
   d. Body awareness facilitates efficient communication.
   e. Promotes an awareness of body parts and relationship of body to other objects and/or persons.
   f. Facilitates efficient organization during class activity.
   g. Knowledge of the transient nature of exercise effects the need for regular participation to develop and maintain the benefits of exercise. Benefits of activity are short-term.
   h. Mere participation in activity does not result in achieving the wide range of benefits possible.
   i. Knowledge of the fact that beneficial effects of activity are specific to the kind, amount, duration, frequency, and intensity of the training.
   j. No physical education program can provide skill in all activities—thus one may benefit from knowing and maintaining something about how to learn a new skill.
   k. Performance improvement is guided by known principles of learning and/or training.

4. *Goal Statement:*

Develop competency in selected *Play, Sport, and Leisure Skills.* Supporting rationale:

   a. Worthy use of leisure time is one of the commonly held goals of general education.
   b. Physical activity can provide for healthful and enjoyable use of leisure time. Sport provides an opportunity for this physical activity.
   c. Participation in sport provides a useful diversion of tensions associated with daily tasks.
   d. The need for biological activity (appropriate kinds, amounts, durations, intensity, and frequency) can be met with the realm of sport and competition.
   e. Leisure sport activities provide a useful and acceptable means for meeting social and sociological as well as physiological needs.
   f. Games and sports provide a context within which behavior can be modified toward that which is socially desirable.
   g. Desire to participate in selected sports may provide sufficient motivation to develop and maintain other health-fitness objectives.

Step 2. Relative Goal Emphasis by Program Level for Each Program Goal

Goals	Kindergarten	Lower Elementary (1–3)	Upper Elementary (4–6)
Develop competence in selected motor skills	50%	40%	35%
Develop and maintain a functional level of physical fitness	20%	20%	20%
Develop competency in body management skills	20%	30%	10%
Develop competency in play, sport, and leisure skills	10%	10%	35%
Total Time	100%	100%	100%

Step 3. Place Selected Program Objectives in Program Levels for Each Program Goal

Program Goal Area	Program Objectives by Program Levels		
	Kindergarten	Lower Elementary (1–3)	Upper Elementary (4–6)
PLAY, SPORT, AND LEISURE SKILLS	directed free play (1)* organized minor games (2)	directed free play (4) organized minor games (1) soccer—trap (3) —pass (2)	*Soccer* throw-in (6) dribble (1) tackle (10) *Basketball* chest pass (2) set shot (5) dribbling (7) *Dance* circle formation (3) *Kickball* fielding (9) running base (4) participation (8)
FUNDAMENTAL MOTOR SKILLS	walk (1) run (2) roll a ball (3) kick a ball (6) throw a ball (4) catch a ball (5) hit a ball (7)	run (1) hit a ball (6) hop (12) ascend stairs (7) gallop (2) descend stairs (8) roll (11) jump down (9) skip (14) jump over (10) slide (13) bounce (4) kick (3) catch (5)	run (1) throw kick (9) —underhand (3) bounce (12) —overhand (4) catch (2) strike move to an even —overhand (8) beat (11) —underhand (6) horizontal jump —forehand (5) (10) —side arm (7)
BODY MANAGEMENT SKILLS	walk on balance beam (3) hang from bar (5) log roll (1) climb on an object (2) pull an object (4)	body actions (1) body parts (2) directions in space (4) shapes and sizes (3) general spaces (5) holding/carrying (6) pulling/pushing (8) lifting (7)	body planes (2) directions in space (1) lifting (4) holding/carrying (5) ascending/descending (6) general space (3)
PHYSICAL FITNESS SKILLS	sit-ups (2) walk/run for endurance (1)	sit-ups/abdominal (2) lifting/lowering objects (4) pushing/pulling (3) stamina and heart/lung endurance (1)	arm/shoulder/chest (5) abdominal strength/sit-ups (4) cardiorespiratory endurance trunk/leg flexibility (6) weight maintenance (2) relaxation (3)

*Priority ranking of the program objective.

Step 4. Calculation of Available Instructional Time
Class/Level: K through 6

1. *Total number* of instructional weeks available: *47 weeks*
   180 day school year = 36 instructional weeks
   230 day school year = 47 instructional weeks
   (Christmas, Spring, Summer vacations already excluded.)

2. Subtract 2 weeks of the total time available to
   allow for *cancelled physical education classes* due
   to: Conference time, psychological testing (Brigance), swimming schedule, snow days, field
   trips, voting days (gym in use), holiday assem-
   blies, beginning and ending school.   *2 weeks*

3. Subtract 1 week of the total time available to
   allow for flex time (unplanned adjustments that
   need to be made to allow for additional instruc-
   tional needs).   *1 week*

4. Total weeks available (item 1 minus 2 and 3)   *44 weeks*

5. Total days available:
   a. Multiply item 4 by the number of gym classes   44 ×   1 days gym/wk
      per week   =   44 days gym/yr
   b. Multiply total number of days by the length   1 ×   30 min gym/day
      (minutes) of your PE class (instructional   = 1320 min gym/yr
      time—not dressing or set up time):

Step 5. Time Estimations for Attainment of Meaningful Performance Gain

Performance Objective	Minutes per Objective
Kindergarten	
Fundamental Motor Skills	180
Body Management Skills	120
Health/Fitness	180
Play, Sport, and Leisure Skills	210
Elementary (Lower)	
Fundamental Motor Skills	180
Body Management Skills	120
Health/Fitness Skills	180
Play, Sport, and Leisure Skills	210
Elementary (Upper)	
Fundamental Motor Skills	150
Body Management Skills	120
Health/Fitness Skills	150
Play, Sport, and Leisure Skills	180

Step 6. Determine Total Number of Program Objectives for Meaningful Performance Gain by Program Level

Kindergarten

$$\frac{1320}{\text{Total Time Available}} \div \frac{180}{\substack{\text{Mins/PO needed} \\ \text{(approximate)}}} \quad \frac{7.34}{\text{total POs}}$$

Lower Elementary

$$\frac{1320}{\text{Total Time Available}} \div \frac{180}{\substack{\text{Mins/PO needed} \\ \text{(approximate)}}} \quad \frac{7.34}{\text{total POs}}$$

Upper Elementary

$$\frac{1320}{\text{Total Time Available}} \div \frac{150}{\substack{\text{Mins/PO needed} \\ \text{(approximate)}}} \quad \frac{8.8}{\text{total POs}}$$

Step 7. Comprehensive Program Plan: Selection of Essential Objectives by Goal and Program Level—Kindergarten through Upper Elementary

Program Goal Area	Kindergarten	Lower Elementary (1–3)	Upper Elementary (4–6)
Play, Sport, and Leisure Skills	PO (1)* Directed free play	PO (1) Organized minor games	POs (3) Soccer dribble, basketball chest pass, dance circle formation
Fundamental Motor Skills	POs (4) Walk, Run, Roll a ball, Throw a ball	POs (3) Run, Gallop, Kick	POs (3) Run, Catch, Underhand throw
Body Management Skills	PO (1) Log roll	POs (2) Body actions, Body parts	PO (1) Directions in Space
Physical Fitness Skills	PO (1) Walk run for endurance	PO (1) Stamina and Heart/Lung Endurance	POs (2) Cardiorespiratory Endurance, Weight Maintenance
Total POs	(7)	(7)	(9)

*Number of program objectives for each program goal.

Step 8A.   Development of Yearly Instructional Units

Level: Kindergarten

Teaching Unit	Time	Weeks
1. Walk/Run for Endurance	30	7
Directed Free Play	50	
Roll a Ball	90	
Log Roll	40	
2. Walk	100	7
Walk/Run for Endurance	20	
Log Roll	60	
Directed Free Play	30	
3. Walk/Run for Endurance	30	7
Roll a Ball	30	
Walk	80	
Run	30	
Directed Free Play	40	
4. Walk/Run for Endurance	30	7
Run	80	
Log Roll	30	
Directed Free Play	70	
5. Walk/Run for Endurance	40	8
Throw a Ball	80	
Log Roll	50	
Run	70	
6. Walk/Run for Endurance	30	8
Directed Free Play	110	
Throw a Ball	100	
	1320	44

Step 8B. Development of Yearly Instructional Units

Level: Lower Elementary

Teaching Unit	Time	Weeks
1. Stamina Heart/Lung Endurance	30	7
Body Parts	90	
Run	60	
Organized Minor Games	30	
2. Stamina Heart/Lung Endurance	30	7
Body Parts	60	
Run	60	
Organized Minor Games	60	
3. Stamina Heart/Lung Endurance	30	7
Body Parts	30	
Body Actions	60	
Run	60	
Organized Minor Games	30	
4. Stamina Heart/Lung Endurance	30	7
Body Actions	90	
Gallop	50	
Organized Minor Games	40	
5. Stamina Heart/Lung Endurance	30	8
Body Actions	30	
Gallop	70	
Kick	50	
Organized Minor Games	60	
6. Stamina Heart/Lung Endurance	30	8
Gallop	60	
Kick	70	
Organized Minor Games	80	
	1320	44

Step 8C. **Development of Yearly Instructional Units**

Level: Upper Elementary

Teaching Unit	Time	Weeks
1. Weight Maintenance	30	7
Cardiorespiratory Endurance	20	
Run	90	
Underhand Throw	70	
2. Weight Maintenance	20	7
Cardiorespiratory Endurance	30	
Run	60	
Underhand Throw	60	
Catch	40	
3. Weight Maintenance	20	7
Cardiorespiratory Endurance	30	
Underhand Throw	20	
Catch	80	
Directions in Space	60	
4. Weight Maintenance	30	7
Cardiorespiratory Endurance	20	
Catch	30	
Basketball Chest Pass	90	
Directions in Space	40	
5. Weight Maintenance	20	8
Cardiorespiratory Endurance	30	
Dance in Circle Formation	60	
Basketball Chest Pass	50	
Directions in Space	20	
Soccer Dribble	60	
6. Weight Maintenance	30	8
Cardiorespiratory Endurance	20	
Dance in Circle Formation	60	
Basketball Chest Pass	40	
Soccer Dribble	90	
	1320	44

Step 9A. Development of Weekly Unit Lesson Plans

		PO's	Min		PO's	Min
Gym: ___1___ Days/Weeks		Walk/Run for Endurance	30		Roll a Ball	90
___30___ Min/Days		Directed Free Play	50		Log Roll	40

Class Level ___Kindergarten___   Unit ___1___   Projected Time Line ___9/7/83–10/19/83___

Walk/Run for Endurance (10) Roll a Ball (15) Directed Free Play (5) Assess 9/7	Walk/Run for Endurance (5) Roll a Ball (15) Directed Free Play (10) Assess/Teach 9/14	Directed Free Play (20) Roll a Ball (10) Teach 9/21	Walk/Run for Endurance (5) Log Roll (15) Assess Roll a Ball (10) Teach 9/28	Walk/Run for Endurance (5) Directed Free Play (10) Roll a Ball (15) Reassess/Teach 10/5
Directed Free Play (5) Log Roll (15) Roll a Ball (10) Teach 10/12	Walk/Run for Endurance (5) Log Roll (10) Roll a Ball (15) Teach/Reassess 10/19			

Step 9B. Development of Weekly Unit Lesson Plans

		PO's	*Min*		*PO's*	*Min*
Gym:	__1__ Days/Weeks	Stamina Heart/Lung Endurance	30	Run		60
	__30__ Min/Days	Body Parts	90	Organized Minor Games		30

Class/Level __Lower Elementary__   Unit ____1_____   Projected Time Line __9/8/83–10/20/83__

Stamina, Heart/
  Lung Endurance
  (10)
Body Parts (15)
Organized Minor
  Games (5)
Assess
 	
9/8
	Run (10)
	Body Parts (15)
	Organized Minor
	  Games (5)
	Assess/Teach
	
	9/15
		Stamina, Heart/
		  Lung Endurance
		  (5)
		Body Parts (10)
		Run (10)
		Organized Minor
		  Games (5)
		Teach
		9/22
			Stamina, Heart/
			  Lung Endurance
			  (5)
			Body Parts (15)
			Run (10)
			Teach
			
			9/29
				Stamina, Heart/
				  Lung Endurance
				  (5)
				Body Parts (15)
				Run (10)
				Reassess/Teach
				
				10/6

Body Parts (5)
Run (10)
Organized Minor
  Games (15)
Teach
 	
10/13
	Stamina, Heart/
	  Lung Endurance
	  (5)
	Run (10)
	Body Parts (15)
	Reassess/Teach
	
	10/20			

Step 9C. Development of Weekly Unit Lesson Plans

	PO's	Min		PO's	Min
Gym: 1 Days/Weeks	Weight Maintenance	30		Run	90
30 Min/Days	Cardiorespiratory	20		Underhand	70
				Throw	

Class/Level __Upper Elementary__   Unit _____1_____   Projected Time Line __9/7/83–10/19/83__

Weight
  Maintenance
  (10)
Run (15)
Cardiorespiratory
  (5)
Assess
 	
         9/7
	Cardiorespiratory
	  (5)
	Underhand Throw
	  (15)
	Run (10)
	Assess/Teach
	
	        9/14
		Weight
		  Maintenance (5)
		Run (15)
		Underhand Throw
		  (10)
		
		     ,9/21
			Weight
			  Maintenance (5)
			Cardiorespiratory
			  (5)
			Run (10)
			Underhand Throw
			  (10)
			Teach 9/28
				Cardiorespiratory
				  (5)
				Underhand Throw
				  (15)
				Run (10)
				Reassess/Teach
				
				       10/5

Weight
  Maintenance (5)
Underhand Throw
  (10)
Run (15)
Teach
 	
     10/12
	Weight
	  Maintenance (5)
	Underhand Throw
	  (10)
	Run (15)
	Reassess/Teach
	
	     10/19			

Glossary

Accommodation: The reasonable adjustments or modifications made in the instructional program so that all children can achieve desired learning outcomes.

Accountability: To hold schools and/or individuals responsible for producing desired learning outcomes on definitive educational goals for all students.

Achievement: Successful performance on objectives of instruction to a specified criterion or standard.

Achievement-Based Curriculum (ABC) Model: A systematic process that sequentially plans, implements, and evaluates an instructional program based on essential educational goals and objectives.

Achievement-Based Curriculum Model Components: The five components of the ABC Model are: planning, assessing, prescribing, teaching, and evaluating.

Adaptation: The modification of program goals, objectives, and/or instruction to meet the students' unique needs and abilities.

Allotted Instructional Time: The time allocated for teaching a program objective: daily, unit, yearly, program level, or any other time period.

Annual Goal: A statement of student expectancies on instructional objectives to be achieved in the yearly program plan.

Appropriateness: Maximizing the degree to which the instructional program and placement meet the needs of students as they progress toward achieving educational goals of the school.

Assessment: A sequential problem-solving process that uses educational measurements (tests) within a decision-making process.

Assistance Levels: A continuum of instructional cues, verbal and nonverbal, ranging from total manipulation to self-directed learning.

Available Instructional Time: The time available in the school schedule for a given subject matter area such as physical education.

Baseline Data: Students' performance data collected over several days and/or trials to determine at what level to initiate instruction.

Class Expectancies: The amount of meaningful gain, units of improvement that the teacher expects a high proportion (90%) of the class members to achieve as the result of instruction.

Class Management: Procedures used by the teacher to decrease discipline problems and increase student active learning time.

Consensus-Building Technique: A four-step systematic process to assist teachers, administrators, and other team members in decision-making.

Class Performance Score Sheet: A record of the assessment and reassessment data of students' achievement of the performance standards for the instructional objectives taught and tested.

Consulting Teacher: A specially trained teacher who provides support services to teachers.

Contingent: When reinforcement is dependent on the existence of a particular designated performance. The reinforcement or reward is never given unless that designated performance occurs.

Contingency Contracts: A learning contract specifying consequences (contingencies) between the student and the teacher. For example, for a completed assigned task, the student is rewarded with a specific privilege such as choice of activities or points.

Corrective Procedures: Task-related feedback procedures to correct student performance or work behavior.

Criterion: Established performance standard used to assess student's level of performance on instructional objectives taught.

Criterion-Referenced Evaluation: Evaluating student's performance by using standardized criterion-referenced tests to compare the student's performance to established performance standards on the instructional objective (content) taught. These tests document the results of instruction focused on student achievement of instructional content.

Design Criteria: Six characteristics of quality instructional programs: accountability, communication, compliance, effectiveness, efficiency, and flexibility.

Disability: Any restriction resulting from an impairment that prevents an individual from performing an activity within the range considered normal for a person of the same size, age, and sex.

Educational Program Goals: The instructional intent or purposes of the school program.

Effective Practices: Instructional practices focused on student achievement that have proved effective based on school improvement studies such as clear statements of educational goals; high expectations; safe, orderly task-related learning environment, leadership, and parent involvement.

Effective Schools: Schools where the expected educational goals are achieved by the students.

Effective Teaching: Teachers impact on student achievement and behaviors by planning, managing, and teaching in ways that keep students involved and successfully achieving instructional objectives taught.

Enabling Objectives: Prerequisite skills that students need to progress toward achieving more complex skills.

Entry Status: The student's initial skill peformance on the instructional objectives to be taught.

Essential Program Objectives: Objectives that define skills and knowledge (program content) that a community wishes their children to achieve as a result of the instructional program.

Evaluation: A systematic process by which program merit can be determined systematically by comparing program expectations with actual program products: student achievement.

Feedback: The information provided about the results of performances or work behaviors.

Functional Competence: Achievement of a performance level that allows the student to participate in active play-leisure, daily living activities and/or enables the student to achieve higher levels of skills consistent with his or her innate abilities.

Game Adaptation: Modification of game activities to meet students' participation needs and abilities such as changing boundaries, type of equipment, or number on sides.

Grouping: A flexible class organization for adjusting the program to the needs and abilities of class members: constant regrouping is necessary as students achieve learning tasks.

Handicapped Children: (P.L. 94-142) Those children evaluated as being mentally retarded, hard of hearing, deaf, speech impaired, visually handicapped, seriously emotionally disturbed, orthopedically impaired, other health impaired, deaf-blind, multihandicapped, or as having specific learning disabilities, who because of those impairments need special education and related services.

Impairment: A permanent or transitory psychological, physiological, or anatomical loss or abnormality of structure or function.

Incidence: Number identified; percentage of occurrence within the entire population.

Individualized Education Program: (P.L. 94-142) A written program plan that specifies requirements with regard to developing, monitoring, evaluating, and reporting on an individual instruction plan (objective based with time lines) for each handicapped student. Annual reporting, evaluating, and updating are specified.

Individualizing Instruction: Maximizing the degree to which each student is actively engaged in learning and successfully achieving the desired learning outcomes.

Individualizing the Program: The selection and/or modification of program objectives based on students' abilities and needs as students' progress toward attaining program goals.

Instructional Objectives: Statements that describe what students will be able to do after a prescribed unit of instruction. Each instructional objective specifies clearly what the student is to learn and how the student is to demonstrate learning, including criteria to evaluate each learner's performance. Other terms used to describe this type of an objective are behavioral objectives or performance objectives.

Instructional Planning: A systematic process to help teachers make decisions before, during, and after instruction to increase the probability of students achieving the desired learning outcomes.

Instructional Unit: Identification of compatible objectives with allotted instructional time sequentially arranged over a period of time such as a semester or a year.

Learning Tasks: Mastery performance criteria for students to achieve as they progress toward achieving mastery of the instructional objective.

Legislative Mandates: Federal and/or state laws, rules, and regulations.

Lesson Plan: Instructional objectives to be taught or reviewed with time lines organized into introductory activities; the body of the lesson including presentation, grouping, and practice activities, and a summary or review activity.

Least Restrictive Environment: (P.L. 94-142) Educating handicapped children with nonhandicapped children "to the maximum extent appropriate" and that removing such children from regular classes occur "only when the nature or severity of the handicap is such that education in regular classes with the use of supplementary aids and services cannot be achieved satisfactory . . ." A continuum of placement options must be available; placement options be reviewed annually, based on the IEP. Such options in physical education as regular classes, special physical education classes or adapted physical education classes in regular school settings; physical education in special settings such as community based school or residential.

Mastery Level Performance Gain: The achievement of continuous performance gain scores to master a given instructional objective upon exit from the school program.

Mastery Performance Criteria: The predetermined performance standards used to evaluate a student's mastery of target instructional objective.

Meaningful Performance Gain: The amount of achievement gain that is judged to make a difference in the student's ability to demonstrate a higher level of competence on the instructional objective taught within a specified time period.

Modeling: The presentation of a standard or example for the student to imitate or make comparison to when learning a skill or to induce new behaviors to take the place of undesirable behaviors in the learning environment.

Monitoring: An arrangement for observing or recording the implementation of the ABC model and/or the performance and needs of students in the class.

Motivation: Students' interest in learning and achieving the target objectives of instruction.

Nondiscriminatory Evaluation: (P.L. 94-142) Nonprejudiced, testing and evaluation of a student. Conducting tests in the student's native language if possible, and not using a single procedure to determine a child's placement or program. Detailed requirements for assessing, administering, and judging such evaluations are provided in the regulations.

Normalization: A principle of human service that addresses the provisions of patterns of life for the handicapped that are as close as possible to those of other members of society.

Norm-Referenced Evaluation: Standardized norm-referenced tests used to compare the scores measured to established statistics such as age and sex norms.

Occupational Therapy: Activities consisting of light exercise to provide diversion and/or to exercise an affected part of the body, to develop daily living skills, and to develop prevocational skills.

Paraprofessional: A person trained as a teacher assistant.

Performance Objective: An instructional objective.

Performance Standard: Mastery performance criteria of the instructional objective which comprise the criterion-referenced test items.

Physical Education: (P.L. 94-142) The development of physical and motor fitness and fundamental motor skills and patterns; and skills in aquatics, dance, and individual and group games and sports (including intramural and lifetime sports). The term includes special physical education, adapted physical education, movement education, and motor development.

Physical Therapy: Physical agents such as manipulation, braces, corrective devices, massage, heat or water therapy dealing with the treatment of diseases or injury.

Positive Reinforcement: The maintenance or increase of a behavior because a particular rewarding stimulus is applied.

Prescription: The effective use of student assessment data in planning daily instructional activities, games, and procedures to enhance each student's acquisition of objectives taught and tested.

Professional Imperative: The skills, knowledges, and commitment to provide quality physical education programs for all students in our nation's schools to achieve desired learning outcomes relevant to the school's program goals; and, to have documented evidence of the effectiveness of our programs.

Program Evaluation: Student evaluation data are used to both document program merit (appropriateness) and improve systematically the procedures of planning, implementing, and evaluating the effectiveness of instruction.

Program Goals: Statements that describe the purposes and instructional intents of the school program.

Program Level: The logical levels or breakpoints in the school program such as elementary, junior (middle) high school, and senior high school.

Program Objectives: Statements of content defining what is taught and when (scope and sequence) in the instructional program to make the program goals operative.

Program Plan: Instruction related to a specific objective, unit, year, instructional program level, or an entire comprehensive program plan K through 12. A comprehensive program plan identifies program goals with objectives organized sequentially by program levels that can be effectively taught for students to achieve desired learning outcomes K through 12. It is sometime called a long-term plan.

Public Law 94-142: Education for all Handicapped Children Act of 1975. Guarantees handicapped children a free, appropriate public education in the least restrictive environment. See Federal Register August 23, 1977.

Quality Instruction: Teachers impact on student behavior and achievement by planning, managing, and teaching so that students are actively engaged in learning and successfully achieve objectives of the program.

Quality School Program: A school program in which the instructional intent is clearly stated in terms of program goals, the scope and sequence by program objectives, and a high proportion (90%) of all students achieve stated expectancies.

Reassessment: The constant evaluation of student performance included as part of instruction that results in feedback to the student and information for the teacher.

Reinforcer: A stimulus that results in the maintenance or increase of a behavior.

Reinforcement: A method by which a stimulus increases or maintains a specific behavior.

Related Services: (P.L. 94-142) Transportation and such developmental, corrective services required to assist a handicapped child to benefit from special education. These services include occupational therapy, physical therapy, and recreation.

Reliability: Ability of a test to produce the same results when repeated.

Section 504: Section 504 of the Rehabilitation Act of 1973, containing requirements designed to guarantee the civil rights of the handicapped (see Federal Register, May 4, 1977).

Short-Term Instructional Objectives: Observable and measurable learning tasks specified for the instructional objective to be taught.

Skill Levels: Skill levels of the instructional objectives are sequential levels of performance that comprise the instructional objective (i.e., run) being taught.

Speech Therapy: Therapy focused on improving the student's articulation and/ or remediating language difficulties.

Special Education: (P.L. 94-142) Specially designed instruction, at no cost to the parent, to meet the unique needs of a handicapped child, including classroom instruction, instruction in physical education, home instruction, and instruction in hospitals and institutions.

State Plan: Public Law 94-142 requires each state department of education to submit to the U.S. Department of Education an annual plan for the implementation and administration of the Law.

Steps in Lesson Design: The five steps that provide a framework for planning effective lessons include: (1) presentation of an overview and statement of objectives; (2) clarity of explanation and demonstration of the skill to be learned; (3) continuous monitoring of students' skills and level of understanding to make appropriate instructional decisions during and after the lesson; (4) providing practice time, an opportunity for students to practice the new skill, both guided and independent; and (5) student and class results being recorded and reviewed by teacher and students.

Student Profile Records: A comprehensive reporting system that incorporates the objectives (content) covered, student entry, exit, and change status on the instructional objectives included in the reporting period.

Student Involvement: The amount of time students are actively engaged in task-related learning.

Student Behaviors: Specific behaviors linked to student achievement such as student's active learning time and success in achieving instructional objectives taught and tested.

Student Evaluation: A systematic process of reassessment of student's performance on instructional objectives taught to enable appropriate changes to be made during and at the end of instruction.

Student Expectancies: The amount of meaningful gain, units of improvement, the teacher expects each student to achieve as the result of instruction.

Student Needs Assessment: Identification of a student's learning, personal-social, and physical and motor strengths, and needs to make appropriate instructional decisions.

Structured Lesson: The organization or design of a lesson and activity to meet the targeted objectives of instruction (i.e., preassessment of students' needs on target objectives of the lesson).

Task Analysis: The process of breaking down an instructional objective into smaller, teachable, and measurable learning tasks that, when acquired, lead to the achievement of the objective.

Teaching: The effective management and instruction of a class, individual student, or group of students so that desired learning takes place.

Time-On-Task: The actual amount of time the student is actively involved in learning the objectives targeted for instruction.

Teacher Behaviors: Procedures that teachers use to plan, manage, and teach that impact on student achievement and behaviors so discipline problems are infrequent and desired learning outcomes are achieved by all students.

Team Teaching: Pairs or small groups of teachers working to plan, manage, and effectively teach to meet students' needs and promote personal satisfaction and professional growth.

Team Assisted Individual Instruction: Heterogeneous grouping of students into teams to assist in planning, managing, coaching, assessing, and recording data on team and individual performance.

Validity: The degree to which a test measures what it was designed to measure.

INDEX

Numerals in *italics* indicate a figure; "t" following a page number indicates a table.